Recent Advances in Therapeutic Diets

**Compiled by the Clinical Staff,
Dietary Department,
University of Iowa
Hospitals and Clinics,
Iowa City**

FOURTH EDITION

IOWA STATE UNIVERSITY PRESS / Ames

©1970, 1973, 1979, 1989 Iowa State University Press, Ames, Iowa 50010

First edition, 1970
Revised printing, 1971
Second edition, 1973
Second printing, 1974
Third printing, 1974
Fourth printing, 1976
Third edition, 1979
Second printing, 1984
Fourth edition, 1989

Library of Congress Cataloging-in-Publication Data

Recent advances in therapeutic diets / compiled by the clinical staff, Dietary Department,
    University of Iowa Hospitals and Clinics, Iowa City. – 4th ed.
        p. cm.

    Bibliography: p.
    Includes index.

    ISBN 0-8138-1064-7

    1. Diet therapy. I. University of Iowa. Hospitals and Clinics.
Dietary Dept.
    [DNLM: 1. Diet therapy. 2. Food Service, Hospital. WB 400 R295]
RM216.R379 1989
615.8'54–dc19
DNLM/DLC
for Library of Congress   89-1766

ii

CONTENTS

iii

PREFACE

THIS DIET MANUAL was developed for use as a reference and guide for members of the health care team. The diets are described in technical terms and are intended for use by professionals.

The diet manual includes the general hospital diet, modifications of the general diet, and all therapeutic diets commonly used at the University of Iowa Hospitals and Clinics and the Veterans Administration Hospital in Iowa City. Patient diet instructions with additional explanatory information are adapted from the diets contained in the manual. Frequently there are combinations of several dietary restrictions. Each diet is adjusted by the clinical dietitians to meet the individual patient's dietary prescription as well as food preferences.

The sample menus are modified from the general menu; the foods listed on these menus are typical of patients' meals at the University of Iowa Hospitals and Clinics. The adequacy of the diets is based on the 1980 revision of the Recommended Daily Dietary Allowances prepared by the Food and Nutrition Board of the National Research Council. Any significant inadequacies of the diet are noted following the description. Some levels of nutrients as calculated from the suggested menu may seem high or low due to the foods used in the sample menu. Each day's menu will afford some variation in the level of nutrients. The nutrients were calculated using USDA Handbook Number 8 for nutrient values. Nutritional value of foods not listed in the handbook were taken from other recognized sources which are listed in the bibliography.

New to the fourth edition of our diet manual are sections on nutritional assessment, nutrition and cancer, sports and exercise, anorexia and bulimia, recommendations for the special needs of burn patients, and a listing of the dietary fiber content of foods. New diets include a protein-phosphorus restricted diet for renal patients, a bland diet for esophageal reflux and hiatal hernia, and a renal diabetic exchange plan. Diets have also been added for oral and maxillofacial surgeries.

Many sections have been revised and expanded, including dietary management of diabetes, vegetarian diets, weight control, postgastrectomy, and diets for VBG patients. The section on maternal nutrition contains information on vegetarianism, pregnancy in adolescents, and high risk (including diabetic) pregnancies. The calcium restricted diet utilizes exchanges and is planned for 4 levels from mild (40 mEq) to very strict (10 mEq). The food allergies section includes the chicken-rice-lamb diet as well as information on salicylates and metabisulfites.

The diet manual represents the time, effort, and composite knowledge of the clinical staff dietitians and the Medical Advisory Committee for Review of the Diet Manual. We extend our thanks to these dedicated professionals from the University of Iowa Hospitals and Clinics who gave so freely of their time.

Special recognition is accorded Elaine Hovet, Assistant Director, Clinical, and Marjorie Caruth, Clinical Dietitian, who coordinated the work of the committee and served as editors of the fourth edition.

Rose Ann Sippy
Director
Dietary Department
University of Iowa Hospitals and Clinics

ACKNOWLEDGMENTS

WE HAVE ATTEMPTED to make this fourth edition of *Recent Advances in Therapeutic Diets* as complete, accurate, and representative of current dietary practice as possible. The diets and procedures outlined in the manual represent the combined efforts of the present and former clinical staff dietitians of the University of Iowa Hospitals and Clinics. We also acknowledge the contribution of Kay Evans, B.S.N., M.A., R.N.

Lois Ahrens, B.S., R.D., L.D.
Joan Bickel, B.A.
Rebecca Biga, B.S., M.S., R.D., L.D.
Lisa Brooks, B.S., M.A., R.D., L.D.
Ann Bruce, B.S., M.A., R.D., L.D.
Susan Carlson, B.S., M.S., R.D., L.D.
Sydne Carlson, B.S., M.S., R.D., L.D.
Marjorie Caruth, B.S., M.S., R.D., L.D.
Catherine Chenard, B.S., R.D., L.D.
Betty Dickinson, B.S., M.S., R.D., L.D.
Cathy Dostal, B.A., R.D., L.D.
Marlys Dunphy, B.A., M.A., Ed.S., R.D., L.D.
Constance Evers, B.S., M.S., R.D., L.D.
Jane Faber, B.S., M.S., R.D., L.D.
Pat Graff, B.S., M.A., R.D., L.D.
Julie Gilmore, B.A., M.S., R.D., L.D.
Donna Hollinger, B.S., M.S., R.D., L.D.
Kristi Hopkins, B.A., R.D., L.D.
Elaine Hovet, B.S., M.S., R.D., L.D.
Laura Iasiello-Vailas, B.A., M.S., R.D.
Teresa Kelly, B.S., R.D., L.D.

Joyce Krause, B.S., R.D., L.D.
Susan Krug-Wispe, B.S., M.S., R.D., L.D.
Kim Lash, B.A., M.A., R.D.
Mary Mardan, B.S., M.P.H., R.D., L.D.
Beverly McCabe, B.S., M.S., Ph.D., R.D., L.D.
Susan MacDowell, B.S., M.P.H., R.D., L.D.
Kathryn Haack Norwood, B.S., M.S., R.D.
Marilyn Bukoff Priddy, B.A., M.A., R.D.
Joetta Redlin, B.S., M.S., R.D., L.D.
Cheryl Richmond, B.S., R.D., L.D.
Nancy Rohde, B.A., R.D., L.D.
Karen Smith, B.A., M.S., R.D., L.D.
Linda Snetselaar, B.S., M.S., Ph.D., R.D., L.D.
Diane Stadler, B.S., M.S., R.D., L.D.
Patti Steinmuller, B.S., M.S., R.D., L.D.
Phyllis Stumbo, B.S., M.S., Ph.D., R.D., L.D.
Ellen Swanson, B.A., M.S., R.D., L.D.
Ellen Wade, B.S., R.D., L.D.
Delores Williamson, B.S., M.S., R.D., L.D.
Louise Wolf-Novak, B.S., M.A., R.D., L.D.
Susan Briggs Vilims, B.S., R.D.

The Medical Advisory Committee for Review of the Diet Manual includes:

Dr. Lloyd J. Filer, Professor Emeritus, Pediatrics, and Chairman of the Medical Advisory Committee for Review of the Diet Manual
Dr. John A. Bertolatus, Assistant Professor, Internal Medicine, Renal
Dr. Joseph D. Brown, Associate Professor, Internal Medicine, Endocrinology
Dr. C. Patrick Burns, Professor, Internal Medicine, Hematology and Oncology
Dr. Samuel Fomon, Professor, Pediatrics
Dr. L.G. Hunsicker, Associate Professor, Internal Medicine, Renal
Dr. G. Patrick Kealey, Assistant Professor, Surgery
Dr. Kenneth Kempf, Assistant Professor, Hospital Dentistry, Oral and Maxillofacial Surgery
Dr. Wilma Krause, Assistant Professor, Pediatrics
Dr. William J. Lawton, Associate Professor, Internal Medicine, Renal
Dr. Julia Lee, Associate, Pediatrics
Dr. Edward Mason, Professor, Surgery
Dr. Michael D. Maves, Associate Professor, Otolaryngology
Dr. Donald M. Mock, Associate Professor, Pediatrics
Dr. Jody Murph, Assistant Professor, Pediatrics
Dr. Hal Richerson, Professor, Internal Medicine, Allergy
Dr. Charles Riggs, Jr., Assistant Professor, Internal Medicine, Oncology
Alan J. Ryan, Research Assistant, Exercise Science/Physical Education

Dr. Harold Schedl, Professor, Internal Medicine, Gastroenterology
Dr. Helmut G. Schrott, Associate Professor, Preventive Medicine and Internal Medicine
Dr. Robert Summers, Professor, Internal Medicine, Gastroenterology
Dr. Thomas Symreng, Associate Professor, Anesthesia
Dr. Ernest Theilen, Professor, Internal Medicine, Cardiology
Dr. Eva Tsalikian, Associate Professor, Pediatrics
Dr. Deborah Turner, Assistant Professor, Obstetrics and Gynecology
Dr. Luis Urdaneta, Associate Professor, Surgery
Dr. Howard Winfield, Assistant Professor, Urology
Dr. Jerold Woodhead, Assistant Professor, Pediatrics
Dr. William Yates, Assistant Professor, Psychiatry
Dr. Kabir Younoszai, Professor, Pediatrics
Dr. Frank Zlatnik, Professor, Obstetrics and Gynecology

GOOD NUTRITION
A Basis for Good Health

A SIMPLE METHOD of food selection to meet the Recommended Dietary Allowances is the Basic Four Food Plan.[1] The nutrient content of a diet based on this plan varies according to which foods within the groups are selected. The recommended number of servings for an adult from each food group provides approximately 1200 kilocalories (kcal). To meet higher caloric needs, as would be the case with most adults, one should select other servings from the basic four food groups plus foods from group five. It should be emphasized that the Recommended Dietary Allowances are intakes of nutrients that meet the needs of healthy people and do not take into account special needs arising from infections, metabolic disorders, chronic diseases, or other abnormalities that require special dietary treatment. These must be considered as unique clinical problems requiring individual attention.[2]

A GUIDE TO GOOD EATING

The Basic Four Food Plan

<u>Milk Group</u>: These foods supply significant amounts of calcium, riboflavin, and protein.
    1 cup milk, plain yogurt, or calcium equivalent:
        1 1/2 oz cheddar cheese
        1 cup pudding
        1 3/4 cups ice cream
        2 cups cottage cheese

<u>Meat Group</u>: These foods supply significant amounts of protein, niacin, iron, and thiamin.
    2 oz cooked lean meat, fish, poultry, or protein equivalent:
        2 eggs
        2 oz cheddar cheese
        1/2 cup cottage cheese
        1 cup cooked, dried beans or peas
        4 tbsp peanut butter

<u>Fruit-Vegetable Group</u>: Orange or dark green leafy vegetables and fruit are recommended 3 or 4 times weekly for vitamin A. A fruit or vegetable rich in vitamin C is recommended daily.
        1/2 cup cooked or juice
        1 cup raw
        Portion commonly served, such as medium-size apple or banana

---

[1] National Dairy Council.

[2] Recommended Dietary Allowances.

<u>Grain Group</u> (whole grain, fortified or enriched): These foods supply significant amounts of carbohydrate, thiamin, iron, and niacin.

       1 slice bread
       1 cup ready-to-eat cereal
       1/2 cup cooked cereal, pasta, or grits

<u>Others</u>: Foods and condiments such as oils and sugars complement but do not replace foods from the four groups. Amounts consumed should be determined by individual caloric needs.

RECOMMENDED DAILY PATTERN

This pattern provides the foundation for a nutritious, healthful diet. The chart below gives recommendations for the number of servings for several categories of people.

Food Group	Recommended Number of Servings				
	Child	Teenager	Adult	Pregnant Woman	Lactating Woman
Milk	3	4	2	4	4
Meat	2	2	2	3	3
Fruit-Vegetable	4	4	4	4	4
Grain	4	4	4	4	4
Other	Amounts should be determined by individual caloric needs				

DIETARY GUIDELINES

The 1985 U.S. Dietary Guidelines are 7 recommendations for good eating habits based on moderation and variety. The general menus at the University of Iowa Hospitals and Clinics are planned so that these guidelines can be followed.

1. Eat a variety of foods.

2. Maintain desirable weight.

3. Avoid too much fat, saturated fat, and cholesterol.

4. Eat foods with adequate starch and fiber.

5. Avoid too much sugar.

6. Avoid too much sodium.

7. If you drink alcoholic beverages, do so in moderation.

SECTION 1

Routine Hospital Diets and Modifications in Consistency and Texture

A. GENERAL DIET

DESCRIPTION: The General Diet is designed for patients who require no special dietary modifications or restrictions. Individual intolerances may necessitate the exclusion of certain food items. Salt, pepper, and sugar are routinely added to the tray.

FOODS ALLOWED: Amounts to use daily are based on the Basic Four Food Plan.

Food Group	Foods Allowed	Amount
Beverages	Milk (any kind), coffee, tea, other beverages	2 or more cups milk, others as desired
Breads	All	3 or more servings, enriched or whole grain
Cereals	All	1 serving
Desserts	All	0-2 servings
Eggs	Any preparation	0-2 per week
Fats	Table spreads, cream, salad dressings	2-6 tsp
Fruits, Fruit Juices	All	2 or more servings (1 should be rich in vitamin C unless a vegetable high in vitamin C is consumed instead)
Meat, Fish, Poultry, Cheese	All	2 servings (5 oz total)
Soups	All	As desired
Sugar, Sweets	All	As needed
Vegetables, Vegetable Juices	All	2 or more servings (1 should be orange or dark green leafy for a source of vitamin A)

1

FOODS ALLOWED (continued):

Food Group	Foods Allowed	Amount
Miscellaneous	Salt, condiments, herbs, spices	As needed

APPROXIMATE COMPOSITION OF SAMPLE MENU:

Calories	2023
Protein, g	97
Fat, g	62
Carbohydrate, g	282

SAMPLE MENU FOR GENERAL DIET:

Breakfast	Luncheon	Dinner
1/2 cup orange juice	1/2 cup grape juice	3 oz roast beef
1/2 cup farina	3/4 cup creamed chicken on	1/2 cup mashed potatoes
1 slice toast, cracked wheat	1 biscuit	1/2 cup cooked carrots
1 tsp butter or margarine	1/2 cup green beans	3/4 cup tossed lettuce salad
1 tbsp grape jelly	1/2 sliced tomato on lettuce	1 tbsp french dressing
1 cup 2% milk	1 tsp mayonnaise	1 slice bread, cracked wheat
1 tsp sugar	1 slice bread, cracked wheat	1 tsp butter or margarine
Coffee or tea	1 tsp butter or margarine	Small banana
	1/2 cup canned peaches	3 vanilla wafers
	1 slice angel food cake	1 cup 2% milk
	1 cup 2% milk	Coffee or tea
	Coffee or tea	

MODIFICATIONS OF THE GENERAL DIET:

1. Ground General

DESCRIPTION: This diet is designed for edentulous patients or for those who have difficulty chewing. Some patients chew quite well in the absence of teeth, while others may experience indigestion or choking if large pieces of food are swallowed. Modifications are made according to the patient's ability to chew. For this diet, the soft menu is utilized with no restriction in seasoning or fat. If a "very soft diet" is necessary, a soft pureed diet may be ordered (see page 10). The following modifications are suggested for the ground general:

Meats: Grind and/or add gravy or broth. Poultry and fish often do not require mechanical tenderizing.

Vegetables: Omit raw vegetables or shred finely. Cooked corn may need to be pureed.

Fruits: Omit raw apple or shred finely.

2. High Protein, High Calorie General

DESCRIPTION: The High Calorie, High Protein Diet is indicated to prevent weight loss and tissue wasting from catabolic conditions, and to renourish patients with protein-calorie malnutrition. Conditions which may lead to a catabolic state include cancer, major burns, infections, surgery, anorexia nervosa, and trauma.

Extra food is added to the meals and 3 high protein, high calorie nourishments are served between meals. In addition to the diet, formula supplements may be used (see chart on pages 288-92). The dietitian may be asked to calculate caloric intake and/or to provide a nutritional assessment to assist in the treatment of these patients.

Although needs will vary according to the patient, a typical diet would include 1000 or more supplemental calories daily and a minimum of 1.5 grams of protein/kg. body weight. For the average adult, the goal would be 3000 to 3700 calories/day and 100 to 120 g protein.

Should a restricted consistency or texture be necessary, the Soft or Full Liquid Diet may be ordered with the high protein, high calorie notation, e.g., "High Protein, High Calorie Soft." Therapeutic diets are also available with the high protein, high calorie modification.

3. High Fiber

DESCRIPTION: This diet may be used to prevent and treat constipation, diverticulosis, or chronic irritable bowel. The increased bulk results in shortened transit time and decreased intraluminal pressure.

Dietary fiber is defined as a mixture of complex carbohydrates that are largely resistant to human digestion such as cellulose, hemicellulose, pectic substances, and a noncarbohydrate, lignin. These are found only in plant foods. The techniques for determining dietary fiber are still being developed, and published data are limited. The recommended level of dietary fiber is 25 to 50 g per day. The lists on pages 18-22 may be used to calculate an approximate level in terms of grams.

On this diet, it is especially important to consume the recommended 6 to 8 cups of water per day.

FOODS ALLOWED AND FOODS TO AVOID:

Food Group	Foods Allowed	Foods to Avoid
Beverages	All	None
Breads	Breads, crackers, and quick breads made from 100% whole wheat or whole rye flour; graham, wheat, and rye crackers	Refined white or rye bread or crackers
Cereals	Bran or whole grain cereals, two 1/2-cup servings daily	Highly refined cereals such as farina or cornflakes
Desserts	All, especially those containing fruits or nuts	None
Eggs	All	None
Fats	All	None
Fruits, Fruit Juices	All, especially fresh or dried, 3 or more servings daily	None
Meat, Fish, Poultry, Cheese	All	None
Potatoes or Substitutes	Baked potato with skin, fibrous sweet potato or yam, brown and wild rice	Hominy, macaroni, noodles, potato chips, spaghetti, white rice
Soups	All	None
Vegetables, Vegetable Juices	All, especially raw, 3 or more servings daily	None

3

APPROXIMATE COMPOSITION OF SAMPLE MENU:

Calories	2126
Protein, g	103
Fat, g	63
Carbohydrate, g	303

SAMPLE MENU FOR HIGH FIBER DIET:

Breakfast

Fresh orange
1/2 cup bran cereal
1 slice toast,
   100% whole wheat
1 tsp butter or
   margarine
1 tbsp jam
1 cup 2% milk
1 tsp sugar
Coffee or tea

Luncheon

3/4 cup creamed chicken on
1 slice toast, 100% whole
   wheat
1/2 cup green beans
1 sliced tomato
3/4 cup lettuce salad
1/2 cup canned peaches
Oatmeal-raisin cookie

Midafternoon
Nourishment

Fresh apple

Dinner

1/2 cup lentil soup
2 oz roast beef
1 baked potato w/skin
1/2 cup cooked carrots
3/4 cup tossed salad
1 tbsp french dressing
1 slice bread, 100% whole
   wheat
1 tsp butter or margarine
Date bar
1 cup 2% milk
Coffee or tea

Evening
Nourishment

1/2 cup bran cereal
1/2 cup 2% milk
1 tsp sugar

4. Maternal Nutrition: Pregnancy and Lactation

INTRODUCTION: Adequate nutrition before and during pregnancy has been found to be an important determinant of the outcome of pregnancy. The Recommended Dietary Allowances (RDA) for pregnant and lactating women are used as the standard for determining the nutrient adequacy of the diet. Based on the general diet for healthy adults, the diet for pregnancy and lactation should include foods from the four food groups in amounts listed on page xi. To supply sufficient calories, larger servings of these foods and/or other foods are needed. Adequate fluid must be consumed to provide for an expanding blood volume, tissue and fetal growth, the demands of lactation, and prevention of constipation. Six to eight cups per day is recommended during pregnancy, and eight or more during lactation.

WEIGHT GAIN DURING PREGNANCY: Weight gain during normal pregnancy should average 11 to 14 kg (24 to 30 lbs). The pattern of gain is as important as the total: 1 to 2 kg (2 to 4 lb) during the first trimester and approximately 0.4 kg (1 lb) per week the second and third trimesters. Overweight women should also follow this pattern, but the underweight woman may need to gain more. (See the prenatal weight gain chart on page 7.) Weight loss by caloric restriction is contraindicated, and a nutritionally adequate intake should be encouraged to prevent ketosis.

DIETARY MANAGEMENT OF HIGH RISK PREGNANCY: Certain factors are associated with increased nutritional risk and require additional dietary intervention. These patients need periodic nutritional assessment and counseling throughout pregnancy.

PREGNANT ADOLESCENT: The pregnant adolescent is at increased risk with the nutritional demands for her own growth superimposed on those of the developing fetus. Protein needs are calculated according to age and ideal body weight (nonpregnant):

Age	Protein needs in grams per kg ideal body weight
Under 15 years	1.7
15 to 17 years	1.5
Over 18 years	1.3

DIABETES AND PREGNANCY: Proper nutritional care for the diabetic woman should begin before pregnancy to have the best outcome for a healthy baby. During the first trimester, there is usually no need for increased calories. Fetal growth is increased starting with the second trimester, and calories should be added to promote normal weight gain. Three meals and three snacks per day are recommended during pregnancy in order to distribute nutrients throughout the day and prevent wide variations in blood glucose levels. The bedtime snack should be high in protein and complex carbohydrate to prevent hypoglycemic episodes at night.

TOXEMIA AND PREGNANCY: Although many nutritional components have been suggested as factors leading to toxemia, the exact role of nutrition in the etiology of toxemia is not known at the present time. The preeclamptic woman experiencing symptoms of edema and hypertension may require a mild sodium restriction of 3 to 4 g/day or a no added salt diet. Salt restriction does not prevent the development of preeclampsia.

PREGNANT VEGETARIAN: The pregnant vegetarian has special needs. At least a quart of milk is recommended in addition to supplements of iron, pyridoxine, and possibly folacin (see Vegetarian Diet, Section 6).

SUPPLEMENTATION: By consuming the recommended servings on page xi, all nutrients for the average pregnant woman with the exception of iron, folate, and possibly calories are provided. At The University of Iowa Hospitals and Clinics, daily supplements of 82 mg iron and 100 mcg folate are prescribed throughout pregnancy as Ircon-FA.

LACTATION: The basic diet for the lactating woman is shown on page xi. An additional 500 calories per day during the first 3 months of lactation is needed. This amount may need to be increased if the mother continues nursing beyond 3 months, suckles more than one baby, or if the maternal weight falls below the ideal weight for height.

APPROXIMATE COMPOSITION OF SAMPLE MENU:

Calories	2339
Protein, g	128
Fat, g	86
Carbohydrate, g	282

SAMPLE MENU FOR PREGNANCY:

Breakfast

1/2 cup orange
   juice
1/2 cup farina
1 egg, soft cooked
1 slice toast,
   whole wheat
1 tsp butter or
   margarine
1 tsp sugar
1 cup 2% milk

Luncheon

3/4 cup creamed chicken on
1 biscuit
1/2 cup green beans
1/2 sliced tomato on lettuce
1 slice angel food cake
1 cup 2% milk

Dinner

3 oz roast beef
1/2 cup mashed potato
1/2 cup cooked carrots
3/4 cup tossed salad
1 tbsp french dressing
1 slice bread, whole wheat
1 tsp butter or margarine
1 cup 2% milk

SAMPLE MENU FOR PREGNANCY (continued):

Midmorning Nourishment	Midafternoon Nourishment	Evening Nourishment
Fresh apple 2 oatmeal raisin cookies 1/2 cup grape juice	1 oz cheddar cheese Fresh peach	1 slice whole wheat bread 1 tbsp peanut butter 1 tsp jelly 1 cup 2% milk

NUTRITION (AMERICAN COLLEGE OF OBSTETRICIANS AND GYNECOLOGISTS): A woman's nutritional status during pregnancy is of great importance to her health and to that of her baby. Ideally, nutritional assessment should be made before conception. Failing that, it should be repeated at regular intervals during and after pregnancy.

Growth is a process requiring energy. Maternal energy sources about 15% above average nonpregnant needs are required during pregnancy. This is equivalent to an additional 300 kcal per day. The actual advisable caloric intake varies within wide limits depending upon maternal age, activity, height, prepregnant weight, stage of pregnancy, and ambient temperature. Caloric needs are greater in the last trimesters than the first. [The caloric value of the diet refers to the physiologically available or metabolizable energy yield of foods actually consumed. The unit of measure is the kilocalorie (kcal).]

The simplest method of evaluating caloric intake is to observe the pattern of weight gain, which is usually minimal (1 to 2 kg) in the first trimester followed by a relatively linear rate of gain of approximately 0.4 kg per week during the last two trimesters. Therefore, caloric intake should be sufficient to support a total weight gain of at least 10 to 12 kg during the entire pregnancy in all patients regardless of the prepregnant weight. Weight reduction diets in pregnancy are not advisable.

Protein requirements in pregnancy should be calculated on a weight basis. This amounts to a total daily protein intake of 1.3 g per kg for the adult woman (approximately 75 g per day), 1.5 g per kg for the adolescent aged 15 to 18, and 1.7 g per kg for younger girls. About two-thirds of the total protein intake should be of high biologic quality such as found in eggs, milk, meat, or soy protein. Adequate total energy intake is essential for optimal protein utilization.

Most women are unable to meet the gestational requirement for iron by diet and iron stores. It is therefore recommended that prophylactic supplements be given in the form of simple ferrous salts in amounts of 30 to 60 mg of elemental iron daily throughout pregnancy and for several months postpartum.

Folic acid is also required in increased amounts during pregnancy. Particularly rich dietary sources of folate include green leafy vegetables, kidney, liver, and peanuts. Since dietary levels of folate may or may not be adequate to meet the demands of pregnancy, some authorities advocate routine supplementation of all patients. If folate supplementation is elected, amounts of 400 to 800 mcg per day are appropriate.

Although other vitamins and minerals are generally required in increased amounts during pregnancy, the advisability of routine supplementation is controversial. If vitamin-mineral supplements are given, they should not be regarded as substitutes for a balanced diet and continued nutritional counseling.

Sodium is required in pregnancy for the expanded maternal tissue and fluid compartments as well as to provide for fetal needs. The normal patient may use the level of sodium intake she prefers. Routine sodium restriction is not advised.

Unless otherwise indicated by complications of the preceding pregnancy and delivery, a well-balanced diet should be provided during the early puerperium. Fluid should neither be restricted nor markedly increased.

For the woman who chooses to breastfeed her infant, nutrition is particularly important. Lactation requires substantial amounts of energy sources, with at least 500 kcal per day above nonpregnant levels recommended. Calcium and protein are also required in greatly increased amounts during lactation inasmuch as 0.2 to 0.3 g of calcium and 8 to 12 g of protein are contained in each day's production of breast milk. Consumption of one quart of milk daily will provide these needs for the nursing mother. In patients for whom milk is physiologically or psychologically unacceptable, alternative sources of protein and calcium will be needed.

If weight reduction is indicated because of pre-gestational obesity or excessive weight gain during pregnancy, weight reduction regimens may be instituted after lactation or, for the nonnursing mother, 2 to 4 weeks postpartum (American College of Obstetricians and Gynecologists 1977).

Prenatal Gain In Weight

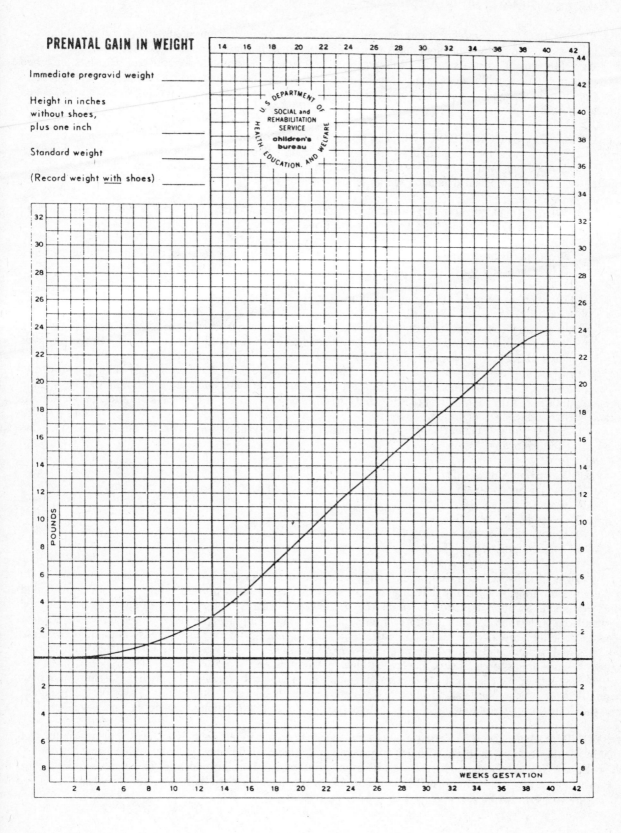

PRENATAL GAIN IN WEIGHT

Immediate pregravid weight _____

Height in inches
without shoes,
plus one inch _____

Standard weight _____

(Record weight with shoes) _____

U S DEPARTMENT OF HEALTH, EDUCATION, AND WELFARE
SOCIAL and REHABILITATION SERVICE
children's bureau

POUNDS

WEEKS GESTATION

5. Diet and Ostomies

DESCRIPTION: Dietary modifications for ostomy patients are based on anatomical/ physiological and aesthetic factors. The amount of small and/or large intestine resected influences fluid, electrolyte, vitamin B_{12}, and folic acid needs. The extent of the ileal resection determines the amount of water and bile salts absorbed and whether renal or gallbladder stones are formed. Flatulence, odor, and discoloration of the output are occasional problems. However, most ostomy patients, especially those with a colostomy, tolerate a normal diet with no difficulty.

FLUID AND ELECTROLYTE NEEDS: The primary function of the terminal ileum is to absorb water and sodium. Consistent with these are studies that show that healthy ileostomy patients have 11% less body water, 7% less body sodium, increased serum aldosterone, and decreased urine volume compared to the normal population. The physiological dynamics are as follows:

- Effluent (ileostomy output) normally contains 60 mEq sodium per 500 cc. When there is more sodium in the effluent, there is less in the urine.

- When the urine contains less than the critical level of 10 mEq sodium, the urine volume declines to less than 600 cc.

- As much as 60 mEq potassium per liter may also be lost.

One to two weeks after surgery, the volume of effluent ranges from 1000 to 1500 cc per day, tapering to 200 to 600 cc. If more than 5 to 10 cm of the ileum has been resected, the volume of effluent remains between 1000 and 1500 cc, proportional to body size. Patients with high outputs may require oral salt and antidiarrheal medications, but all patients are advised to consume 1 to 2 extra cups of fluid per day, and more after exercise or in very hot weather. Because most Americans consume large amounts of salt, sodium supplementation is not routinely necessary, but there may be a need for extra salt after an ileostomy. Potassium needs are also increased.

Diarrhea and subsequent dehydration can occur suddenly in ileostomy patients. The cause can be one or more of the following:

1. Recurrent Crohn's disease
2. Partial or complete intestinal obstruction which can lead to vomiting, bloating, cramping, and reduced output
3. Intra-abdominal sepsis
4. Emotional distress
5. Dietary indiscretion(s)

Signs of dehydration include a dry tongue, decreased skin turgor, and low intraocular pressure. A 70 kg patient who appears clinically dehydrated may need at least 4 liters normal saline for both sodium and water repletion. Sodium depletion is often the greater problem. Symptoms of sodium depletion include lightheadedness, headache, nausea, anorexia, and/or leg cramps. Rapidly transfused saline increases effluent volume and sodium, but decreases the concentration of potassium. Corticosteroids increase potassium excretion and intestinal sodium and water absorption. However, potassium depletion occurs infrequently and can be treated by consuming foods and/or beverages high in this mineral.

Some patients can treat short-term dehydration at home by alternating high potassium and high sodium drinks. Orange juice and strong tea are readily available sources of potassium. Palatable high sodium beverages can be made by adding 1/4 tsp salt to 1 cup cola, or 1 tsp baking soda to 1 cup of water.

MAGNESIUM: Magnesium excretion is about the same in ileostomy effluent as in feces, but deficiency can develop if the output is high. Clinical signs of magnesium deficiency include tetany and secondary hypocalcemia. The recommended treatment is to prescribe magnesium, not calcium. If magnesium deficiency is severe, magnesium sulfate in normal saline should be given. The standard daily dose should equal the RDA, 300 mg for adults, plus 20 mg magnesium sulfate.

VITAMIN B$_{12}$ AND FOLIC ACID: During the first year after surgery, vitamin B$_{12}$ absorption will be low, even in the absence of ileal resection. Resection of the distal ileum may cause malabsorption of both vitamin B$_{12}$ and folic acid. If the resection is appreciable, monthly vitamin B$_{12}$ injections may be required.

FOODS THAT CAUSE OBSTRUCTION: Fruit stones such as pits or seeds of apricots, cherries, dates, prunes, or olives can cause obstruction and should be avoided. Poultry skin or tough sausage casings can also cause blockages as can any high fiber food that is consumed in large amounts or not chewed well. The following foods have been reported as common sources of problems:

Beans and peas, dried
Berries
Cabbage family vegetables
Carrots
Celery
Citrus fruit membranes
Coconut
Corn, particularly "on-the-cob"
Fruit, dried
Green beans
Lettuce
Mushrooms

Nuts
Olives
Onions
Oriental vegetables
Peas
Persimmons
Pickles
Pineapple
Popcorn
Potato skins
Skins and seeds of fruits
  and vegetables
Wild rice

The following symptoms may indicate obstruction:

1. Effluent change from semisolid to thin liquid
2. Increased volume of effluent, with continuous discharge
3. Cramps, usually followed by thin liquid discharge
4. Bloating
5. Vomiting
6. No drainage for 4 to 6 hours

If these occur, the patient is advised to stop eating solid foods and to increase fluid intake. If the obstruction is not relieved within 3 hours, the physician should be contacted.

UROLITHIASIS AND CHOLELITHIASIS: Compared to 4% of the general population, 7% to 18% of ileostomy patients develop renal stones. The most common type is uric acid.

An increased risk for cholelithiasis exists only if the terminal ileum is resected. Its absence has an adverse effect on the enterohepatic circulation of bile acids, increasing the formation of gallstones.

FOODS THAT CAUSE FLATULENCE, ODOR, OR DISCOLORATION: Ostomy bags currently on the market should not leak or emit odor if they fit properly. Therefore dietary precautions regarding odor are usually not necessary. Flatulence may be a problem for some individuals if certain foods are consumed. Other factors such as swallowing extra air during meals, emotional distress, or illness can be the reason.

Beets can produce a reddish effluent similar to the color of blood.

B. SOFT DIET

DESCRIPTION: The Soft Diet, sometimes used as a progression from the liquid to the general diet, consists of foods that are moderate in spice and fiber content. Foods allowed and foods to avoid are the same as for the Low Fiber, Low Residue Diet on page 16, except that milk is not restricted.

    The Soft Diet is *not* designed for the edentulous patient who needs a ground general diet (page 2). For a "very soft diet" which offers a selection of ground and pureed foods that are easily swallowed, the Pureed Soft Diet (pages 10-12) may be ordered. If a greater reduction in residue is required, a minimum residue diet should be ordered (pages 23-25).

MODIFICATION OF THE SOFT DIET:

1. Soft Pureed

DESCRIPTION: This diet is composed of foods that are especially easy to masticate and swallow. It is suitable for patients who have mechanical difficulty in chewing and swallowing. All meats are pureed or ground and served in broth or cream sauce. Vegetables and fruits, except banana, are pureed. Soft cakes, cookies, and other desserts are included.

FOODS ALLOWED AND FOODS TO AVOID:

Food Group	Foods Allowed	Foods to Avoid
Beverages	Milk and milk drinks, carbonated beverages, coffee, tea, decaffeinated coffee, cereal beverages	None
Breads	Enriched white bread or toast, saltine and graham crackers	Bread or rolls with tough crusts, bread or other crackers containing whole grain flour or bran
Cereals	Refined cooked cereals such as cornmeal, farina, rice, oatmeal; refined prepared cereals such as corn or rice flakes, puffed rice	Whole grain cereals except oatmeal, other prepared cereals unless tolerated
Desserts	Plain cornstarch, rice, and tapioca puddings; custards; ice cream; sherbet; plain or flavored yogurt; gelatin desserts; fruit whips; thinly iced or plain soft cakes and cookies	Pastries; pies, any dessert containing nuts, raisins, coconut, or fruit that is not pureed
Eggs	Baked, creamed, poached, soft or hard cooked, scrambled, made into soufflé or fondue	Fried eggs

FOODS ALLOWED AND FOODS TO AVOID (continued):

Food Group	Foods Allowed	Foods to Avoid
Fats	Butter, margarine, cream, vegetable shortening and oils, bland salad dressings, white sauce	Fried foods
Fruits, Fruit Juices	All fruit juices, raw ripe banana, all other fruit that is cooked and pureed	Tart fruit juices if irritating to mouth or throat, raw fruit except banana, fruit that is not pureed
Meat, Fish, Poultry, Cheese	Beef, lamb, veal, liver, pork, chicken, turkey, fish without bones (all should be pureed or finely ground and served in broth or cream sauce); cottage cheese, cream cheese, mild cheddar or processed cheese	Meat, fish, or poultry not prepared as indicated; fatty meat or bacon; spiced or smoked meat or fish; sharp or strongly flavored cheese
Potatoes or Substitutes	Mashed or well-cooked white potatoes, mashed sweet potato, hominy, rice, spaghetti, macaroni, noodles (if able to masticate)	Highly seasoned potatoes or substitutes, fried potatoes or potato chips, wild or brown rice
Soups	Cream soups made with pureed foods, broth soups	Spicy soups or those containing pieces of whole meat or vegetables
Sugar, Sweets	Sugar, syrup, honey, clear jelly, plain candies	Jams, preserves, and candies containing nuts, seeds, coconut, or tough skins
Vegetables, Vegetable Juices	All vegetable juices; cooked and pureed asparagus, beets, green and wax beans, carrots, corn, lima beans, peas, pumpkin, spinach, squash, tomatoes	All raw vegetables, all others
Miscellaneous	Salt, mild flavorings, dilute vinegar, cinnamon, chocolate and cocoa in moderation, smooth peanut butter, cream sauce, nongreasy gravy	Horseradish, pepper, nuts, coconut, olives, pickles, relish, catsup, mustard, popcorn, chili sauce, excessive amounts of spices and herbs[1]

---

[1]Inclusion of spices and seasonings may be modified according to the tolerance of the patient.

APPROXIMATE COMPOSITION OF SAMPLE MENU:

Calories	3007
Protein, g	123
Fat, g	101
Carbohydrate, g	402

SAMPLE MENU FOR SOFT PUREED DIET:

Breakfast	Luncheon	Dinner
1/2 cup orange juice	1/2 cup tomato juice	3 oz ground roast beef
1/2 cup farina	3/4 cup creamed ground chicken on	1/2 cup mashed white potato
1 egg, soft cooked	1/2 cup rice	1/4 cup beef broth gravy
1 slice bread, white enriched	1/2 cup pureed green beans	1/2 cup pureed carrots
1 tsp butter or margarine	1 slice bread, white enriched	1 slice bread, white enriched
1 tbsp grape jelly	1 tsp butter or margarine	1 tsp butter or margarine
1 cup milk	1/2 cup pureed peaches	1/2 cup sherbet
1 tsp sugar	1 slice angel food cake	3 vanilla wafers
Coffee or tea	1 cup milk	1 cup milk
	1 tsp sugar	1 tsp sugar
	Coffee and tea	Coffee or tea

Midmorning Nourishment	Midafternoon Nourishment	Evening Nourishment
1 cup milkshake	1/2 cup vanilla pudding	1 cup chocolate milk

2. Supraglottic

DESCRIPTION: The purpose of the supraglottic diet is to provide a method of eating with minimal aspiration following the removal of the patient's epiglottis and false vocal cords. The diet is also prescribed after a partial or total glossectomy, partial pharyngectomy, or any procedure in which the potential for aspiration exists. The consistency of food is modified to assist the patient in relearning the swallowing process and/or until swelling and soreness subside. The diet includes foods of pureed consistency that are heavy and moist that will form a bolus.

After surgery the patient is maintained on a nasogastric feeding for 10 to 14 days. When the patient starts to eat, the diet is restricted to the following foods: applesauce, farina, pureed fruit, puddings, custard, and mashed potatoes with gravy or butter. If these feedings are tolerated with minimal aspiration, small amounts of fluids are offered orally under the nurse's supervision, and may be added to the tray if only minimal aspiration occurs. Carbonated beverages or thickened liquids such as milkshakes are often tolerated better than other fluids. Water is probably the most difficult fluid for these patients to swallow and should be introduced only some weeks or months after initiation of oral feedings. Small frequent feedings are recommended in order to provide adequate calories.

FEEDING PROCEDURE: The nasogastric tube may or may not be removed before the procedure is initiated. If the patient has a tracheotomy tube with an inflatable cuff, the cuff may be inflated (do not use full cork if the cuff is inflated). The physician or nurse should assist with initial feedings and thereafter as needed. The patient is instructed to sit with the upper trunk of the body in an upright position and to extend the neck backwards to facilitate the flow of food by gravity. The patient is then instructed to:

a. Take a deep breath and hold it.
b. Take a bite of food.
c. Swallow 3 times.
d. Clear the throat.
e. Swallow 3 times and clear the throat again.
f. Take another deep breath before repeating steps a through e.

INITIAL FOODS ALLOWED:

Applesauce   Pureed Fruit
Farina   Mashed Potatoes
Pudding   Custard

FOODS ALLOWED AND FOODS TO AVOID:
(Advance to this level of diet only when there is minimal aspiration.)

Food Group	Foods Allowed	Foods to Avoid
Beverages	As tolerated: carbonated beverages, milk, milk beverages, thick milkshakes, supplemental formulas	Any not tolerated (coffee, tea, water)
Breads	None	All
Cereals	Refined cooked cereals	Oatmeal and all others
Desserts	Pudding, custard, ice cream, sherbet, gelatin	All others
Eggs	Soft cooked, poached, scrambled, plain omelet, custard	Fried, hard cooked
Fats	Butter, margarine, mayonnaise, oil, cream, sour cream	All others
Fruits, Fruit Juices	Fruit juices as tolerated, pureed fruit	All others
Meat, Fish, Poultry, Cheese	Pureed meat, poultry, fish, melted cheese, pureed casseroles made with allowed foods	All others
Potatoes or Substitutes	Mashed white or sweet potatoes, pureed pasta and rice	All others
Soups	Pureed cream soups as tolerated	Broth, bouillon, broth-based soup
Sugar, Sweets	Sugar, syrup, honey, jelly	All others
Vegetables, Vegetable Juices	Vegetable juice as tolerated, pureed vegetables	All others
Miscellaneous	Herbs, spices, salt, vinegar, gravy, sauces, cocoa powder	All others

APPROXIMATE COMPOSITION OF SAMPLE MENU:

Calories	2022
Protein, g	67
Fat, g	72
Carbohydrate, g	292

SAMPLE MENU FOR ADVANCED SUPRAGLOTTIC DIET:

Breakfast

1/2 cup farina
1 egg, soft cooked
1 tsp butter or
  margarine
1/2 cup applesauce
2 tsp sugar

Midmorning
Nourishment

1/2 cup custard

Luncheon

3/4 cup pureed macaroni and
  cheese
1/2 cup pureed green beans
1 tsp butter or margarine
1/2 cup peaches
1/2 cup chocolate pudding

Midafternoon
Nourishment

1/2 cup pureed fruit

Dinner

3 oz pureed beef
1/2 cup mashed potatoes
1/4 cup beef broth gravy
1/2 cup carrots
1 tsp butter or margarine
1/2 cup pureed pears

Evening
Nourishment

1/2 cup vanilla pudding

3. Diets for Oral, Maxillofacial, and Pharyngeal Surgeries

a. Oral and Maxillofacial Surgeries

1. Mandibular or Maxillary Osteotomies and Fractures

The University of Iowa Hospitals and Clinics Oral and Maxillofacial Surgery Department is presently using two types of procedures for mandibular or maxillary osteotomies. The intermaxillary fixation (IMF) is a procedure in which the jaws are tightly wired for 6 to 8 weeks. This is routinely used for fractures and occasionally for osteotomies. Rigid fixation, a procedure in which screws and metal plates are placed permanently in the jaw to fixate it, is used more often for osteotomies. For the initial 1 to 2 weeks following the rigid fixation, the jaws may be wired. The diet progression for both procedures is listed in the chart on page 15.

2. Vestibuloplasty

This is a surgical procedure altering the vestibule of the mouth in preparation for dentures. A skin graft is placed and covered by a splint. No mastication is possible for 4 weeks until the graft is healed. Dentures will be fitted 2 to 3 months after surgery.

3. Temporal Mandibular Joint (TMJ)

Arthroscopy and/or implantation of artificial meniscus are procedures done for TMJ disorder. The patient has extreme pain and headaches from the temporal mandibular joint, especially when eating. The diet following surgery is a cup liquid for the first 3 days and then advances to mechanical soft for 3 months. Hard foods and those difficult to chew should be avoided.

14

Type of Surgery	Diet Type/Rationale	Time Period Post Surgery
Maxillary Osteotomy (IMF) Mandibular Osteotomy (IMF) Fracture (IMF)	Cup liquid - jaws are wired No mastication is possible	6-8 weeks
Mandibular and/or Maxillary Osteotomy (rigid fixation)	Full cup liquid - patient unable to masticate	2-4 weeks
	Soft ground - patient can do minimal mastication	2-4 weeks
	General diet - patient able to chew	4-6 weeks
Vestibuloplasty	Full liquid/full cup liquid No mastication is possible Spoons are allowed	10 days
	Pureed - no mastication allowed	4 weeks
	Soft ground - minimal mastication	1-2 months (until dentures)
TMJ	Full liquid/full cup liquid	3-10 days
	Soft ground or diet as tolerated. Avoid hard foods	3 months

b. Uvulopalato-Pharyngealplasty (UPPP)

The uvulopalato-pharyngealplasty is used to treat sleep apnea. After surgery the UPPP diet is ordered to reduce irritation to the nasal and oral pharynx. Clear liquids consisting of noncitrus juices and cool liquids are allowed. When the diet is progressed to soft, the meals and snacks include the following:

Breakfast: Noncitrus juices, cooked cereal (no ready-to-eat), soft egg, bread (no toast), margarine, jelly, milk

Lunch and Dinner: Noncitrus juices, casseroles, soup, soft meat, mashed potatoes, soft vegetables, canned fruit, gelatin, soft desserts, bread, margarine, milk, iced tea

Nourishments: Shakes, ice cream, sherbet, pudding

C. LOW FIBER, LOW RESIDUE DIET

DESCRIPTION: The Low Fiber, Low Residue Diet provides food that will result in a reduced amount of fecal material in the lower bowel, and produce only a moderate amount of intestinal residue. This diet is designed for the patient receiving radiation therapy on or near the intestines or for the patient with partial bowel obstruction. The diet may also be helpful for patients with acute gastroenteritis, or postoperatively for those who have undergone anal or hemorrhoid surgery. For partial bowel obstruction, the diet should be given as six small meals to decrease the size of the food bolus. Fluids should be encouraged to decrease the possibility of constipation.

The optimal types and levels of fiber for these conditions have not yet been established. Considerable individual tolerance is possible. The fiber content of plant foods differs according to variety and state of maturity. For these reasons, a gram level or range is not specified for this diet. Rather, individual foods are listed in order of fiber content for the following categories: grains, nuts, legumes, fruits, and vegetables. Patients are advised to choose foods they have traditionally tolerated, and to gradually increase the number and variety of servings. Certain foods low in dietary fiber may not be tolerated because of their texture and/or gas-forming properties.

The following suggestions are made for each of the four food groups. Tender meat or meat made tender in the cooking process is used to decrease the amount of connective tissue. Nuts and legumes should be avoided. Milk is restricted to 1 pint daily since it produces a bulky residue in the colon due to bacterial overgrowth with lactose. In individual cases, more milk may be tolerated. Refined breads and cereals which contain little fiber are recommended, but some patients will be able to tolerate whole grains. It is suggested that patients choose 2 fruits and 2 vegetables, thus meeting the basic four recommendations for this food group. Paring fruits and vegetables will reduce the fiber content. Fruits and vegetables which have traditionally been well tolerated are noted.

If a greater reduction in residue is required, a minimum residue diet should be ordered.

ADEQUACY: This diet meets the Recommended Dietary Allowances for all nutrients except iron for women of childbearing age.

FOODS ALLOWED AND FOODS TO AVOID:

Food Group	Foods Allowed	Foods to Avoid
Beverages	Milk and milk drinks (no more than 1 pint daily including that used in cooking), carbonated beverages, coffee, tea, decaffeinated coffee, cereal beverages, nondairy creamer	Milk in excess of 1 pint
Breads	Enriched white and light rye breads or rolls, saltine crackers, melba toast, rusk, zwieback	Bread or crackers containing whole grain flour, bran, or seeds

FOODS ALLOWED AND FOODS TO AVOID (continued):

Food Group	Foods Allowed	Foods to Avoid
Cereals	Cooked refined wheat, corn, or rice cereal; cooked oatmeal; prepared cereals made from corn, rice, or oats	Whole grain cereals
Desserts	Candies, cakes, gelatin, pie, ice cream, pudding, sherbet (all made from milk allowed)	All products containing coconut, seeds, nuts, tough skins, or other foods not tolerated
Eggs	Any	None
Fats	Butter, margarine, vegetable oils, lard, cream or half-and-half (no more than 1/2 cup daily), crisp bacon, mild salad dressings	None
Fruits, Fruit Juices	Choose 2 or more servings from the low and moderate group	Those not tolerated
Meat, Fish, Poultry, Cheese	Tender beef, chicken, fish, lamb, liver, pork, ham, turkey, veal; cottage cheese, cream cheese, mild natural or processed cheese	Unless tolerated: spicy meats and strong cheeses
Potatoes or Substitutes	Hominy, macaroni, noodles, polished rice, spaghetti	Brown or wild rice
Soups	Cream soups (made from milk allowance), broth-based soups made from foods tolerated	All others
Sugar, Sweets	Candy, fruit butter, honey, jelly, molasses, sugar, syrup, (all used in moderation)	Unless tolerated: candy containing fruits or nuts, jam or marmalade containing fruit seeds or skins
Vegetables, Vegetable Juices (including potatoes)	Choose 2 or more servings from the low and moderate groups	Legumes, dried beans and peas, or other vegetables not tolerated
Miscellaneous	Catsup, gravy, smooth peanut butter, mild spices, vinegar, white sauce	Unless tolerated: chili sauce, coconut, horseradish, nuts, olives, pickles, popcorn, relish

Food	Portion	Wt.(g)	Dietary Fiber (g)
Grains: Cereals, Ready-to-eat or Cooked			
Rice Krispies	3/4 cup	21	0.04
Cornflakes	3/4 cup	21	0.2
Farina	1/2 cup	120	0.4
Cornmeal, degermed	1/2 cup	121	0.5
Wheat germ, raw	1/4 cup	19	0.5
Cheerios	3/4 cup	17	0.7
Wheat germ, toasted	1/4 cup	28	0.8
Puffed wheat	1 1/2 cup	18	1.4
Oatmeal, cooked	1/2 cup	116	1.5
Wheaties	3/4 cup	22	1.5
Rice bran	1/2 oz	14	1.6
Whole grain wheat	1/2 cup	75	1.6
Shredded wheat	1 biscuit	24	2.2
Cornmeal, whole grain	2 tbsp	15	2.3
Rolled wheat	1/2 cup	120	2.6
Bulgur wheat	1/2 cup	68	3.5
Oat bran	1/2 oz	14	3.9
40% bran flakes	3/4 cup	34	5.0
Wheat bran	1/2 oz	14	5.6
Corn bran	1/2 oz	14	9.3
All Bran	1/2 cup	42	11.8
100% bran	1/2 cup	42	12.2
Grains: Pasta and Rice, Cooked			
Macaroni	1/2 cup	65	0.5
Spaghetti	1/2 cup	70	0.6
Egg noodles	1/2 cup	80	0.8
Rice, white	1/2 cup	98	0.8
Rice, brown	1/2 cup	98	2.1
Grains: Breads, Crackers, and Popcorn			
Bagel, plain	1 whole	55	0.5
French bread	1 slice	28	0.5
Taco shell	1 shell	11	0.7
White bread	1 slice	28	0.7
Saltine crackers	6 squares	17	0.7
Raisin bread	1 slice	28	0.8
Muffin, plain	1	40	1.1
Rye bread, light	1 slice	28	1.1
Whole wheat crackers	1 oz	28	1.0-1.4
Cornmeal muffin	1	40	1.4
Popcorn, popped	1 cup	6	1.5
Rye bread, dark	1 slice	28	1.7
Cracked wheat bread	1 slice	28	1.7
Bran muffin	1	40	1.8
Mixed grain bread	1 slice	28	1.9
Graham crackers	2 squares	28	2.8
Whole wheat bread	1 slice	28	3.2
Fruits and Fruit Juices			
LOW			
[a]Peach nectar	1/2 cup	125	0.2
[a]Pineapple juice	1/2 cup	125	0.4

Note: Values were obtained from ESHA Research (1985), Lanza and Butrum (1986), and Anderson.
[a]Fruits and vegetables that have traditionally been well tolerated.

Food	Portion	Wt.(g)	Dietary Fiber (g)
[a]Apple juice	1/2 cup	120	0.4
[a]Apricot nectar	1/2 cup	125	0.4
[a]Orange juice	1/2 cup	120	0.5
[a]Tangerine juice	1/2 cup	124	0.5
[a]Grapefruit juice	1/2 cup	120	0.5
[a]Grape juice	1/2 cup	120	0.6
[a]Pear nectar	1/2 cup	125	0.8
[a]Papaya nectar	1/2 cup	125	0.8
Cantaloupe	1/2 cup	80	0.8

MODERATE

Food	Portion	Wt.(g)	Dietary Fiber (g)
Papaya	1/3 medium	101	1.2
Pineapple, canned	1/2 cup	125	1.2
Kiwi fruit	1 average	76	1.2
Cherries, sweet or sour, fresh	10 cherries	68	1.2
Cherries, sour, canned	1/2 cup	122	1.3
Apricots, canned	3 halves	84	1.4
Pineapple, fresh	1/2 cup	78	1.4
[a]Fruit cocktail	1/2 cup	126	1.4
[a]Prune juice	1/2 cup	126	1.5
Apricots, raw	2 medium	71	1.5
[a]Grapefruit, canned	1/2 cup	122	1.5
Grapefruit, fresh	1/2 medium	120	1.5
Rhubarb, cooked, unsweetened	1/2 cup	61	1.5
[a]Avocado	1/4 cup	58	1.6
Dates, dry	2 medium	18	1.6
Grapes	1/2 cup	80	1.6
[a]Mandarin oranges	1/2 cup	100	1.6
Strawberries, fresh	1/2 cup	75	1.7
Tangerine, raw	1 small	84	1.7
Nectarine, raw	1 small	69	1.7
Plums, canned, syrup pack	3	95	1.8
Mango	1/2 cup	83	1.9
Fig, fresh	1 medium	50	1.9
[a]Cherries, sweet, canned	1/2 cup	124	1.9
Peaches, raw	1 medium	87	2.0
Cranberries, raw	1/2 cup	48	2.0
Cranberry sauce	1/4 cup	69	2.0
Plums, canned, juice pack	3	95	2.1
Watermelon, diced	1 cup	160	2.1
[a]Applesauce	1/2 cup	122	2.3
Currants, zante, dried	1/4 cup	124	2.4
Apple, cooked	1/2 cup	85	2.4
Gooseberries, raw	1/2 cup	75	2.4
Blueberries, raw	1/2 cup	73	2.5
[a]Pear, canned	1/2 cup	122	2.5
Rhubarb, cooked, sweetened	1/2 cup	120	2.6
Figs, canned	3 medium	85	2.6
Plum, fresh	1	66	2.6
Raisins, seedless	1/4 cup	41	2.8
Passion fruit, raw	1	18	2.9
Gooseberries, canned	1/2 cup	126	3.0

HIGH

Food	Portion	Wt.(g)	Dietary Fiber (g)
Apple, peeled	1 average	128	3.4
Strawberries	1 cup	149	3.4
Orange, raw	1 average	131	3.5
[a]Banana	1 medium	108	3.6
[a]Peaches, canned	2 halves	162	3.7
Fig, dried	1 medium	20	3.7
Currants, white, raw	1/2 cup	56	3.8
Blackberries, frozen	1/2 cup	76	3.9
Prunes, dried	3	25	4.1
Apple, raw, whole	1 average	138	4.3

19

Food	Portion	Wt.(g)	Dietary Fiber (g)
Raspberries, red, raw	1/2 cup	61	4.5
Loganberries	1/2 cup	74	4.6
Currants, red, raw	1/2 cup	56	4.6
Pear, fresh	1 medium	164	4.7
Currants, black, raw	1/2 cup	56	4.9
Boysenberries, canned	1/2 cup	128	5.3
Blackberries, raw	1/2 cup	72	5.3
Guava	1 medium	90	5.3
Lemons	1 medium	108	5.6
Prunes, canned	1/3 cup	71	5.7
Raspberries, canned	1/2 cup	123	6.1
Blackberries, canned	1/2 cup	128	6.5

Vegetables and Vegetable Juices

LOW

Food	Portion	Wt.(g)	Dietary Fiber (g)
Cucumber, raw, pared	1/2 cup	70	0.3
aTomato juice, canned	1/2 cup	122	0.3
Vegetable juice, canned	1/2 cup	121	0.4
Cucumber, raw, unpared	1/2 cup	53	0.5
Alfalfa sprouts	1/2 cup	17	0.5
Watercress, chopped	1/2 cup	17	0.6
Radishes, red	5 medium	25	0.6
Lettuce, shredded	3/4 cup	42	0.6
Pickle, dill	1 medium	65	0.7
Bean sprouts, raw	1/2 cup	53	0.8
Spinach, chopped, raw	1/2 cup	28	0.8
Mushrooms, sliced, raw	1/2 cup	35	0.9
aPotato, mashed	1/2 cup	105	1.0
Kohlrabi, raw	1/2 cup	70	1.0
Peppers, green or red, sweet	1/2 cup	50	1.0
Asparagus, raw	1/2 cup	67	1.0
Cauliflower, raw	1/2 cup	50	1.1
Green pepper, cooked	1/2 cup	68	1.1
Chinese or savory cabbage, raw	1/2 cup	38	1.1
aGreen beans, canned, drained	1/2 cup	68	1.1
Turnip greens, raw	1/2 cup	28	1.1
Kohlrabi, cooked	1/2 cup	82	1.2
Summer squash, raw	1/2 cup	65	1.2
Celery, raw, chopped	1/2 cup	60	1.2
Cabbage, red, raw	1/2 cup	35	1.2
Bean sprouts, canned	1/2 cup	62	1.3
Soybeans	1/2 cup	90	1.4
Water chestnuts	1/2 cup	70	1.4
Onions, cooked	1/2 cup	105	1.4
Summer squash, cooked	1/2 cup	90	1.4
Tomato, raw	1/2 cup	90	1.5
Cauliflower, fresh cooked	1/2 cup	62	1.6
aAsparagus, cooked	1/2 cup	90	1.6
aPotato, french fried	10 pieces	50	1.6
Broccoli, raw	1/2 cup	44	1.6
Carrots, grated	1/2 cup	55	1.6
Rutabaga	1/2 cup	70	1.6
Turnip, cooked	1/2 cup	78	1.7
Olives	10 large	46	1.7
Cabbage, cooked	1/2 cup	70	1.8
Rutabaga, cooked	1/2 cup	85	1.8
aGreen beans, frozen cooked	1/2 cup	68	1.9

MODERATE

Food	Portion	Wt.(g)	Dietary Fiber (g)
Sauerkraut, canned	1/2 cup	103	2.2
Peas, edible pod, raw	1/2 cup	73	2.2
Parsnips, cooked slices	1/2 cup	78	2.2

Food	Portion	Wt.(g)	Dietary Fiber (g)
Cabbage, savory, raw	1/2 cup	35	2.2
aBeets, canned	1/2 cup	85	2.2
Cauliflower, frozen cooked	1/2 cup	90	2.3
Spinach, fresh cooked	1/2 cup	90	2.3
Carrot, raw	1 medium	81	2.4
aPumpkin, canned	1/2 cup	123	2.4
Tomatoes, canned	1/2 cup	120	2.5
Beans, green, raw	1/2 cup	55	2.5
Broccoli, fresh cooked	1/2 cup	78	2.5
Mixed vegetables, frozen cooked	1/2 cup	91	2.5
Okra, cooked	1/2 cup	87	2.6
aCarrots, fresh cooked	1/2 cup	73	2.6
aCarrots, canned	1/2 cup	73	2.7
aPotato chips	14 chips	28	2.7
Turnip greens, cooked	1/2 cup	72	2.8
aGreen beans, fresh cooked	1/2 cup	63	2.8
aSweet potato, baked, mashed	1/2 cup	100	2.8
Yam, white, cooked cubes	1/2 cup	68	2.8
Brussels sprouts	1/2 cup	78	2.8
aEggplant, cooked	1/2 cup	100	3.0
Broccoli, frozen cooked	1/2 cup	93	3.0
aSweet potato, baked, peeled	1	114	3.0
aMushrooms, canned	1/2 cup	78	3.0
aSweet potato, canned	1/2 cup	128	3.1
Peas, edible pod, cooked	1/2 cup	80	3.2
Corn-on-the-cob	1 small ear	70 (corn only)	3.3
aSquash, winter, boiled or mashed	1/2 cup	123	3.4
aSweet potato, boiled, peeled, mashed	1/2 cup	128	3.4
Lentils, cooked	1/2 cup	100	3.5
Parsnips, raw slices	1/2 cup	78	3.5
aSweet potato, boiled, peeled	1	151	3.6
Peas, black-eyed, fresh cooked	1/2 cup	83	3.6
Peas, raw	1/2 cup	73	3.8
aPotato, baked, no skin	1 average	156	3.9
Corn, frozen cooked	1/2 cup	82	3.9

HIGH

Food	Portion	Wt.(g)	Dietary Fiber (g)
Peas, fresh or frozen cooked	1/2 cup	80	4.2
Succotash, frozen cooked	1/2 cup	85	4.3
Butter beans, cooked	1/2 cup	85	4.4
Lima beans, cooked	1/2 cup	84	4.4
Potato, baked with skin	1 average	202	4.4
aSquash, winter, baked	1/2 cup	103	4.6
Garbanzo beans, cooked	1/2 cup	85	4.8
Spinach, frozen cooked	1/2 cup	95	5.0
Spinach, canned	1/2 cup	103	5.3
Peas, canned, drained	1/2 cup	85	6.0
Peas, black-eyed, dry cooked	1/2 cup	125	6.1
Great northern beans, cooked	1/2 cup	90	6.2
Artichoke, whole, cooked	1/2 globe	190	6.3
Corn, canned, creamed	1/2 cup	128	7.3
Corn, whole kernel, canned	1/2 cup	128	7.3
Broad beans, cooked	1/2 cup	100	9.3
Black beans, cooked	1/2 cup	100	9.7
Kidney beans, cooked	1/2 cup	93	9.7
Pinto beans, cooked	1/2 cup	95	10.0

Nuts, Seeds, and Related Products

Food	Portion	Wt.(g)	Dietary Fiber (g)
Pumpkin/squash kernels, dried	2 tbsp	17	0.4
Pine nuts	1 oz	28	0.4

Food	Portion	Wt.(g)	Dietary Fiber (g)
Pistachios, shelled	2 tbsp	16	0.4
Macadamia nuts	2 tbsp	17	0.7
Almonds, blanched, slivered	2 tbsp	15	0.7-1.7
Walnuts, english	2 tbsp	15	0.7
Soybeans, roasted/toasted	2 tbsp	14	0.8
Tahini (sesame butter)	1 tbsp	15	0.8
Walnuts, black	2 tbsp	16	0.8
Filberts (hazelnuts), chopped	2 tbsp	14	0.9
Sunflower seeds	2 tbsp	18	1.0
Cashews	2 tbsp	16	1.0
Cashew butter	1 tbsp	16	1.0
Peanut butter	1 tbsp	9	1.2
Almonds, dried, whole	2 tbsp	18	1.3-2.5
Peanuts, roasted, salted	2 tbsp	18	1.5
Peanuts, dried	2 tbsp	18	1.7
Sesame seed kernels, hulled	2 tbsp	19	1.1
Chestnuts, roasted	2 tbsp	18	1.2
Brazil nuts	6 large	28	2.5
Coconut, fresh	1/4 cup	20	2.7
Chestnuts, raw	1 oz	28	3.2
Coconut, dried sweetened	1/4 cup	21	4.9

D. MINIMUM RESIDUE DIET

DESCRIPTION: The purpose of the Minimum Residue Diet is to supply food that will provide more complete nourishment than the Clear Liquid Diet while producing a minimum of fecal residue in the lower bowel. This diet may be used for patients before and after abdominal surgery, or as a transitional diet between clear liquid and soft diets. To reduce indigestible carbohydrate to a minimum, all fruits and vegetables are omitted except strained fruit juice and tomato juice. Eggs, tender meat, or meat made tender in the cooking process are used. Milk as a beverage is not allowed.

If no residue is desired, an elemental diet with predigested protein can be used. However, similar results can be obtained with better acceptance using the minimum residue diet.

ADEQUACY: This diet does not meet the Recommended Dietary Allowances for calcium, iron, vitamin A, riboflavin, or vitamin D. If used for a long period, it should be supplemented with vitamins and minerals or a minimum residue formula (see chart on pages 288-94).

FOODS ALLOWED AND FOODS TO AVOID:

Food Group	Foods Allowed	Foods to Avoid
Beverages	Coffee, tea, decaffeinated coffee, cereal beverages, carbonated beverages, nondairy creamer, 1 oz cream/day	Milk, milk drinks
Breads	Saltine crackers, melba toast, rusk, zwieback; refined, enriched white bread	Bread or crackers containing whole grain flour or bran
Cereals	Cooked refined wheat, corn, or rice cereal; strained oatmeal; prepared cereals made from refined corn or rice	Whole grain cereals, barley
Desserts	Arrowroot and plain sugar cookies, angel food and sponge cakes, plain gelatin desserts, puddings made with strained fruit juice or water, popsicles, fruit ices and frappés made without milk; sugar and vanilla wafers	All products containing seeds, nuts, coconut, fruit, fruit pulp, and other foods to avoid
Eggs	Any except fried	Fried eggs
Fats	Butter, margarine, crisp bacon, bland salad dressings	None

FOODS ALLOWED AND FOODS TO AVOID (continued):

Food Group	Foods Allowed	Foods to Avoid
Fruits, Fruit Juices	Strained fruit juices	All others
Meat, Fish, Poultry, Cheese	Tender beef, chicken, lamb, liver, turkey, pork, veal, fish; cottage cheese; cream cheese; American cheese (used only in cooking)	Fried meat, fish, poultry; cheese other than that allowed
Potatoes or Substitutes	Macaroni, noodles, refined rice, spaghetti	Potatoes, hominy, whole grain or wild rice
Soups	Bouillon, broth, consommé	All others
Sugar, Sweets	Plain candy, honey, jelly, marshmallows, sugar, syrup (all used in moderation)	Jam, marmalade, candy containing fruits or nuts
Vegetables, Vegetable Juices	Tomato juice	All others
Miscellaneous	Salt, mild spices in moderation, dilute vinegar, gravy in moderation	Catsup, chili sauce, peanut butter, coconut, garlic, horseradish, nuts, olives, pickles, relish, popcorn, herbs

APPROXIMATE COMPOSITION OF SAMPLE MENU:

Calories	2477
Protein, g	82
Fat, g	56
Carbohydrate, g	406

SAMPLE MENU FOR MINIMUM RESIDUE DIET:

Breakfast

1/2 cup strained orange juice
1/2 cup farina
1 egg, soft cooked
2 slices refined white bread, enriched
2 tsp butter or margarine
1 tbsp grape jelly
2 tsp sugar
1/4 cup nondairy creamer

Luncheon

1/2 cup tomato juice
2 oz sliced chicken
1 cup rice
2 slices refined white bread, enriched
2 tsp butter or margarine
1 tbsp honey
1 slice angel food cake
1 tsp sugar
Coffee or tea

Dinner

3 oz roast beef
1/2 cup noodles
1/2 cup beef broth
2 slices refined white bread enriched
2 tsp butter or margarine
1 tbsp apple jelly
1/2 cup orange gelatin
3 vanilla wafers
1/2 cup lemon pudding
1 tsp sugar
Coffee or tea

SAMPLE MENU FOR MINIMUM RESIDUE DIET (continued):

Midmorning Nourishment	Midafternoon Nourishment	Evening Nourishment
3 arrowroot cookies	1 popsicle	1/2 cup apple juice
1/2 cup grape juice		

E. BLAND DIET

DESCRIPTION: This diet may be used for esophageal reflux (heartburn), hiatal hernia, and as a treatment for acute or chronic peptic ulcer disease.

1. Bland Diet for Esophageal Reflux or Hiatal Hernia

DESCRIPTION: Esophageal reflux refers to regurgitation of gastric contents into the esophagus. Chronic reflux may lead to esophagitis and subsequent ulceration, hemorrhage, and/or stricture. Normally the esophageal sphincter prevents reflux, but in relation to hormonal, drug, mechanical, or dietary factors, the sphincter pressure may become low with resulting regurgitation. It may also occur late in pregnancy when an increase in progesterone results in muscle relaxation. Intra-abdominal pressure in relation to obesity and constipation or even constricting garments can also result in regurgitation. Nicotine exposure is reported to be a factor.

When the esophagus is ulcerated by reflux of digestive juices, heartburn is made worse by acidic fruits and juices such as citrus juices. The patient can identify these and avoid them. Dietary manipulation cannot eliminate the cause (digestive juice reflux), but may reduce the symptoms.

Hiatal hernia refers to a rupture in which a portion of the stomach protrudes through the diaphragm at the esophagus. Initial symptoms are often similar to reflux with mild to severe pain. Small volumes of food are usually better tolerated than larger ones. Moderation in fat, caffeine, and spice intake is recommended and food temperature extremes should be avoided. Although small amounts may be tolerated in a meal, the following foods should generally be avoided.

FOODS TO AVOID:

Food Groups	Foods to Avoid
Beverages	Coffee, decaffeinated coffee, carbonated beverages, and chocolate
Fats	Excessive amounts
Fruits, Fruit Juices	Citrus fruits and juices
Vegetables, Vegetable Juices	Tomato, tomato juice
Miscellaneous	Dill, peppermint, spearmint, and foods prepared with excess spices

2. Bland Diet for Peptic Ulcer

DESCRIPTION: When the Bland Diet is used for the treatment of acute or chronic peptic ulcer disease, the following principles are used as guidelines.

1. The diet should be as liberal as possible and individualized to fit the needs of the patient in regard to food intolerance, life-style, work schedule, and education.

2. Broth, coffee (both regular and decaffeinated), caffeine, and pepper are usually avoided since they stimulate gastric secretion.

3. Three to five feedings of moderate volume are advocated as a means of lowering the acidity of the gastric contents and to promote the physical comfort of the patient. (Three feedings are often recommended for the patient of normal weight. By restricting the number of meals and taking antacids, total acid production is reduced. For the patient who needs to gain weight or who cannot tolerate normal volumes of food, five feedings may be required. A bedtime snack is specifically not recommended in order to decrease gastric acid production at night.)

4. Selection of a varied diet is encouraged by the use of educational materials and the selective menu.

5. It is recognized that a milk-rich diet may be contraindicated when certain other conditions are present such as milk allergy, lactose intolerance, or hypercalcemia.

When a bland diet is requested for the patient with peptic ulcer disease, the Soft Diet (pages 10-12) is offered to the patient with the following conditions:

1. Coffee is omitted. (Pepper and other strong spices are not included on the Soft Diet.)

2. Three meals of moderate volume are encouraged.

3. Individualization of the diet is emphasized. A diet with general consistency is often tolerated.

Should a more restricted consistency or texture be necessary, the Low Fiber, Low Residue; Pureed Soft; or Full Liquid diets may be ordered with the bland notation, e.g., "Full Liquid, Bland." The appropriate diet will be offered to the patient with the conditions listed above. Therapeutic diets are also available with the bland modification.

F. FULL LIQUID DIET

DESCRIPTION: The Full Liquid Diet includes a variety of foods that are liquid or will become liquid at body temperature. The diet is recommended for short-term use when a patient cannot tolerate solid food. Nourishments served between meals and at bedtime increase the caloric and nutrient intake.

The diet is high in lactose unless acidophilus milk or lactose-free formulas are used instead of milk. The diet is also high in cholesterol and fat. Although this is not usually a problem for short-term use, the diet can be modified to be low in cholesterol and fat.

ADEQUACY: This diet will meet the Recommended Dietary Allowances for all nutrients, except iron for women of childbearing age, only if the diet includes more than the recommended number of servings from the Basic Four Food Plan. The most difficult foods to include are those from the meat, fish, poultry, and cheese group (3 1/2 oz jar pureed meat = 2 oz meat).

FOODS ALLOWED AND FOODS TO AVOID:

Food Group	Foods Allowed	Foods to Avoid
Beverages	Coffee, tea, decaffeinated coffee, cereal beverages, milk, milk drinks, carbonated beverages, fruit drinks	All others
Breads	None	All
Cereals	Cooked refined cereal, cereal gruel	All others
Desserts	Custard, gelatin desserts, rennet dessert, ice cream, sherbet, cornstarch pudding, popsicles	All products containing seeds, nuts, coconut, fruit, and other foods not allowed
Eggs	Soft custard, eggnog	All others
Fats	Butter, margarine, cream, vegetable oils	All others
Fruits, Fruit Juices	All fruit juices, pureed fruit	All others
Meat, Fish, Poultry, Cheese	Mild cheese sauce, pureed meat added to broth or cream soup	All others
Potatoes or Substitutes	Mashed white potato used in cream soup	All others

FOODS ALLOWED AND FOODS TO AVOID (continued):

Food Group	Foods Allowed	Foods to Avoid
Soups	Consommé, broth, bouillon, strained cream soup made from foods allowed	All others
Sugar, Sweets	Honey, sugar, syrup, hard candy	Jam; marmalade; candy containing coconut, fruit, or nuts
Vegetables, Vegetable Juices	All vegetable juices, pureed vegetables in cream soup	All others
Miscellaneous	Salt, flavorings, chocolate syrup, cocoa powder, cinnamon, nutmeg	All others

APPROXIMATE COMPOSITION OF SAMPLE MENU:

Calories	2528
Protein, g	82
Fat, g	82
Carbohydrate, g	372

SAMPLE MENU FOR FULL LIQUID DIET:

Breakfast	Luncheon	Dinner
1/2 cup orange juice	1/2 cup tomato juice	1/2 cup pineapple juice
1/2 cup farina	3/4 cup cream of potato soup	3/4 cup strained cream of chicken soup (1/2 cup soup with 1/4 cup pureed chicken)
1 cup milk	1/2 cup pureed peaches	
2 tsp sugar	1/2 cup vanilla ice cream	
1 cup eggnog	1 cup milk	3/4 cup chocolate milkshake
Coffee or tea	1 tsp sugar	1/2 cup flavored gelatin
1/2 oz half-and-half	Coffee and tea	1/2 cup pureed pears
	1/2 oz half-and-half	1 cup milk
		1 tsp sugar
		Coffee and tea
		1/2 oz half-and-half

Midmorning Nourishment	Midafternoon Nourishment	Evening Nourishment
1/2 cup pureed banana	1/2 cup vanilla flavored yogurt	1 cup chocolate milk

MODIFICATIONS OF THE FULL LIQUID DIET:

1. High Protein, High Calorie Liquid

DESCRIPTION: If a patient's nutritional status is compromised, or if a liquid diet is needed for more than a week, the high protein, high calorie modification should be ordered. Calories will be increased by approximately 800 and protein by 30 g when additional liquids are added to the 3 meals and snacks. For additional calories, butter or margarine may be added to hot liquids, powdered glucose polymers may be dissolved in fruit juices, and stick candy may be added to the tray.

For additional protein in the diet, dry milk powder or powdered protein supplements may be added to foods. Protein, vitamins, minerals, and calories may be increased by the addition of supplemental formulas or milk-based nourishments. Adequate water must be provided to excrete the daily urinary solute load and to avoid dehydration. Urinary specific gravity should be maintained at a level below the maximum for that person.

APPROXIMATE COMPOSITION OF SAMPLE MENU:

Calories	3251
Protein, g	102
Fat, g	105
Carbohydrate, g	483

SAMPLE MENU FOR HIGH PROTEIN, HIGH CALORIE LIQUID DIET:

Breakfast	Luncheon	Dinner
1 cup orange juice	1/2 cup tomato juice	1 cup pineapple juice
1 cup farina	3/4 cup cream of potato soup	3/4 cup strained cream of
1/4 cup half-and-half	1/2 cup pureed peaches	chicken soup (1/2 cup soup
1 cup eggnog	1/2 cup chocolate custard	with 1/4 cup pureed
1 cup milk	1/3 cup vanilla ice cream	chicken)
2 tsp sugar	1 cup milk	1/2 cup sherbet
Coffee and tea	1 tsp sugar	3/4 cup chocolate milkshake
1 oz half-and-half	Coffee and tea	1/2 cup flavored gelatin
	1 oz half-and-half	1/2 cup pureed pears
		1 cup milk
		1 tsp sugar
		Coffee and tea
		1 oz half-and-half

Midmorning Nourishment	Midafternoon Nourishment	Evening Nourishment
1/2 cup pureed banana	1 cup vanilla flavored yogurt	1 cup chocolate milk

2. Cup Full Liquid

DESCRIPTION: This diet consists of foods that can be drunk from a cup. Drinking straws and eating utensils are omitted from the tray. The diet is commonly ordered for patients unable to chew due to injury and/or surgery. Spices and seasonings that cause sneezing should be avoided to prevent potential damage to the repaired tissues. Many patients lose weight on this diet due to difficulty in consuming large volumes of liquids. To prevent excess weight loss, the following recommendations are made:

Eat small frequent meals, 5 to 6 times a day.

Plan variety in temperature, color, and flavor.

Limit empty calorie foods such as coffee, tea, alcohol, and soft drinks.

If the patient's nutritional status is compromised or if the diet is needed for more than 1 week, the high protein, high calorie modification is recommended.

FOODS ALLOWED AND FOODS TO AVOID:

Food Group	Foods Allowed	Foods to Avoid
Beverages	Milk, thinned milkshakes, eggnog, cocoa, supplemental formulas, carbonated beverages, coffee, tea, decaffeinated coffee	Alcoholic beverages; coffee, tea, and carbonated beverages in excess of 2-3 cups
Breads	None	All
Cereals	Thinned, blended, cooked cereal	All others
Desserts	Thinned, blended desserts, puddings, custard, ice cream, sherbet, yogurt; liquid gelatin	Desserts with seeds, nuts, or coconut
Eggs	Eggnog, blended egg dishes	All others
Fats	Melted butter or margarine, cream, mayonnaise, salad dressings, oils, gravy	All others
Fruits, Fruit Juices	All fruit juices; thinned, pureed fruit without skins or seeds	Fruits prepared other than as indicated
Meats, Fish, Blended Cheese, or Substitutes	Blended, thinned meat, fish, poultry, cottage cheese, casseroles made with allowed foods, cooked dried beans or peas	Any prepared other than as indicated
Potatoes or Substitutes	Blended, thinned, mashed sweet potatoes, rice, and pasta	All others
Soups	Blended, strained vegetable and cream soups; broth, bouillon, consommé	All others
Sugar, Sweets	Sugar, syrup, honey, chocolate syrup	All others
Vegetables, Vegetable Juices	All vegetable juices; thinned, pureed vegetables without skins and seeds	Vegetables with skins or seeds
Miscellaneous	Salt, cinnamon, spices, seasonings, cocoa powder, lemon juice, vinegar, sauces	Pepper, spices, or seasonings that cause sneezing

APPROXIMATE COMPOSITION OF SAMPLE MENU:

Calories	2602
Protein, g	113
Fat, g	79
Carbohydrate, g	364

SAMPLE MENU FOR CUP FULL LIQUID DIET:

Breakfast

1/2 cup orange
  juice
1 cup thinned
  farina
1 cup eggnog
1 cup milk
Coffee or tea
2 tsp sugar
1/2 oz half-and-
  half

Luncheon

1/2 cup tomato juice
3/4 cup strained cream of
  potato soup
1/2 cup blended, thinned,
  green beans
1 tsp butter or margarine
1/2 cup thinned yogurt
1 cup milk

Dinner

1/2 cup pineapple juice
1 cup strained cream of
  chicken soup (3/4 cup soup
  with 1/4 cup pureed
  chicken)
3/4 cup blended, thinned
  goulash
1/2 cup pureed, thinned
  applesauce
1 cup milk

Midmorning Nourishment

1 cup Instant
  Breakfast
1/2 cup pureed,
  thinned banana

Midafternoon Nourishment

1 cup strawberry milkshake
1/2 cup pureed, thinned
  peaches

Evening Nourishment

1 cup chocolate milk
1/2 cup pureed, thinned
  pears

G. CLEAR LIQUID DIET

DESCRIPTION: This diet provides clear fluids that are easily absorbed with a minimum of digestive activity and leave little residue. Nearly all of the calories are provided as carbohydrate, unless a minimum residue formula is given (see pages 288-94; lactose-free, partially predigested, and elemental). No milk products are included. The foods are liquid or will become liquid at body temperature. The clear liquid diet is used only for short periods of time: preoperatively to minimize the risk of regurgitation and/or aspiration during surgery; postoperatively to test the patient's tolerance to food; during acute illnesses when nausea, vomiting, or diarrhea is severe; and prior to certain tests, such as the barium enema.

Due to its high concentration of simple carbohydrates, the Clear Liquid Diet may be contraindicated following gastric surgery because the high concentration of simple sugars may cause osmotic diarrhea. The diet must be modified for the patient with diabetes mellitus or hypoglycemia and in these cases should be ordered as "Diabetic Clear Liquid" or "Hypoglycemia Clear Liquid."

ADEQUACY: This diet does not meet the Recommended Dietary Allowance for any nutrient except ascorbic acid. It is especially low in protein, and few patients who need the diet are able to consume adequate calories. Its continued use leads to weight loss, tissue wasting, and multiple nutritional deficiencies, particularly if instituted in individuals with increased caloric needs or in those whose nutritional status is marginal. Thus the diet is not recommended for more than 3 days without supplementation. A high protein clear liquid diet can be ordered (see page 34) which is supplemented with various minimum residue formulas. The adequacy of the patient's diet would then depend upon the quantity of formula consumed.

FOODS ALLOWED AND FOODS TO AVOID:

Food Group	Foods Allowed	Foods to Avoid
Beverages	Carbonated beverages, coffee, tea, decaffeinated coffee, fruit-flavored drinks, minimum residue formulas	Milk, milk drinks
Breads	None	All
Cereals	None	All
Desserts	Clear, flavored gelatin; popsicles	All others
Eggs	None	All
Fats	None	All
Fruits, Fruit Juices	Fruit juices (apple, cherry, cranapple, pineapple, cranberry, grape, orange)	Fruit juices with excess pulp, all fruit
Soups	Clear broth, consommé	All others
Sugar, Sweets	Sugar, honey, syrup, stick candy, clear sugar candy	All others

33

APPROXIMATE COMPOSITION OF SAMPLE MENU:

Calories	1189
Protein, g	43
Fat, g	1
Carbohydrate, g	256

SAMPLE MENU FOR CLEAR LIQUID DIET:

Breakfast	Luncheon	Dinner
1/2 cup orange juice	1/2 cup grape juice	1/2 cup apple juice
3/4 cup broth	3/4 cup broth	3/4 cup broth
1/2 cup flavored gelatin	1/2 cup flavored gelatin	1/2 cup flavored gelatin
1 tsp sugar	2 sticks hard candy	2 sticks hard candy
Coffee or tea	1 tsp sugar	1 tsp sugar
	Coffee or tea	Coffee and tea

Midmorning Nourishment	Midafternoon Nourishment	Evening Nourishment
1 cup high protein liquid supplement[1]	1/2 cup high protein gelatin	1 cup high protein clear liquid supplement[1]

MODIFICATIONS OF CLEAR LIQUID DIET:

1. High Protein, High Calorie Clear Liquid

DESCRIPTION: If a patient's nutritional status is compromised, or if a clear liquid diet is needed for more than a week, the high protein, high calorie modification should be ordered. Calories will be increased by approximately 800 and protein by 30 g when a minimum residue formula and supplement are added to the 3 meals and snacks. (See pages 288-94; lactose-free, partially pre-digested and elemental.) Adequate water must be provided to excrete the daily urinary solute load and to avoid dehydration. Urinary specific gravity should be maintained at a level below the maximum for that person.

APPROXIMATE COMPOSITION OF SAMPLE MENU:

Calories	2529
Protein, g	92
Fat, g	30
Carbohydrate, g	476

---

[1]Citrotein (Sandoz Nutrition, 5320 W. 23rd St., P.O. Box 370, Minneapolis, MN 55440), SLD (Ross Laboratories, 625 Cleveland Ave., Columbus, OH 43215), or Nutrex Drink (Nutrex Corporation, 1168 Aster Ave., Bldg. C., Sunnyvale, CA 94086).

SAMPLE MENU FOR HIGH PROTEIN, HIGH CALORIE CLEAR LIQUID DIET:

Breakfast	Luncheon	Dinner
1/2 cup orange juice	1/2 cup grape juice	1/2 cup apple juice
1/2 cup broth	3/4 cup broth	3/4 cup broth
1/2 cup high protein gelatin[1]	1/2 cup high protein gelatin[1]	1/2 cup high protein gelatin[1]
1 cup high protein clear liquid supplement[2]	1 cup high protein clear liquid supplement[2]	1 cup high protein clear liquid supplement[2]
1 tsp sugar	2 sticks hard candy	2 sticks hard candy
Coffee or tea	1 tsp sugar	1 tsp sugar
	Coffee or tea	Coffee or tea

Midmorning Nourishment	Midafternoon Nourishment	Evening Nourishment
1/2 cup cranberry juice	1/2 cup high protein gelatin[1]	1/2 cup high protein gelatin[1]
1 cup minimum residue formula[3]	1 cup minimum residue formula[3]	1 cup minimum residue formula[3]

2. Surgical Clear Liquid

DESCRIPTION: This diet consists only of tea, broth, and noncola carbonated beverages. It may be ordered for postoperative patients and those in acute stages of many illnesses. It is inadequate in calories and all nutrients.

3. Cup Clear Liquid

DESCRIPTION: All allowed clear liquids that can be drunk from a cup will be used. Drinking straws and eating utensils are omitted from the tray.

---

[1]Recipe in Appendix J.

[2]Citrotein (Sandoz Nutrition, 5320 W. 23rd St., P.O. Box 370, Minneapolis, MN 55440, SLD (Ross Laboratories, 625 Cleveland Ave., Columbus, OH 43215), or Nutrex Drink (Nutrex Corporation, 1168 Aster Ave., Bldg. C., Sunnyvale, CA 94086).

[3]Ensure (Ross Laboratories, 625 Cleveland Ave., Columbus, OH 43215) was used in this sample menu.

SECTION 2

Modification in Mineral Content

MILLIEQUIVALENT (mEq) CONVERSION TABLE

To Determine mEq Values of	Divide Milligrams by mEq Weight[a]
Sodium	23
Potassium	39
Magnesium	12
Phosphorus	15.5
Calcium	20
Chlorides (as Cl)	35.5
Chloride (as NaCl)	58.5

Example: 1000 mg sodium $= \dfrac{1000}{23} = 43.4$ mEq sodium

[a]mEq weight of an element is the atomic weight divided by the valence.

FORMULA FOR CONVERTING MILLIGRAMS TO MILLIEQUIVALENTS

$$\frac{\text{Milligrams}}{\text{Atomic weight}} \times \text{Valence} = \text{Milliequivalents}$$

Example: $\dfrac{300 \text{ mg calcium}}{40.07} \times 2 = 15$ milliequivalents

or

Milligrams X Conversion Factor = Milliequivalents
Example: 300 mg calcium X 0.05 = 15 milliequivalents

Mineral	Atomic Weight	Valence	Conversion Factor
Calcium	40.07	2	0.05
Chlorine	35.46	1	0.0282
Phosphorus	31.04	2	0.06443
Potassium	39.1	1	0.02557
Sodium	23	1	0.0435
Magnesium	24.32	2	0.08141

A. CALCIUM RESTRICTED DIETS

DESCRIPTION: Although contraindicated for most cases of hypercalcemia, idiopathic hypercalciuria, and metastatic cancer, the calcium restricted diet is occasionally used. For diagnostic purposes, the 200 mg calcium diet is sometimes used during a limited period to assure a minimum relatively constant intake of calcium while calcium metabolism is being studied.

These diets are ordered in terms of milligrams or milliequivalents of calcium, the level varying with the patient's condition, drug therapy, and individual response. Common levels of calcium restriction are:

Mild - 800 mg (40 mEq)

Moderate - 600 mg (30 mEq)

Strict - 400 mg (20 mEq)

Very Strict - 200 mg (10 mEq)

Many different combinations of foods are possible within the calcium restricted diet, especially for the higher levels. The suggested exchanges constitute a pattern typical of patients at University of Iowa Hospitals and Clinics. However, individualization of the diet is recommended, and changing the pattern by calculation and substitution will improve adherence.

The estimated calcium content of a diet that includes a variety of food, but no milk or milk products, is 500 to 600 mg. Although milk and milk products are the richest sources of calcium in American diets, soft edible fish bones, quick breads, dark green leafy vegetables, and foods or supplements fortified with calcium can contribute significant amounts. Many antacids also contain calcium. Labels for food and medications should be read carefully.

Hard water can contain considerable calcium. To determine the amount, the patient should check with the local dietitian or municipal water company. Foods may be cooked with tap water, unless the calcium content is more than 200 mg per liter. If the calcium content is less than 25 mg per liter, the tap water may be used for drinking. Because Iowa City water contains 50 to 100 mg calcium per liter, distilled water is recommended for preparing beverages for all low calcium diets.

ADEQUACY: The nutritional adequacy of the calcium restricted diet depends upon the patient's appetite, food preferences, and level of calcium restriction. With careful selections from the basic four food groups, the Recommended Dietary Allowances (except for calcium) can be met at the 800 and 600 mg levels for most age and sex groups. Because of the limited selections, diets restricted to 400 mg or less are often inadequate in iron, riboflavin, folic acid, and magnesium. Supplementation of these vitamins and minerals may be necessary.

1. Mild Low Calcium Diet (800 mg or 40 mEq)

DESCRIPTION: A general hospital diet is used with 200 to 300 mg calcium permitted in milk or milk products (see table on page 38). A diet history is taken to determine the average calcium content of the patient's diet and to determine if other calcium-rich foods are consumed in sufficient quantity or frequency to warrant calculation. Foods highly fortified with calcium should be avoided.

300 mg Calcium	200 mg Calcium	100 mg Calcium
1 cup whole, 2%, chocolate, or skim milk	1 oz cheese, cheese spreads, or cheese foods	1/2 cup cottage cheese
1 cup buttermilk		1/2 cup ice cream
1 cup yogurt		1/3 cup pudding
1/3 cup nonfat dry milk		1/3 cup custard
1/2 cup evaporated milk		1/6 of 9 in. cream pie
		1/2 cup cream soup
		1/2 cup cream or half-and-half

2. Moderate Low Calcium Diet (600 mg or 30 mEq)

DESCRIPTION: A general diet is used with no milk, milk products, or fish with soft edible bones. Foods containing considerable calcium as a supplement or additive are also restricted. Exceptions may be permitted in some cases based on the patient's individual food preferences and habits.

FOODS ALLOWED AND FOODS TO AVOID:

Food Group	Foods Allowed	Foods to Avoid
Beverages	Coffee, tea, or decaffeinated coffee, carbonated beverages. Limit Kool-Aid, Tang, and similar powdered fruit drink mixes to 1 cup per day[1]	Milk, milk beverages; Kool-Aid, Tang, and similar powdered fruit drink mixes in excess of 1 cup per day
Breads	Limit to 200 mg calcium/day using the following bread exchange lists:	Breads or crackers made with significant amounts of cheese (check labels)

Breads: (Since the USRDA for calcium is 1000 mg, 2% is 20 mg, 4% is 40 mg and so on. Labels for commercial foods may be used to determine the amount of calcium per serving, and therefore the category to which the food belongs.)

LIST A: Average 5 mg/serving

Biscuit from refrigerated dough (2 in. diam)	1
Bread, any made without milk products and not enriched with calcium such as most italian, french, and vienna breads	1 slice
Breadsticks, plain	2
Graham crackers	2
Saltine or soda crackers	4
Goldfish cheese crackers	12
Rusk	1

---

[1]Calcium phosphates are added to powdered soft drink mixes to regulate tartness and prevent caking. The amounts added vary according to flavor and type of mix, i.e., sugar-sweetened, unsweetened, and aspartame-sweetened. The calcium content of the beverages varies from negligible to 70 mg per cup, averaging 18 mg per cup for prepared beverage mixes containing sugar, 27 mg per cup prepared beverage for mixes containing aspartame, and 14 mg per cup prepared beverage for unsweetened mixes to which the consumer adds sweetener.

LIST B: Average 25 mg/serving

Bagel half	1
Biscuit made from mix with water (2 in. diam)	1
Bread, any kind, except as noted in List A	1 slice
Doughnut (3 in. diam)	1
English muffin, medium	1 whole
Sweet roll	1 medium or 2 oz

LIST C: Average 50 mg/serving

Bagel, medium	1 whole
Biscuit made from mix with milk (2 in. diam)	1
Coffeecake (no nuts)	2 in. sq
Cornbread (2 in. cube)	1
Muffin, any kind (3 x 2 x 1/2 in.)	1
Taco shell or corn tortilla	1

LIST D: Average 100 mg/serving

Pancake (6 in. diam)	1
Waffle (4 in. sq)	1

<u>Cereals</u>: One to two servings containing <20 mg calcium per serving (check labels for nutrient analysis of products not listed--less than 2% USRDA means <20 mg) per serving.

Dry Cereals (3/4 cup)	Cooked Cereals (1/2 cup)
Bran flakes	Cornmeal (degerminated)
Corn flakes	Cream of Rice
Puffed rice	Cream of Wheat
Puffed wheat	Farina
Rice Krispies	Hominy grits
Shredded wheat	Malt-O-Meal
Wheaties	Oatmeal
	Pettyjohns
	Ralston
	Wheatena

Avoid: Any containing more than 20 mg calcium per serving including Cheerios, Life, Total, most granolas, and quick or instant cooked cereals.

<u>Desserts</u>: Limit to 100 mg calcium per day using the following dessert exchange lists:

Free:

Fruit ice
Gelatin

LIST A: Average 15 mg/serving

Brownie (2 x 2 x 1 in.)	1
Cake, angel food (homemade only), pound, shortcake, or sponge cake	1 oz slice
Cookies	
Any kind, except molasses (3 in. diam)	2
Ladyfingers	3
Macaroons	3
Oreos	4
Sugar wafers	5
Vanilla wafers	9
Pie, fruit (all except rhubarb, raisin, and mincemeat)	1/6-1/8 of 8-9 in. pie
Lemon pudding made with water	1/2 cup
Sherbet	1/2 cup

LIST B: Average 75 mg/serving

Cake made from commercial mix, frosted (check labels for 8% or less of USRDA) (3 x 2 x 1)	1 slice
Cookies, molasses (3 in. diam)	2
Fruitcake	1 oz
Pie, pecan or pumpkin	1/6-1/8 of 8-9 in. pie

LIST C: Average 100 mg/serving

Cream pie	1/6 of 8-9 in. pie
Custard	1/3 cup
Ice cream	1/2 cup
Pudding	1/3 cup
Rhubarb pie	1/6 of 8-9 in. pie

    Avoid: Cheesecake

Fruits, Fruit Juices: Limit to 75 mg calcium per day using the following fruit exchange lists:

LIST A: (1/2 cup) (3-7 mg Ca, average 5 mg/serving)

Applesauce
Banana, fresh (1 medium)
Blueberries
Casaba melon
Cranberries, fresh
Cranberry juice cocktail
Cranberry sauce
Fruit drinks
Honeydew
Nectarine (1 medium)
Peach, fresh or canned,
Peach nectar
Pear, fresh or canned
Pear nectar
Plums, fresh (2 medium)
Watermelon

LIST B: (1/2 cup) (8-16 mg Ca, average 10 mg/serving)

    Apple, fresh (1 medium)
    Apple juice
    Apricot nectar
    Apricots, fresh or canned
    Cantaloupe
    Cherries, fresh or canned
    Fruit cocktail, canned
    Grape juice, canned or frozen
    Grapefruit, fresh (1/2 medium) or canned
    Grapefruit juice
    Grapes, fresh or canned
    Mango
    Orange juice, fresh, canned, or frozen
    Papaya, cubed
    Papaya nectar
    Persimmon, fresh (1 medium)
    Pineapple, fresh, frozen, or canned
    Prune juice
    Raspberries, fresh
    Strawberries, fresh
    Tangerine, fresh (1 medium)

LIST C: (1/2 cup) (17-34 mg Ca, average 25 mg/serving)

    Blackberries, fresh or canned
    Currants, fresh
    Dates
    Figs, fresh or canned
    Gooseberries, fresh or canned
    Kiwi fruit, fresh (1 medium)
    Pineapple juice
    Prunes, dried, cooked (5 whole)
    Raspberries, canned or frozen
    Strawberries, frozen
    Tangerine (mandarin oranges), canned
    Tangerine juice, canned

LIST D: (35-65 mg Ca, average 50 mg/serving)

    Orange, fresh (1 medium)
    Raisins, packed (1/2 cup)

    Avoid: Rhubarb

Food Group	Foods Allowed	Foods to Avoid
Eggs	Egg whites as desired	Limit egg yolk (30 mg calcium) to 1/day
Fats	Butter, margarine, bacon, gravy made with broth; french, italian, russian, or thousand island dressing; mayonnaise, shortening, vegetable oils	Limit milk-based gravy to 1/4 cup per day

FOODS ALLOWED AND FOODS TO AVOID (continued):

Food Group	Foods Allowed	Foods to Avoid
Meat, Fish, Poultry, Cheese	All except those to avoid; three oz shellfish may be substituted for 100 mg calcium from the bread group	Any containing milk or milk solids; cheese, shellfish; fish with soft edible bones such as canned sardines or salmon
Potatoes or Substitutes	All prepared without milk or cheese	Any prepared with milk or cheese unless calculated in diet; limit sweet potato (25-41 mg calcium) to 1/2 cup per week
Soups	Limit to 20 mg calcium/day using broth-based soup prepared with allowed vegetables or canned condensed cream soup made with water (check labels for 2% or less of USRDA per serving)	Any containing milk, cheese, shellfish, or vegetable to avoid; salad dressing made with cheese such as roquefort
Sugar, Sweets	All except those to avoid (1 oz chocolate may be substituted for 75 mg calcium from dessert exchange lists)	Molasses, maple syrup, brown sugar, corn syrup, candy containing nuts

Vegetables, Vegetable Juices: Limit to 75 mg calcium/day using the following vegetable exchange lists:

LIST A: (3-7 mg Ca, average 5 mg/serving)

Avocado	1/4 cup
Bamboo shoots, canned	1/2 cup
Bean sprouts, fresh	1/2 cup
Corn, fresh, frozen, or canned	1/2 cup
Green pepper, fresh or cooked	1/2 cup
Lettuce, iceberg	1/2 cup
Mushrooms, raw or cooked	1/2 cup
Radishes, raw	5 medium
Tomato, fresh	1 small
Water chestnuts	1/2 cup

LIST B: (1/2 cup) (8-16 mg Ca, average 10 mg/serving)

Asparagus, fresh
Bamboo shoots, raw slices
Bean sprouts, cooked or canned
Beets, fresh, cooked or canned
Cabbage, green, fresh
Carrot, fresh, grated, or 6 to 8 1/4 x 3 in. sticks
Cauliflower, fresh
Cucumber, pared, 1/4 medium
Eggplant
Leeks, cooked

Lettuce, butterhead or romaine
Squash, summer, fresh or cooked
Tomato, fresh cooked or juice
Vegetable juice

LIST C: (1/2 cup) (17-34 mg Ca, average 25 mg/serving)

Asparagus, fresh or frozen, cooked or canned
Artichoke, fresh or frozen, cooked
Black beans, cooked
Black-eyed peas, fresh, frozen, or canned
Broccoli, fresh
Brussels sprouts, fresh or frozen cooked
Cabbage, green or red, cooked
Cabbage, red, fresh
Carrots, fresh or frozen, cooked, canned
Carrot juice
Cauliflower, fresh or frozen cooked
Celery, raw or cooked, or six 6 x 1/2 in. sticks
Green beans, fresh, frozen, or canned
Kidney beans, cooked or canned, drained
Kohlrabi, fresh or cooked
Leeks, raw
Lentils
Lettuce, looseleaf
Lima beans, fresh, frozen, or canned
Mixed vegetables, canned or frozen
Onions, raw or cooked
Parsnips
Peas, fresh, frozen, or canned
Pumpkin, canned
Rutabaga, fresh or cooked
Scallions, fresh or cooked
Split peas, cooked
Squash, winter, cooked
Tomato, canned or sauce
Turnips, fresh or cooked
Watercress, fresh

LIST D: (1/2 cup) (35-65 mg Ca, average 50 mg/serving)

Broccoli, frozen, cooked
Cabbage, chinese (bok choy)
Fresh garbanzo beans, cooked
Great northern beans, cooked
Navy beans, cooked
Okra, fresh or frozen cooked
Pinto beans, cooked
Sauerkraut

Avoid: All others, including baked beans, soybeans, green leafy vegetables (beet greens, swiss chard, collards, dandelion, kale, mustard, spinach, turnip greens), white mustard cabbage, and fresh cooked broccoli.

Food Group	Foods Allowed	Foods to Avoid
Miscellaneous	Salt, catsup, herbs and spices, coffee whitener[1], horseradish, sweet pickles, soy sauce, popcorn, vinegar, sauce made without milk or milk products (Limit prepared mustard to 1 tbsp/day)	Supplements containing calcium, tofu (soybean curd), nuts, brewer's yeast, olives

APPROXIMATE COMPOSITION OF SAMPLE MENU:

Calories	2672
Protein, g	88
Fat, g	60
Carbohydrate, g	452
Calcium, mg	511

SAMPLE MENU FOR 600 mg (30 mEq) CALCIUM DIET:

Breakfast	Luncheon	Dinner
1 cup orange juice	1 cup grape juice	1 cup apple juice
1/2 cup farina	3 oz sliced chicken	3 oz roast beef
1 egg, soft cooked	1/2 cup rice	1/2 cup cubed white potato
2 slices bread, cracked wheat	1/2 cup green beans	1/4 cup beef broth gravy
1 tsp butter or margarine	1/2 sliced tomato	1/2 cup cooked carrots
1 tbsp grape jelly	1 tsp mayonnaise	2 slices bread, cracked wheat
1 tsp sugar	2 slices bread, cracked wheat	2 tsp butter or margarine
Coffee or tea	2 tsp butter or margarine	Banana
	1 cup canned peaches	9 vanilla wafers
	Coffee or tea	Coffee or tea

Midmorning Nourishment	Midafternoon Nourishment	Evening Nourishment
1 cup Kool-Aid	1 cup Hi-C drink	1/2 cup tomato juice
Plain muffin	2 molasses cookies	
1 tsp butter or margarine		

---

[1]Most brands of coffee whitener contain approximately 1 mg calcium per level teaspoon of powder so should be used only in limited quantities. Check labels or product information literature.

3. Strict Low Calcium Diet (400 mg or 20 mEq)

DESCRIPTION: This diet is the same as the 600 mg (30 mEq) diet on pages 38-44 with the following *additional* restrictions:

Food Group	Foods Allowed	Foods to Avoid
Beverages		Kool-Aid, Tang, and similar powdered fruit drink mixes
Breads	Limit to 100 mg calcium/day	
Desserts	Limit to 75 mg calcium/day	
Fruits, Fruit Juices	Limit to 50 mg calcium/day	
Vegetables, Vegetable Juices	Limit to 50 mg calcium/day	
Miscellaneous		More than 1 tbsp cocoa powder/day

APPROXIMATE COMPOSITION OF SAMPLE MENU:

Calories	2467
Protein, g	88
Fat, g	71
Carbohydrate, g	370
Calcium, mg	373

SAMPLE MENU FOR 400 mg (20 mEq) CALCIUM DIET:

Breakfast	Luncheon	Dinner
1/2 cup orange juice	1/2 cup grape juice	1/2 cup apple juice
1/2 cup farina	3 oz sliced chicken	3 oz roast beef
1 egg, soft cooked	1/2 cup rice	1/2 cup cubed white potato
2 slices bacon	1/2 cup green beans	1/4 cup beef broth gravy
1 slice bread, cracked wheat	1/2 sliced tomato	1/2 cup cooked carrots
1 tsp butter or margarine	1 tsp mayonnaise	1 slice bread, cracked wheat
1 tbsp grape jelly	1 slice bread, cracked wheat	2 tsp butter or margarine
1 tsp sugar	2 tsp butter or margarine	Banana
Coffee or tea	1/2 cup canned peaches	1/2 cup sherbet
	Brownie	9 vanilla wafers
	Coffee or tea	Coffee or tea

Midmorning Nourishment	Midafternoon Nourishment	Evening Nourishment
1/2 cup gelatin	1 cup Hi-C drink	1/2 cup tomato juice
2 graham crackers	2 sugar cookies	4 saltine crackers

4. Very Strict Low Calcium Diet (200 mg or 10 mEq)

DESCRIPTION: This diet is the same as the 400 mg (20 mEq) diet on page 45 with the following *additional* restrictions:

Food Group	Foods Allowed	Foods to Avoid
Breads	Limit to 50 mg calcium/day	
Cereals	Limit to 1 serving/day	
Desserts	Limit to 30 mg calcium/day	
Fruits, Fruit Juices	Limit to 15 mg calcium/day	
Soups	Plain broth or bouillon (Broth-based soup containing vegetable may be substituted for appropriate vegetable exchange)	Cream soups made with water *or* milk
Eggs		Egg yolk
Sugar, Sweets		Chocolate
Vegetables, Vegetable Juices	Limit to 25 mg calcium/day	

APPROXIMATE COMPOSITION OF SAMPLE MENU:

Calories	2426
Protein, g	92
Fat, g	55
Carbohydrate, g	366
Calcium, mg	224

SAMPLE MENU FOR 200 mg (10 mEq) CALCIUM DIET:

Breakfast	Luncheon	Dinner
1/2 cup orange juice	1/2 cup grape juice	1/2 cup cranberry juice cocktail
1/2 cup farina	3 oz sliced chicken	3 oz roast beef
2 slices bacon	1/2 cup rice	1/2 cup cubed white potato
2 slices italian bread	1/2 cup zucchini	1/4 cup beef broth gravy
2 tsp butter or margarine	1/2 sliced tomato	1/2 cup cooked beets
1 tbsp grape jelly	1 tsp mayonnaise	2 slices italian bread
1 tsp sugar	2 slices italian bread	Banana
Coffee or tea	2 tsp butter or margarine	9 vanilla wafers
	1/2 cup canned peaches	Coffee or tea
	Brownie	
	Coffee or tea	

SAMPLE MENU FOR 200 mg (10 mEq) CALCIUM DIET (continued):

Midmorning Nourishment	Midafternoon Nourishment	Evening Nourishment
1/2 cup gelatin 2 graham crackers	1/2 cup Hi-C drink	1/2 cup fruit ice 4 saltine crackers 1 tsp butter or margarine

SUGGESTED MEAL PATTERNS FOR CALCIUM RESTRICTED DIETS

Food Group	Portion	Average Calcium Content (mg)	600 (mg)	400 (mg)	200 (mg)
Beverages					
Powdered soft drink	1 cup	20	1	0	0
Breads					
List A	Varies	5	--	--	5
List B	Varies	25	2	2	1
List C	Varies	50	1	1	0
List D	Varies	100	1	0	0
Cereals	Varies	15	2	1-2	1
Desserts					
Free		0	As desired	As desired	As desired
List A	Varies	15	--	--	2
List B	Varies	75	--	1	0
List C	Varies	100	1	0	0
Meat, Fish, Poultry	1 oz	5	6-8	6-8	6-8
Potatoes or Substitutes	1/2 cup	10	2	2	2
Soups	1/2 cup	10	1-2	1-2	0-1
Eggs	1	30	1	1	0
Fats	Varies	2	As desired	As desired	As desired
Fruits, Fruits Juices					
List A	1/2 cup	5	--	--	1
List B	1/2 cup	10	--	--	1
List C	1/2 cup	25	1	2	0
List D	1/2 cup	50	1	0	0
Sugars, Sweets	Varies	1	As desired	As desired	As desired
Vegetables					
Lists A	Varies	5	--	--	1
List B	1/2 cup	10	--	--	2
List C	1/2 cup	25	1	2	0
List D	1/2 cup	50	1	0	0
TOTAL AVERAGE CALCIUM, using 7 oz meat			605 using 2 soups	395 using 1 cereal and 2 soups	200 using 1 soup

48

B. HIGH IRON DIET

DESCRIPTION: A high iron diet is recommended for persons who have iron deficiency anemia or who are at risk for developing it. The following four groups are especially at risk:

1. Infants: Iron stores of normal full-term babies are sufficient only for approximately 6 months. The iron content of human milk and formula without supplemental iron is low.

2. Children and Adolescents: During periods of rapid growth, iron needs are high.

3. Women of Childbearing Age: Iron is lost during menstruation.

4. Pregnant Women: Iron needs are increased due to expanded blood volume, demands of the placenta and fetus, and blood loss at childbirth.

The elderly, as well as chronic alcoholics, may also be at risk due to low iron intakes. Because adding high iron foods to the diet may not be sufficient to correct iron deficiency anemia, a supplement is recommended in addition to the diet. When the supplement is discontinued, the diet can maintain iron stores.

The Recommended Dietary Allowances for iron are 10 mg/day for men and postmenopausal women and 18 mg/day for women of childbearing age. The RDA for iron is set at these levels to provide replacement of iron losses from the body, and because, on the average, only 10% of ingested iron is absorbed. The average American diet provides approximately 6 mg iron/1000 calories. Three factors are important when considering the iron value of foods in a diet: iron content, iron availability, and the influence of foods ingested simultaneously. The heme form of iron is most readily absorbed. Since fiber interferes with the absorption of iron and other minerals, it is important to consume extra iron with a high fiber intake.

To increase iron intake and absorption, the following guidelines are recommended:

1. Eat foods high in iron daily.

2. Use foods that are iron fortified. Read labels, particularly of breads, cereals, and pastas.

3. Substitute iron-fortified dry cereal for flour when appropriate in meatloaf, casseroles, or baked products.

4. Cook foods in small amounts of liquids to retain iron content, and use the liquid in soups and gravies.

5. Avoid large amounts of tea with meals containing eggs and vegetables, since the tannic acid in tea inhibits the absorption of iron from these foods.

6. Eat a food rich in ascorbic acid (vitamin C) with iron-containing foods. The presence of ascorbic acid may increase iron absorption up to fivefold.

7. Cook acidic foods in iron utensils. The amount of iron released from the utensil increases with the acidity of the cooked food.

8. Include heme iron sources (meat, fish, poultry) in the same meal with nonheme sources (eggs and vegetable products). This enhances the absorption of the nonheme iron.

FOODS HIGH IN IRON
(1.5 mg or more per serving)

	Weight (g)	Serving Size	Iron (mg)
Meat and Meat Substitutes			
Beef, cooked	100	3 1/2 oz	2.6
Beef, dried	85	3 oz	4.3
Bologna	84	3 slices	1.5
Chicken, cooked			
Dark meat	100	3 1/2 oz	1.7
Light meat	115	4 oz	1.5
Clams, canned	100	1/2 cup	4.1
Ham, cooked	100	3 1/2 oz	2.5
Heart, cooked			
Beef	100	3 1/2 oz	5.9
Calf	100	3 1/2 oz	4.4
Chicken	100	3 1/2 oz	3.6
Kidney, beef, cooked	100	3 1/2 oz	13.1
Liver, cooked			
Beef	100	3 1/2 oz	8.9
Calf	100	3 1/2 oz	14.2
Chicken	100	3 1/2 oz	8.5
Pork	100	3 1/2 oz	29.1
Liver sausage	28	1 slice	1.5
Mackerel, canned	100	3 1/2 oz	2.2
Oysters, canned or raw	100	3 1/2 oz	5.5
Pork, cooked	100	3 1/2 oz	4.4
Salami	84	3 slices	2.1
Sardines, canned	100	3 1/2 oz	5.2
Scallops, steamed	100	3 1/2 oz	3.0
Shrimp, canned	100	3 1/2 oz	3.1
Tongue	100	3 1/2 oz	2.2
Tuna			
Oil pack, drained solids	80	1/2 cup	1.5
Water pack, solids and water	85	1/2 cup	1.4
Turkey			
Dark meat	100	3 1/2 oz	2.3
Light meat	125	4 1/2 oz	1.5
Veal, cooked	100	3 1/2 oz	3.5
Beans, dry, cooked			
Cowpeas	80	1/2 cup	1.7
Kidney	100	2/5 cup	2.4
Lima	100	5/8 cup	2.5
Tofu (soybean curd)	100	3 1/2 oz	1.9
Brazil nuts	45	12 nuts	1.5
Cashew nuts	45	21 nuts	1.8
Egg, cooked	96	2 medium	2.2
Peanuts	45	3 tbsp	1.5
Peanut butter	100	7 tbsp	1.9

	Weight (g)	Serving Size	Iron (mg)
Fruits and Vegetables			
Apple juice	245	1 cup	1.5
Apricots, dried	30	5 halves	1.6
Greens			
Beets, cooked	100	1/2 cup	1.9
Chard, cooked	100	3/5 cup	1.8
Dandelion, cooked	100	1/2 cup	1.8
Kale, cooked	100	3/4 cup	1.6
Mustard, cooked	100	1/2 cup	1.8
Spinach			
Cooked	90	1/2 cup	2.0
Raw	100	2 cups	3.1
Turnips, cooked	150	1 cup	1.7
Peas			
Cooked	100	2/3 cup	1.8
Dried, cooked	100	3/5 cup	1.7
Peaches, dried	44	3 large halves	2.6
Prunes, cooked	100	4 medium	1.5
Prune juice	180	3/4 cup	7.4
Raisins	72	1/2 cup	2.5
Strawberries, whole	150	1 cup	1.5
Tomato juice	180	3/4 cup	1.6
Cereal and Grain Products			
Baby cereals			
Ready-to-serve	14-18	6 tbsp	10.6-14.0
Bread			
White, wheat, enriched	70	3 slices	1.8
Cereals			
Iron-fortified	--	--	Variable[a]
Other			
Corn syrup			
Light and dark	40	2 tbsp	1.6
Molasses			
Light	40	2 tbsp	1.8
Medium	40	2 tbsp	2.4
Dark	40	2 tbsp	4.6
Wheat germ	20	3 tbsp	1.8

[a]The amount of iron in iron-fortified cereals will vary with brand and type. Refer to labels for specific information.

C. PHOSPHORUS RESTRICTED DIET

DESCRIPTION: The purpose of the phosphorus restricted diet is to reduce serum phosphorus to normal levels. Conditions such as hypoparathyroidism, renal insufficiency, and renal failure often result in hyperphosphatemia. A protein restriction may be needed for all conditions listed except hypoparathyroidism; however, protein is inevitably restricted on a low phosphorus diet, because foods high in protein are also high in phosphorus.

The usual American diet provides 1.5 to 2.0 g phosphorus per day. Because phosphorus is so widely distributed in foods, a restriction of less than 800 mg per day is not easily achieved and is rarely prescribed. Phosphates are currently added to a wide variety of processed foods, including carbonated beverages, meats, cheeses, salad dressings, and refrigerated bakery products. Labels should be read carefully.

See the Protein-Phosphorus Restricted Diet calculation, sample menu, and exchange lists on pages 69-77.

ADEQUACY: This diet will not meet the Recommended Dietary Allowances for iron, calcium, phosphorus, and the following vitamins: thiamin, riboflavin, niacin, folic acid, B_6, and D. A multivitamin-mineral supplement is generally recommended.

D. POTASSIUM CONTROLLED DIETS

DESCRIPTION: Dietary potassium may be decreased or increased according to the needs of the patient. It is decreased when potassium is not being excreted properly, and it is increased in hypokalemia. A general diet provides from 2340 mg (60 mEq) to 3900 mg (100 mEq) or more per day depending upon the kind and amount of food consumed.

The potassium content of foods varies according to growing conditions, processing, and cooking methods. To allow for greater variety within the diet, foods have been categorized into various exchange lists (pages 84-98). Some special low sodium dietetic foods such as broth, baking powder, cheese, and salt substitutes are higher in potassium than their sodium-containing counterparts. These hidden sources of potassium should be considered when a sodium restriction is ordered in conjunction with the potassium restriction.

ADEQUACY: The level of potassium restriction will determine the nutritional adequacy of the diet.

1. High Potassium Diet (5070 mg or 130 mEq or more)

DESCRIPTION: This diet is given to replenish potassium reserves. An increase in urinary potassium loss can be anticipated when certain diuretics or adrenal corticosteroids are prescribed. An increased endogenous production of steroids in such conditions as primary hyperaldosteronism, cirrhosis, congestive heart failure, Cushing's disease, and Bartter's syndrome may also cause potassium deficiency due to urinary loss. Severe diarrhea and/or vomiting can lead to hypokalemia if intake is not adequate.

All foods are allowed, but foods rich in potassium should be consumed daily. If the patient's diet is restricted in sodium, the physician may wish to prescribe a potassium-containing salt substitute. The salt substitute used at the University of Iowa Hospitals and Clinics contains 527 mg or 13.5 mEq potassium per packet.

FOODS ALLOWED:

Food Group	Foods High in Potassium
Beverages	Milk (at least 3 cups per day), percolated coffee, strong tea, fruit juices (especially from List B, page 92)
Breads	Whole grain breads such as whole wheat, pumpernickel, and boston brown bread
Cereals	Bran and whole grain cereals
Desserts	Fruits, especially from List B (page 91), ice cream, puddings, custard, gingerbread, gingersnaps
Fruits, Fruit Juices	At least 2 servings from List B (page 91), dried fruits

FOODS ALLOWED (continued):

Food Group	Foods High in Potassium
Meat, Fish, Poultry, Cheese, Substitutes	All meat, fish, and poultry, especially scallops and veal; peanut butter; dried peas and beans
Soups	Split pea, lentil
Sugar, Sweets	Milk chocolate, candy bars, sorghum, molasses, brown sugar, pure maple syrup
Vegetables, Vegetable Juices	At least 2 servings from List B (pages 89-90)
Miscellaneous	Nuts, catsup, potassium-based salt substitutes

APPROXIMATE COMPOSITION OF SAMPLE MENU:

Calories	2054
Protein, g	109
Fat, g	62
Carbohydrate, g	277
Potassium, mg	5510

SAMPLE MENU FOR HIGH POTASSIUM DIET:

Breakfast	Luncheon	Dinner
1 cup orange juice	3/4 cup creamed chicken on	3 oz roast beef
1/2 cup bran flakes	1 biscuit	Baked potato
1 tbsp brown sugar	1/2 cup lima beans	1/2 cup cooked carrots
1 slice toast, whole wheat	1 sliced tomato on lettuce	3/4 cup tossed lettuce salad
	1 slice bread, whole wheat	1 tbsp french dressing
1 tsp butter or margarine	1 tsp butter or margarine	1 slice bread, pumpernickel
1 tbsp grape jelly	Banana	1 tsp butter or margarine
1 cup 2% milk	1 cup 2% milk	1/2 cup vanilla ice cream
Percolated coffee	Percolated coffee	1 cup 2% milk
		Percolated coffee

2. Potassium Restricted Diet (390-3120 mg or 10-80 mEq)

DESCRIPTION: The physician may prescribe this diet for the patient who is not excreting potassium adequately. The level of restriction depends upon the patient's blood and urine biochemistries. Adequate calories are necessary to prevent body catabolism and a subsequent rise in serum potassium. Protein, sodium, and fluids are other nutrients that may also be restricted (see renal diets pages 78-80).

In order to allow the patient greater variety of choice within restrictions, the diet is calculated by using exchange lists beginning on page 84.

ADEQUACY: At the lower levels of potassium restriction, the diet will not meet the Recommended Dietary Allowances for protein, iron, calcium and the vitamins thiamin, riboflavin, niacin, B_6, B_{12}, folic acid, and D.

APPROXIMATE COMPOSITION OF SAMPLE MENU:

Calories	2001
Protein, g	74
Fat, g	65
Carbohydrate, g	286
Potassium, mg	1921

SAMPLE MENU FOR POTASSIUM RESTRICTED DIET (2340 mg or 60 mEq):

Breakfast

1/3 cup orange
  juice
1/2 cup farina
1 egg, soft cooked
1 slice toast,
  white enriched
2 tsp butter or
  margarine
1 tbsp grape jelly
1 cup milk
1 tsp sugar
1 cup instant
  coffee

Luncheon

2 oz sliced chicken
1/2 cup rice
1/2 cup green beans
1 slice bread, white enriched
3 tsp butter or margarine
1 tbsp honey
1/3 cup royal anne cherries
1 puffed rice bar
1 cup Kool-Aid

Dinner

3 oz roast beef
1/3 cup cubed white potato
1/3 cup cooked carrots
1/2 cup lettuce salad
1 tbsp french dressing
1 slice bread, white
  enriched
3 tsp butter or margarine
1 tbsp apple jelly
2 canned pear halves
1 cup Kool-Aid

E. SODIUM RESTRICTED DIETS

DESCRIPTION: The purpose of sodium restricted diets is to reduce the sodium content of tissues and promote loss of body water. These diets are prescribed for cirrhosis with ascites, congestive heart failure, hypertension, Meniere's disease, certain renal diseases, and other conditions associated with retention of extracellular fluid. Sodium restrictions are contraindicated in normal pregnancy, for patients who have ileostomies, and for some patients on very restricted protein diets (i.e., 20-30 g/day) who are also taking diuretics.

These diets are ordered in terms of milligrams or milliequivalents of sodium, the level varying with the patient's condition, drug therapy, and individual response. Common levels of sodium restriction are:

Mild (no added salt) - 2500-4000 mg (109-173 mEq)

Moderate - 2000 mg (87 mEq)

Moderately strict - 1000 mg (43 mEq)

Strict - 500 mg (22 mEq)

Very strict - 250 mg (11 mEq)

Salt is the most common source of sodium, but baking soda, baking powder, sodium nitrite, and monosodium glutamate also contribute significant amounts to processed foods. A variety of "reduced sodium," "unsalted," "no-added-salt," and "low sodium" convenience foods are available, but the sodium content differs considerably. To determine the amount per serving, labels should be read carefully. The chart below lists the terms that food processors may use according to Food and Drug Administration regulations:

Description	Amount of Sodium
Sodium free	less than or equal to 5 milligrams per serving
Very low sodium	35 milligrams or less per serving
Low sodium	140 milligrams or less per serving
Reduced sodium	processed to reduce the usual level of sodium by at least 75%
Unsalted	processed without the normally used salt

The patient should be cautioned to check for "hidden" sodium from sources other than food such as alkalizers for indigestion (e.g., Alka Seltzer or bicarbonate of soda); chewing tobacco; some cough medicines, laxatives, pain relievers, and other over-the-counter drugs. Drinking water, especially if softened by ion exchange, can contain considerable sodium. To determine the amount, the patient should check with the local dietitian or municipal water company. Unless the diet is restricted below 1000 mg Na, it is usually not necessary to obtain other drinking water.

Because sodium is typically replaced by potassium in most salt substitutes, they are usually contraindicated when renal function is impaired or potassium-sparing diuretics are used. When potassium-wasting diuretics are used, high potassium foods and a salt substitute may be recommended to avoid hypokalemia. For the patient to receive a salt substitute at UIHC, a physician's order is required. (The potassium content is 13.5 mEq per packet.)

Palatability of the diet may be enhanced through the use of various herbs and spices. Several commercial combinations are low in both sodium and potassium.

ADEQUACY: The nutritional adequacy of the sodium restricted diet depends upon the patient's appetite, food preferences, and level of sodium restriction. With careful selections from the basic four food groups, the Recommended Dietary Allowances can be met. Because of the limited selections and the unpalatability of many low sodium products, diets restricted to 500 milligrams or less are often inadequate in iron, calcium, vitamin B$_6$, and magnesium. Supplementation of these vitamins and minerals may be necessary.

1. Mild Low Sodium Diet (No-Added-Salt) (2500-4000 mg or 109-174 mEq)

DESCRIPTION: A general hospital diet is used without salt packets; highly salted foods are omitted. In some cases a food item not ordinarily allowed may be included in a meal plan. Some "reduced sodium," "no-salt-added," or "unsalted" foods may also be included; however, the amounts and frequency of use must be determined by a dietitian.

FOODS TO AVOID:

Food Group	Foods to Avoid
Beverages	Commercial buttermilk, instant cocoa mixes
Breads	Breads, rolls, and crackers with salted toppings
Cereals	Instant hot cereals
Desserts	Instant pudding mixes
Fats	Bacon drippings, salted gravy, regular peanut butter in excess of 1 tbsp per day
Meat, Fish, Poultry, Cheese	Smoked and salt cured meats or fish such as bacon, bologna, chipped beef, corned beef, frankfurters, ham, kosher meats, luncheon meats, pickled meats, salt pork, sausage, anchovies, caviar, pickled herring; regular canned tuna, salmon, sardines; cheese and most commercial entrees
Soups	Regular canned soups, instant soup mixes, bouillon and consommé
Vegetables, Vegetable Juices	Sauerkraut or other vegetables in brines; regular canned tomato and vegetable juices
Miscellaneous	
Seasonings	Salt and salt-based seasonings such as celery salt, garlic salt, lemon pepper, meat tenderizers, monosodium glutamate, onion salt, seasoned salt, sea salt
Sauces	Barbecue sauce, catsup, chili sauce, horseradish, Kitchen Bouquet, meat sauce, prepared mustard, soy sauce, steak sauce, worcestershire sauce
Others	Olives; pickles; party dips and spreads, salted snack foods such as cheese puffs, corn chips, potato chips; salted nuts or salted popcorn

2. Moderate Low Sodium Diet (2000 mg or 87 mEq)

DESCRIPTION: This diet is similar to the mild low sodium (NAS) diet with limited amounts of milk, bread, and regular desserts. The quantities allowed are based on the patient's individual food preferences. See a suggested meal pattern on page 65. Some "no-salt-added," "unsalted," or "reduced sodium" products may be allowed in some cases.

FOODS ALLOWED AND FOODS TO AVOID:

Food Group	Foods Allowed	Foods to Avoid
Beverages	4 cups milk per day (whole, skim, 2%, chocolate), homemade unsalted buttermilk; coffee, tea, or decaffeinated coffee; carbonated beverages labeled as "very low sodium" (35 mg or less per serving)	Commercial cultured buttermilk, instant cocoa mixes, malted milk, milkshakes, milk mixes, carbonated beverages containing over 35 mg of sodium per serving
Breads	Regular yeast bread and rolls in limited amounts; quick breads made without salt, baking powder, or baking soda (low sodium baking powder may be used); crackers with unsalted tops; holland rusk; zwieback; melba toast; tortilla shells	Bread, rolls, or crackers with salted topping, quick breads
Cereals	Unsalted cooked whole grain and enriched cereals, 1 serving per day of regular cooked or dry cereal, puffed rice, shredded wheat, specially prepared low sodium cereals	Instant hot cereals, regular cooked or dry cereals in excess of 1 serving per day
Desserts	Ice cream, sherbet, ice milk, pudding, or fruit flavored yogurt when used as part of milk allowance; 1 serving per day of baked dessert made with salt, baking powder, baking soda	Instant pudding mixes; baked desserts made with salt, baking powder, or baking soda in excess of 1 serving per day

FOODS ALLOWED AND FOODS TO AVOID (continued):

Food Group	Foods Allowed	Foods to Avoid
Fats	Regular butter or margarine, salad oil, lard or vegetable shortening; unsalted gravy, sour cream, low sodium mayonnaise and salad dressings; low sodium peanut butter; 1 tbsp of one of the following per day: mayonnaise, commercial salad dressings, or regular (salted) peanut butter	Salt pork, bacon drippings, salted gravy More than 1 tbsp per day: mayonnaise, commercial salad dressings, or regular (salted) peanut butter
Fruits, Fruit Juices	All	None
Meat, Fish, Poultry, Cheese, Eggs	Fresh, frozen, or canned meat, fish, poultry, and eggs processed or prepared without salt or sodium compounds, low sodium cheeses	Meat, fish, poultry, eggs processed or prepared with salt or sodium compounds; smoked, salt cured meats or fish such as bacon, bologna, chipped beef, corned beef, frankfurters, ham, kosher meat, luncheon meat, pickled meat, salt pork, sausage; anchovies, caviar, pickled herring, canned tuna, salmon, sardines; shellfish such as clams, crabs, oysters, scallops, and shrimp; all cheese except low sodium cheese
Potatoes or Substitutes	Fresh, frozen, and canned white or sweet potatoes without added salt or sodium compounds; low sodium potato chips; macaroni, spaghetti, noodles, rice	Potato chips; frozen, canned or instant potatoes or substitutes to which salt or sodium compounds have been added; canned hominy
Soups	Any homemade low sodium broth or soup made with allowed foods; low sodium commercial soups or bouillon	All regular commercial broth, soup, bouillon, consommé (instant, canned, or frozen)
Sugar, Sweets	White and brown sugar, honey, jelly, jam, marmalade, maple syrup, molasses, unsalted candies	Any sweets with salt added

FOODS ALLOWED AND FOODS TO AVOID (continued):

Food Group	Foods Allowed	Foods to Avoid
Vegetables, Vegetable Juices	All fresh, frozen, or canned vegetables and juices prepared without salt or sodium compounds	Regular canned vegetables and vegetable juices, frozen peas or lima beans, tomato sauce, sauerkraut and other vegetables in brine
Miscellaneous	Spices and herbs, lemon juice, vinegar, cocoa powder, salted nuts, unsalted popcorn and tortilla chips; low sodium catsup or mustard, low sodium pretzels or potato chips	*Seasonings*: salt and salt-based seasonings such as celery salt, garlic salt, lemon pepper, meat tenderizer, monosodium glutamate, onion salt, seasoned salt, sea salt
		Sauces: barbecue sauce, meat sauce, catsup, chili sauce, prepared mustard, horseradish
		Others: pickles, olives, salted snack foods such as popcorn, nuts, corn chips, or pretzels

APPROXIMATE COMPOSITION OF SAMPLE MENU:

Calories	1984
Protein, g	88
Fat, g	60
Carbohydrate, g	279
Sodium, mg	1604

SAMPLE MENU FOR MODERATE SODIUM RESTRICTED DIET (2000 mg or 87 mEq):

Breakfast	Luncheon	Dinner
1/2 cup orange juice	2 oz sliced chicken, unsalted	2 oz roast beef, unsalted
1/2 cup farina	1/2 cup rice, unsalted	1/2 cup mashed potatoes, unsalted
1 egg, soft cooked	1/2 cup green beans, unsalted	1/2 cup cooked carrots, unsalted
1 slice toast, cracked wheat	1/2 sliced tomato on lettuce	3/4 cup tossed lettuce salad
1 tsp butter or margarine	1 tsp mayonnaise	1 tbsp french dressing
1 tbsp grape jelly	1 slice bread, cracked wheat	1 slice bread, cracked wheat
1 cup 2% milk	1 tsp butter or margarine	1 tsp butter or margarine
2 tsp sugar	1/2 cup canned peaches	1/2 cup sherbet
Coffee or tea	1 slice angel food cake	1 cup 2% milk
Pepper	1 cup 2% milk	Coffee or tea
	Coffee or tea	Pepper
	Pepper	

3. Moderately Strict Low Sodium Diet (1000 mg or 43 mEq)

DESCRIPTION: All foods allowed on this diet are processed and prepared without salt, baking soda, or regular baking powder. Low sodium baking powder may be substituted, if a potassium restriction is not also prescribed. Foods high in natural sodium are restricted. Regular bread and butter or margarine may be permitted in some cases. Refer to the suggested meal plan on page 65.

FOODS ALLOWED AND FOODS TO AVOID:

Foods allowed and foods to avoid are the same as those listed for the 2000 mg Na (87 mEq) diet on pages 58-60 with the following *additional* restrictions:

Food Group	Foods Allowed	Foods to Avoid
Beverages	Limit milk to 3 cups per day	Milk in excess of 3 cups per day
Breads	Low sodium breads and baked products	More than 1 serving per day of breads or baked products made with salt, baking soda, or regular baking powder
Cereals	Low sodium cereals	All others
Desserts	Low sodium baked desserts	All baked desserts made with salt, baking soda, or regular baking powder
Fats	Limited amounts of regular butter or margarine (See suggested meal pattern page 65)	Regular salad dressings, regular peanut butter

APPROXIMATE COMPOSITION OF SAMPLE MENU:

Calories	2013
Protein, g	84
Fat, g	72
Carbohydrate, g	260
Sodium, mg	1087

SAMPLE MENU FOR MODERATELY STRICT LOW SODIUM DIET (1000 mg or 43 mEq):

Breakfast	Luncheon	Dinner
1/2 cup orange juice	2 oz sliced chicken, unsalted	3 oz roast beef, unsalted
1/2 cup farina, unsalted	1/2 cup rice, unsalted	1/2 cup cubed white potato, unsalted
1 egg, soft cooked	1/2 cup green beans, unsalted	1/2 cup cooked carrots, unsalted
1 slice toast, cracked wheat	1/2 sliced tomato on lettuce	3/4 cup tossed lettuce salad
1 tsp butter or margarine	2 tsp mayonnaise, unsalted	1 tbsp french dressing, low sodium
1 tbsp grape jelly	1 slice bread, low sodium	1 slice bread, low sodium
1 cup 2% milk	2 tsp butter or margarine	2 tsp butter or margarine
2 tsp sugar	1/2 cup canned peaches	1/2 cup sherbet
Coffee or tea	1 slice low sodium white cake	1 cup 2% milk
Pepper	1 cup 2% milk	Coffee or tea
	Coffee or tea	Pepper
	Pepper	

4. Strict and Very Strict Low Sodium Diets (500 mg or 22 mEq and 250 mg or 11 mEq)

DESCRIPTION: These diets may be indicated for such acute conditions as severe ascites, congestive heart failure, or hypertension. Because selections are limited and low sodium substitutes are often not well accepted, compliance is a major problem, especially for home use. The diet is rarely prescribed for outpatients, but if required, ongoing counseling is particularly important. Distilled water may be indicated if the sodium content of the patient's usual drinking water is too high.

These diets are often inadequate in iron, calcium, vitamin B_6, and magnesium. Frequent monitoring of the patient's nutritional status is recommended.

a. Strict Low Sodium Diet (500 mg or 22 mEq)

FOODS ALLOWED AND FOODS TO AVOID:

Foods allowed and foods to avoid are the same as those listed for the 1000 mg (43 mEq) diet on page 60 with the following *additional* restrictions:

Food Group	Foods Allowed	Foods to Avoid
Beverages	Low sodium milk (limit regular milk to 2 cups per day)	Regular milk in excess of 2 cups per day
Desserts	All milk used in desserts should be subtracted from the daily milk allowance	
Vegetables, Vegetable Juices	Fresh, frozen, and canned without salt or sodium compounds except for vegetables listed under foods to avoid	Artichokes, beets, beet greens, carrots, celery, swiss chard, kale, spinach, dandelion greens, turnips

APPROXIMATE COMPOSITION OF SAMPLE MENU:

Calories	1782
Protein, g	79
Fat, g	58
Carbohydrate, g	239
Sodium, mg	456

SAMPLE MENU FOR STRICT LOW SODIUM DIET (500 mg or 22 mEq):

Breakfast	Luncheon	Dinner
1/2 cup orange juice	2 oz sliced chicken, unsalted	2 oz roast beef, unsalted
1/2 cup farina, unsalted	1/2 cup rice, unsalted	1/2 cup cubed white potato, unsalted
1 egg, soft cooked	1/2 cup green beans, unsalted	1/2 cup asparagus, unsalted
1 slice toast, low sodium	1/2 sliced tomato on lettuce	3/4 cup tossed lettuce salad
1 tsp butter or margarine, unsalted	1 tsp mayonnaise, low sodium	1 tsp french dressing, low sodium
1 tbsp grape jelly	1 slice bread, low sodium	1 slice bread, low sodium
1 cup 2% milk	2 tsp butter or margarine, unsalted	2 tsp butter or margarine, unsalted
2 tsp sugar	1/2 cup canned peaches	1/2 cup canned pears
Coffee or tea	1 slice low sodium white cake	1 cup 2% milk
Pepper	Coffee or tea	Coffee or tea
	Pepper	Pepper

b. Very Strict Low Sodium Diet (250 mg or 11 mEq)

FOODS ALLOWED AND FOODS TO AVOID:

Foods allowed and foods to avoid are the same as those listed for the 500 mg Na diet on page 62 with the following *additional* restrictions:

Food Group	Foods Allowed	Foods to Avoid
Beverages	3-4 cups low sodium milk	All regular milk
Desserts		All milk-containing desserts, regular gelatin desserts
Eggs	None	All

APPROXIMATE COMPOSITION OF SAMPLE MENU:

Calories	2031
Protein, g	88
Fat, g	75
Carbohydrate, g	253
Sodium, mg	206

SAMPLE MENU FOR VERY STRICT LOW SODIUM DIET (250 mg or 11 mEq):

Breakfast

1/2 cup orange
  juice
1/2 cup farina,
  unsalted
1 slice toast, low
  sodium
1 tsp butter or
  margarine,
  unsalted
1 tbsp grape jelly
1 cup low sodium
  milk
2 tsp sugar
Coffee or tea
Pepper

Luncheon

2 oz sliced chicken, unsalted
1/2 cup rice, unsalted
1/2 cup green beans, unsalted
1/2 sliced tomato on lettuce
2 tsp mayonnaise, low sodium
1 slice bread, low sodium
2 tsp butter or margarine,
  unsalted
1/2 cup canned peaches
1 slice low sodium white cake
1 cup low sodium milk
Coffee or tea
Pepper

Dinner

3 oz roast beef, unsalted
1/2 cup cubed white potato,
  unsalted
1/2 cup asparagus, unsalted
3/4 cup lettuce salad
1 tbsp french dressing,
  low sodium
1 slice bread, low sodium
2 tsp butter or margarine,
  unsalted
1/2 cup canned pears
1 cup low sodium milk
Coffee or tea
Pepper

SUGGESTED MEAL PATTERNS FOR SODIUM RESTRICTED DIETS

Food Group	Portion	Average Sodium Content (mg)	2000 mg (87 mEq)	1000 mg (43 mEq)	500 mg (22 mEq)	250 mg (11 mEq)
Beverages						
Milk						
Fresh	1 cup	120	3	3	2	0
Low sodium	1 cup	6	0	0	0	3
Breads						
Regular bread	1 slice	150	4	1	0	0
Low sodium bread	1 slice	10	0	4	4	4
Cereals						
Regular ready-to-eat or	3/4 cup	250	--	0	0	0
Regular cooked	1/2 cup	200	1	0	0	0
Low sodium ready-to-eat or	3/4 cup	5	0	--	--	--
Low sodium cooked	1/2 cup	5	0	1	1	1
Desserts						
Baked desserts (cake or pie)	Varies	200	1	0	0	0
Low sodium baked desserts	Varies	10	1	1	1	1
Gelatin or ice cream	1/2 cup	50	1	1	0	0
Fats						
Regular butter or margarine	1 tsp	50	4	2	0	0
Unsalted butter or margarine	1 tsp	0	--	As Desired	As Desired	As Desired
Regular salad dressing	1 tbsp	150	1	0	0	0
Low sodium salad dressing	1 tbsp	10	As Desired	As Desired	As Desired	As Desired
Fruits	Varies	2	As Desired	As Desired	4	4
Meat and Substitutes						
Unsalted meats, fish, poultry	1 oz	25	6	5	4	5
Egg	1	60	1	1	1	0
Potatoes and Substitutes						
Unsalted	1/2 cup	5	2	2	2	2
Vegetables						
I Fresh, frozen, or canned without salt	1/2 cup	10	3	3	3	3
II Fresh, frozen, or canned without salt; beets, carrots, celery, spinach	1/2 cup	50	1	1	0	0
TOTAL AVERAGE SODIUM			1978 mg Using 4 Portions Fruit	973 mg Using 4 Portions Fruit	503 mg	246 mg

APPROXIMATE SODIUM CONTENT OF SELECTED FOODS
THAT MAY BE CALCULATED INTO SODIUM RESTRICTED DIETS

	50 mg	100 mg	150 mg	200 mg	250 mg	500 mg
GRAINS	Regular graham cracker		1/2 english muffin	1 bagel 1/2 c regular cooked cereal	1 biscuit from mix 3/4 c regular ready-to-eat cereal	
CONDIMENTS	2 tsp mayonnaise	1 1/2 tsp prepared mustard	1 tbsp regular catsup 1 tbsp regular salad dressing	1 tbsp horseradish		
DAIRY	1/2 c sherbet 1/2 c ice cream 1 1/2 tbsp cream cheese	1 oz neufchatel or mozzarella cheese 1 oz natural swiss 1/2 c ricotta cheese	1 oz brick cheese 1/2 c buttermilk	1/4 c cottage cheese 1/2 oz processed cheese 1 oz natural cheddar cheese	1/2 c cooked pudding from mix 1 c cocoa from mix (water added)	1/2 c instant pudding from mix
DESSERTS	1 sugar cookie 1/2 c flavored gelatin 6 vanilla wafers			1 avg serving baked dessert (cake or pie)		
MEAT/FISH	1 oz steamed clams 1 oz fresh oysters	1 thin strip bacon 1 oz crab 2 oz shrimp 1 oz regular canned tuna	2 oz lobster or scallops	2 oz canned tuna	3/4 oz sliced bologna 2 sausage links	1 1/2 oz frankfurter 1 1/2 oz ham
VEGETABLES	1 artichoke 1/2 c frozen mixed vegetables 1/2 c fresh, frozen, or low sodium canned beets, carrots, celery, kale, swiss chard, spinach	1/2 c frozen lima beans or frozen peas		1/2 c regular canned vegetables (except tomato)	1/2 c regular canned tomato 1/2 c instant mashed potatoes (reconstituted)	1/3 c sauerkraut
MISC		1 tbsp regular peanut butter				1/2 c regular canned soup

SECTION 3

Modification of Protein

A. PROTEIN RESTRICTED DIET (0-60 GRAMS)

DESCRIPTION: A low protein diet is used to control or prevent the symptoms of hyperammonemia and acute or chronic hepatic encephalopathy, and to control symptoms of uremia or possibly delay progression of renal disease. When this diet is used for renal disease, it is usually combined with a phosphorus restriction (See the Protein-Phosphorus Restricted Diet on page 69). Hepatic disease can cause decreased urea synthesis and portal shunting of ammonia into the systemic circulation, producing encephalopathic symptoms. The use of parenteral and enteral branched chain amino acid supplements may be useful, since patients with hepatic encephalopathy exhibit a reduction in the brain and plasma amino acid concentration of these amino acids. Hepatic-Aid II, Travasorb Hepatic, and Nutrisource HBC formula are enteral branched chain amino acid formulas currently available (see chart on pages 294-99).

Essential amino acids and adequate calories must be provided in amounts necessary to maintain nitrogen balance and to prevent body catabolism. High biological value proteins such as eggs, milk, meat, poultry, and fish should provide two-thirds to three-fourths of the protein allowance and be distributed among all 3 meals. The level of dietary protein is prescribed by the physician and adjusted according to the patient's response. In the presence of advanced liver disease, the restriction generally ranges from 30 to 60 grams, and is 20 grams[1] or less for the patient who is rapidly approaching hepatic coma. In renal insufficiency a protein restriction of 0.8 g/kg/day may be prescribed (See the Protein-Phosphorus Restricted Diet on pages 69-77 and Renal Diets, pages 78-98).

During the acute stage of hepatic encephalopathy, a no-protein diet is often required, but should be used with extreme caution for only a few days. The 20 to 30 g of protein needed to maintain nitrogen balance should be provided as a branched chain amino acid formula. As the patient's condition improves, dietary protein may be gradually increased by 10 to 20 grams every 2 to 5 days until a protein intake of 1 g per kg ideal body weight is achieved.

Dietary compliance is difficult, especially if sodium and/or fluid is restricted also. Making the diet as liberal and individualized as possible within necessary modifications is important for achieving optimal nutritional status. The diet pattern is developed using exchange lists in which foods are categorized according to protein content. The protein-phosphorus exchange lists are used, ignoring the phosphorus values unless necessary. Because the composition of manufactured products is subject to change, labels and company literature should be checked periodically.

---

[1]The protein in a diet restricted to 20 g protein should be provided in the form of 1 egg (8 g protein) and 6 oz milk (6 g protein) to supply the essential amino acids. The remaining 6 g protein may be selected from the bread, vegetable, or fruit exchange groups.

To increase calories, methods of food preparation incorporating fats and oils should be used. Fruit-flavored beverage powders, carbonated beverages, sugar, jellies, and hard candy provide additional calories from carbohydrate. Dietary supplements of carbohydrate and fat (see chart on pages 296-99) and special low protein products may be utilized to increase caloric intake.

ADEQUACY: At the lower levels of restriction, this diet will not meet the Recommended Dietary Allowances for protein, iron, calcium, and the following vitamins: thiamin, riboflavin, niacin, folic acid, B_6, B_{12}, and D. A multivitamin-mineral supplement is generally recommended.

APPROXIMATE COMPOSITION OF SAMPLE MENU:

Calories	2353
Protein, g	44
Fat, g	85
Carbohydrate, g	358

SAMPLE MENU FOR RESTRICTED PROTEIN DIET (calculated for a 40 g protein diet with no other restrictions):

Breakfast

1/2 cup orange
  juice
1/2 cup farina
1 slice low
  protein toast[1]
3 tsp butter or
  margarine
1 tbsp grape jelly
1/2 cup milk
2 tsp sugar
Coffee or tea

Luncheon

1 oz (30 g) sliced chicken
1/2 cup cubed white potato
1/2 cup green beans
1 slice low protein toast[1]
3 tsp butter or margarine
1 tbsp honey
2 halves sweetened canned
  peaches
1 cup Kool-Aid

Dinner

2 oz (60 g) roast beef
1/2 cup cooked carrots
1 slice low protein bread[1]
3 tsp butter or margarine
1 tbsp apple jelly
2 halves sweetened canned
  pears
Coffee or tea
1 tsp sugar

Midmorning
Nourishment

Low protein rusk
2 tsp butter or
  margarine
2 tsp cherry jelly
1 cup peach nectar

Midafternoon
Nourishment

1/2 cup sherbet
6 low protein caramels[1]

Evening
Nourishment

1/2 cup milk
2 low protein cookies[1]

---

[1]Recipe in Appendix J.

B. PROTEIN-PHOSPHORUS RESTRICTED DIET

DESCRIPTION: The purpose of the Protein-Phosphorus Restricted Diet is to control symptoms of uremia and consequences of hyperphosphatemia. The diet may also be useful in slowing the progression of chronic renal disease to end stage renal failure. The levels of protein and phosphorus prescribed are determined according to the patient's renal function, as well as the baseline nutritional status. See the table on page 80 to determine other nutrient needs for these patients. A practical restriction is 800 mg phosphorus per day with a protein level no higher than 50 g per day, since it is difficult to provide more protein from food without increasing the phosphorus allowance. If diet alone does not result in appropriate serum levels, a phosphate binder (aluminum hydroxide or calcium carbonate) should be prescribed in addition to the diet. Frequent monitoring of serum phosphorus is necessary to prevent hypophosphatemia.

    Essential amino acids and adequate calories must be provided in amounts necessary to maintain nitrogen balance and to prevent body catabolism. High biological value proteins such as egg white, meat, poultry, and fish should provide one-half to three-fourths of the protein allowance and be distributed among all 3 meals. The diet is calculated using exchange lists in which foods are categorized according to their composition of protein and phosphorus. See the table below.

ADEQUACY: This diet will not meet the Recommended Dietary Allowances for iron, calcium, phosphorus, and the following vitamins: thiamin, riboflavin, niacin, folic acid, B_6, and D. A multivitamin-mineral supplement is generally recommended.

EXCHANGE VALUES FOR PROTEIN-PHOSPHORUS RESTRICTED DIET

Food Group	Protein (g)	Phosphorus (mg)
Meat and Meat Substitutes	8	70
Dairy Products	4	120
Breads	2	40
Vegetables	1.5	40
Fruits and Fruit Juices	trace[a]	20
Fats	--	--
Other Phosphorus Containing Beverages	--	5

[a]Protein per fruit exchange = 0.5 g/serving and must be calculated for protein restricted diets of 20 g or less.

APPROXIMATE COMPOSITION OF SAMPLE MENU:

Calories	2409
Protein, g	55
Fat, g	53
Carbohydrate, g	433
Phosphorus, mg	658

SAMPLE MENU FOR PROTEIN-PHOSPHORUS RESTRICTED DIET (50 g protein, 50 mEq phosphorus):

Breakfast	Luncheon	Dinner
1/2 cup orange juice	2 oz (60 g) sliced chicken	2 oz (60 g) roast beef
1/2 cup farina	1/2 cup rice	1/2 cup cubed white
1 slice toast, white	1/2 cup green beans	potatoes
enriched	1 slice bread, white	1/2 cup cooked carrots
2 tsp butter or	enriched	1 slice bread, white
margarine	2 tsp butter or margarine	enriched
1 tbsp grape jelly	1 tbsp honey	2 tsp butter or margarine
2 tsp sugar	2 halves canned peaches	1 tbsp apple jelly
1 cup coffee	1/2 cup cranberry sauce	5 arrowroot cookies
	1 cup Hi-C grape drink	2 halves canned pears
		1 cup lemonade

Midmorning Nourishment	Midafternoon Nourishment	Evening Nourishment
1/2 cup apricot nectar	2 sugar cookies	6 saltine crackers
	10 jelly beans	1 tsp butter
		1 cup 7-Up

SAMPLE PROCEDURE FOR CALCULATING A PROTEIN-PHOSPHORUS RESTRICTED DIET:

Diet Prescription

Protein	50 g
Phosphorus	50 mEq

1. Convert the milliequivalents of phosphorus in the prescription to milligrams (multiply the number of milliequivalents by the atomic weight ÷ valence, see page 36).

2. Determine the amount of high biological value protein the patient should have, between 50% and 75% of the amount prescribed. (The lower the protein restriction, the higher the percentage of high biological value protein).

3. Divide the high biological value protein between dairy exchanges and meat and meat substitute exchanges.

4. Divide the remaining protein between bread exchanges and vegetable exchanges.

5. Total the amount of phosphorus (P) in these exchanges. Subtract this amount from the total amount of phosphorus allowed.

6. Divide the remaining phosphorus among the fruits, juices, and other beverages.

Example	Amount	Protein (g)	P (mg)
Step 1: 50 mEq P X 31 ÷ 2 = 755 mg P			
Step 2: Protein, 50 g x 50% = 25 g			
50 g x 75% = 37.5 g			
25-38 g high biological value protein			
Step 3: Dairy products exchanges	0		
Meat and meat substitute exchanges	4	32	280
Total protein from dairy and meat exchanges		32	

Example (continued):	Amount	Protein (g)	P (mg)
Step 4: 50 g protein in prescription			
32 g protein from dairy and meat			
18 g protein for bread and vegetables			
Bread exchanges	7	14	280
Vegetable exchanges	3	4.5	120
Total protein		50.5	
Step 5: Total phosphorus from sources other			680
than fruit and beverages			
775 mg phosphorus in prescription			
-680 mg phosphorus from sources other			
than fruit and beverages			
95 mg phosphorus for fruit and beverages			
Step 6: Fruit exchanges	4	0	80
Fats	3	0	0
Other beverages	3	0	15
Total phosphorus			775

<u>Meat and Meat Substitute Exchange List</u>: Each exchange contains approximately 8 g protein and 70 mg phosphorus. Portion sizes of meat, poultry, and fish refer to cooked weights without bone.

Meat
Bacon[1]	4 slices or 1 oz
Beef, lamb, pork, veal, poultry, wild game	1 oz (30 g)
Dried[1] or corned beef[1]	1 oz (30 g)
Frankfurter[1]	1 oz (30 g)
Ham[1] or canadian bacon[1]	1 oz (30 g)
Luncheon meat[1], bologna[1], sausage[1]	1 oz (30 g)

Fish
Shrimp, scallops, lobster, crab, clams, oysters	1 oz (30 g)
Canned, regular[1] or water-pack, low sodium tuna or salmon	1/4 cup

Cottage cheese[1], regular, creamed	1/4 cup
Egg, large[1,2]	1

Avoid liver, cheese (other than cottage), and peanut butter.

---

[1] High in sodium and should be avoided on any sodium restricted diet.

[2] Limit to 1 whole egg per day due to high phosphorus content (85 mg) of yolk. Egg white contains 5 mg phosphorus and may be used to add protein without adding significant phosphorus.

Dairy Products Exchange List: Use only if a more liberal phosphorus restriction is allowed. Each exchange contains approximately 4 g protein and 120 mg phosphorus. One serving per day of cheese or buttermilk is allowed on diets of 2 g Na or more, or a lower sodium diet may be calculated in order to include these foods.

Milk
Whole, 2%, or skim	1/2 cup
Buttermilk[1]	1/2 cup
Evaporated	1/4 cup
Instant nonfat dry	1 1/2 tbsp

Cream
Half-and-half	1/2 cup
Heavy (whipping), before whipping	3/4 cup

Desserts
Custard	1/4 cup
Ice cream or ice milk, any flavor (no nuts or fruit)	3/4 cup
Yogurt, plain or flavored	1/2 cup
Pudding[1], boxed or canned	1/2 cup
Pudding, cornstarch, made without salt	1/2 cup

Miscellaneous
Cheese[1]	1/2 oz
Cream soup[1]	1/2 cup

Bread Exchange List: Each exchange contains approximately 2 g protein and 40 mg phosphorus. If the diet is restricted to less than 2 g sodium, the food should be made without salt (see sodium restricted diets, pages 56-66).

Breads and Crackers[2]
Regular white, vienna, french, italian, raisin	1 slice
Dinner roll (2 in. diam)	1
Hot dog or hamburger bun	1 (12/pkg); or 1/2 (8/pkg)
Doughnut, cake or yeast	3 in. diameter
Sweet roll or danish pastry, medium	1/2 or 1 oz
English muffin, medium	1/2
Bagel, medium	1/2
Tortilla, plain or corn	1
Saltines[1]	6 squares
Crackers with unsalted tops	6 squares
Oyster crackers[1]	20 medium or 30 small
Graham crackers	2 squares
Zwieback	2 pieces
Rusk	1
Melba toast	4
Biscuit, homemade (2 in. diam)	1

---

[1]High in sodium and should be avoided on any sodium restricted diet.

[2]Avoid whole grain, bran, and those with nuts.

Cereals, cooked[1]
    Cream of Rice, Cream of Wheat, cornmeal, farina,
      hominy grits, Malt-O-Meal   1/2 cup

Cereals, dry, processed without fruits or nuts[2]
    Puffed cereals   1 cup
    All others   3/4 cup

Desserts	
Gelatin	1/2 cup
Lemon pudding	1/2 cup
Cake, plain or frosted (3 x 2 x 1 in.)	1 slice
Fruitcake, pound cake (3 x 3 x 1 in.)	1 slice
Cupcake, medium	1
Angel food or sponge cake (1 1/2 in. wedge)	1
Brownie or bar cookie (2 x 2 x 1 in.)	1
Marshmallows	10 large
Arrowroot cookies	5
Pie crust, single (made with salt)	1/8 of 9-in. crust
Vanilla wafers	10
Rice Krispie bar (3 x 2 x 1 in.)	1
Sugar wafers, small	8
Cookies (3 in. diam)	2
Shortbread cookies	4
Gingersnaps	5
Sherbet	1/2 cup
Ladyfingers	1 large or 2 small

Grains	
Flour	2 1/2 tbsp
Cornmeal, dry	2 1/2 tbsp
Masa harina, uncooked	3 tbsp
Pearl barley, cooked	3 tbsp

Pastas and Rice	
Macaroni, cooked	1/2 cup
Spaghetti, cooked	1/2 cup
Egg noodles, cooked	1/3 cup
Rice, white, cooked	1/2 cup

Miscellaneous	
Popcorn, average kernel	1 cup popped
Pretzels, regular[3]	4
Pretzels, low sodium	4

---

[1] Avoid quick-cooking or instant cereals and whole grain cereals such as oatmeal or rolled wheat.

[2] Avoid whole grain cereals such as bran flakes, Cheerios, Wheaties, and shredded wheat.

[3] High in sodium and should be avoided on any sodium restricted diet.

Vegetable Exchange List: Each exchange contains approximately 1.5 g protein and 40 mg phosphorus. If the diet is restricted to 2 g sodium or less, the vegetables must be fresh or frozen or canned without salt.

Asparagus, cut	1/3 cup
Asparagus, spears	4
Avocado, cubed	1/2 cup
Bean sprouts, fresh or cooked	1/2 cup
Beets, fresh cooked or canned	1/2 cup
Beet greens, fresh or cooked	1/2 cup
Broccoli, fresh or cooked	1/2 cup or 1 3-in. stalk
Cabbage, fresh or cooked	1/2 cup
Carrots, cooked	1/2 cup
Carrots, fresh (1/4 x 3 in.)	6-8 sticks
Cauliflower, fresh or cooked	1/2 cup
Celery, fresh (6 x 1/2 in.)	8 sticks
Celery, chopped or cooked	1 cup
Chard, swiss, cooked	1/2 cup
Chard, swiss, fresh	1 cup
Collards, fresh or cooked	1/2 cup
Corn-on-the-cob (4 x 2 in.)	1 ear
Corn, whole kernel or cream style	1/3 cup
Cress, garden	1/2 cup
Cucumber	1/2 medium or 1/2 cup
Dandelion greens, fresh or cooked	1/2 cup
Eggplant, fresh or cooked	1/2 cup
Endive, fresh	1 cup
Escarole, fresh	1 cup
Green beans	1/2 cup
Green pepper	1 cup or 1 medium shell
Kale, fresh or cooked	1/3 cup
Kohlrabi	1/2 cup
Lettuce, chopped	1 cup
Mixed vegetables	1/3 cup
Mushrooms, fresh or canned	1/2 cup
Mustard greens, fresh or cooked	1/2 cup
Okra, fresh or frozen cooked	1/2 cup
Onion, fresh or cooked	1/2 cup
Onions, green (5 x 1/2 in.)	3
Parsley, fresh chopped	4 tbsp
Parsnips, fresh cooked or mashed	1/2 cup
Peas, canned, fresh or frozen cooked	1/4 cup
Potatoes, mashed, boiled, or baked	1 small or 1/2 cup
Potatoes, french fried (3 1/2 in. long)	8 strips
Radishes	10 large or 1 cup sliced
Rutabaga, fresh or cooked	1/2 cup
Spinach, fresh	1 cup
Spinach, cooked	1/3 cup
Squash, summer or winter	1/2 cup
Sweet potatoes, baked	1/2 small
Sweet potatoes, mashed or canned	1/2 cup
Tomato, fresh	1 medium
Tomatoes, cooked	1/2 cup
Tomato paste	3 tbsp
Tomato sauce or puree	1/3 cup
Tomato juice or vegetable juice cocktail	3/4 cup
Turnips, cooked	1 cup
Turnip greens	1/2 cup

Vegetables (continued)

Watercress	1 cup or 10 sprigs
Watercress, chopped	1/2 cup
Wax beans	1/2 cup
Zucchini	1/2 cup

Avoid: Dry beans, lima beans, kidney beans, soybeans, pork and beans, lentils, split peas, and black-eyed peas.

<u>Fruit and Fruit Juice Exchange List</u>: Each exchange contains negligible protein and approximately 20 mg phosphorus (protein averages 0.5 g per exchange and is not counted unless the diet is restricted to 20 g or less protein). Fruits can be fresh, frozen, or canned. If canned with fruit juice, the juice must be drained or counted as part of the exchange as indicated.

Fruit

Apple, fresh	1 medium (3 1/4 in. diam)
Applesauce, fresh or canned	1 cup
Apricots, fresh or canned	2 medium or 4 halves
Banana	1/2 medium or 1/2 cup sliced
Blackberries, fresh, frozen, or canned	1/2 cup
Blueberries, fresh, frozen, or canned	1/2 cup
Boysenberries, fresh, frozen, or canned	1/2 cup
Cantaloupe, cubed	3/4 cup
Cantaloupe wedge (5 in. diam)	1/4 melon
Casaba melon, cubed	3/4 cup
Cherries	1/2 cup
Currants, dried	2 tbsp
Currants, fresh	1/3 cup
Dates, fresh or dried	3 medium
Elderberries, fresh	1/3 cup
Figs, fresh, dried, or canned	2 medium
Fruit cocktail	1/2 cup
Gooseberries, fresh or canned	1 cup
Grapefruit, fresh (4 in. diam)	1/2
Grapefruit sections, fresh or canned	1/2 cup
Grapes	1/2 cup
Honeydew melon, cubed	3/4 cup
Lemon, fresh	1 medium
Lime, fresh	1 medium
Mandarin oranges, canned	1/2 cup
Mango, diced or sliced	1 cup
Mulberries, fresh	3/4 cup
Nectarine, fresh	1/2 medium
Orange	1 medium (2 1/2 in. diam)
Papaya, cubed	1 cup
Peach, canned	2 halves or 1/2 cup sliced
Peach, fresh	1 medium
Pear, fresh or canned	1 small or 2 halves
Persimmon	1 small
Pineapple, fresh, frozen, or canned	1 cup
Plums, fresh or canned	2 medium
Pomegranate	1 medium
Prunes	2 medium
Raisins	2 tbsp
Raspberries, fresh, frozen, or canned	1/2 cup
Rhubarb	1/2 cup
Strawberries, fresh or frozen	1/2 cup
Tangelo	1 medium
Tangerine	1 large

Fruit (continued)

Watermelon, cubed	1 cup
Watermelon wedge (5 in. diam, 1 in. thick)	1

Fruit Juices

Apple juice	1 cup
Apricot nectar	1/2 cup
Cranapple juice	1 cup
Cranberry juice	1 cup
Grape juice	1/2 cup
Grapefruit juice	1/2 cup
Orange juice	1/2 cup
Peach nectar	1/2 cup
Pear nectar	1 cup
Pineapple juice	1/2 cup
Prune juice	1/3 cup

Fat List: The following foods contain negligible protein and phosphorus. If the diet is severely restricted in sodium, all of the fats must be salt-free. If the diet is more liberal, some fats can be regular (salted) and some will be salt-free (see sodium restricted diets page 56).

Butter or margarine
Mayonnaise
Salad dressing, mayonnaise-type
French dressing
Italian dressing
Thousand island dressing

Avoid: Salad dressings with milk or cheese, peanut butter, cream cheese.

Beverage Exchange List: Each exchange contains negligible protein and approximately 5 mg phosphorus.

Coffee or decaffeinated coffee, instant	1 tsp powder
Coffee, percolated or drip	1 cup
Hawaiian punch	1/2 cup
Hi-C fruit drinks	1 cup
Tea, brewed	1 cup
Tea, instant	1 tsp powder
Lemonade or limeade, frozen, diluted	1 cup
Wine	2 oz

Avoid: Beer, Tang, powdered beverage mixes, or carbonated beverages that contain phosphoric acid.

Soft Drinks: The kinds of soda pop allowed depend on the phosphorus content. Complete information was not available from some bottlers. These soft drinks contain negligible phosphorus.

Fanta: ginger ale, grape, orange, diet orange, root beer
Fresca
Mello Yello
Mountain Dew
Ramblin' Root Beer, sugar-free Ramblin' Root Beer
Shasta
Slice
Sprite, diet Sprite
7-Up, diet 7-Up

Additional Foods List: The following foods are low in protein and phosphorus and most add calories to the diet.

List A. Free (Any amount may be eaten each day.)

Butterballs
Chewing gum
Cornstarch
Cotton candy
Gumdrops
Cranberry relish
Herbs
Lard
Lollipops, unfilled
Mints
Oil
Popsicle
Rich's Whip Topping
Shortening
Spices
Sugar, confectioners
Sugar, granulated
Twist powdered soft drink mix
Vinegar, distilled

List B. Limit to 5 servings per day.

Catsup[1]	1 tsp
Catsup, low sodium	1 tsp
Coffee-mate	1 tbsp
Cool Whip	1 tbsp
Cranberries, fresh	1/2 cup
Cranberry relish	1/3 cup
Cranberry sauce	1/2 cup
D-Zerta whipped topping	1 tbsp
Fondant	1-2 pieces
Hard candy	6 pieces
Horseradish	1 tsp
Honey	1 tbsp
Jam or preserves	1/2 tbsp
Jelly beans	10 pieces
Jellies	1 tbsp
Mustard[1]	1/2 tsp
Mustard, low sodium	1/2 tsp
Syrups	1 tbsp
Tapioca, granulated	1 tbsp
Vinegar, cider	1 tbsp

Avoid: Other powdered coffee whiteners, liquid cream substitutes, brown sugar, molasses, imitation sour cream, chocolate, and straight phosphate baking soda.

---

[1]High in sodium and should be avoided on any sodium restricted diet.

C. RENAL DIETS

DESCRIPTION: The purpose of the Renal Diet is to minimize the complications associated with the metabolic changes of acute and chronic kidney disease. The levels of protein, sodium, potassium, phosphorus, and fluid prescribed are determined according to the patient's renal function and method of treatment (see page 80). Making the diet as liberal and individualized as possible is important for achieving optimal nutritional status. The diet is calculated using exchange lists in which foods are categorized according to their composition of protein, sodium, potassium, and phosphorus (see pages 84-98). Because the composition of manufactured products is subject to change, labels and company literature should be checked periodically.

Multiple dietary restrictions make the maintenance of adequate nutrition difficult. If essential amino acids and calories are not provided in amounts necessary to maintain nitrogen balance, body catabolism will take place, increasing serum urea nitrogen and potassium. Enteral nutrition support is the method of choice; however, many of these patients are so ill that they do not have adequate gastrointestinal function, and total parenteral nutrition must be provided.

Frequent monitoring of serum urea nitrogen, creatinine, albumin, sodium, calcium, and phosphorus, as well as of urinary creatinine, sodium, and volume is necessary. Weight loss or gain and the presence of anemia or acidosis are other important variables that require surveillance.

PROTEIN: The level of protein restriction varies according to the glomerular filtration rate, the method of treatment, and the patient's estimated ideal body weight. The symptoms associated with elevated serum urea nitrogen levels (anorexia, nausea, vomiting, fatigue, itching, diarrhea, and general malaise) are partially controlled by protein restriction. Although symptoms may improve more rapidly, the serum urea nitrogen level will not stabilize until two or three weeks after the protein intake has been decreased. Lowering the level of protein in the diet when the glomerular filtration rate is below 4 to 5 ml/minute will not control uremic symptoms, and may cause wasting. There is some evidence that protein restriction may slow the progression of chronic renal failure. Until this issue is resolved more clearly, restriction of dietary protein to 0.8 g/kg/day is safe and prudent for patients with early insufficiency.

Amino acids are lost with hemodialysis treatment, while both amino acids and protein are lost with peritoneal dialysis treatment. Therefore the protein allowance must be increased once therapy has been initiated and the patient is stable. Patients on peritoneal dialysis need more protein if peritonitis occurs, due to increased losses. The filtering efficiency of the peritoneum decreases dramatically in peritonitis, resulting in protein losses 10 to 20 times normal. Patients with acute renal failure undergoing hemodialysis may require normal or above normal levels of protein and calories.

To provide adequate amounts of essential amino acids, high biological value proteins such as eggs, milk, meat, poultry, and fish should provide one-half to three-fourths of the protein allowance and be distributed among all three meals. Travasorb Renal, Amin-Aid, and ProMix Protein are low electrolyte, high biological value protein supplements that may be taken orally.

CALORIES: Energy intake must be maintained in patients with renal disease. Adequate calories from carbohydrate and fat spare dietary protein for tissue synthesis and repair. If insufficient calories are ingested, body catabolism takes place, increasing serum urea nitrogen and potassium levels. Therefore, calories must be adequate to minimize the use of exogenous and endogenous protein for energy. The patient on continuous ambulatory peritoneal dialysis or continuous cyclic peritoneal dialysis treatments will absorb glucose from the dialysate. The amounts vary with the glucose concentration of the dialysate and the frequency of exchanges. Thus, the caloric contribution of the dialysate must be considered in determining the calories needed from the diet.

SODIUM: Sodium restriction is often necessary to control or prevent fluid retention, hypertension, pulmonary edema, or congestive heart failure. Because requirements vary, each patient must be managed individually. A level of 1 to 3 g sodium per day is usually adequate to control hypertension and edema (see sodium restricted diets, pages 56-66). In both acute and chronic renal failure, sodium intake is usually adjusted to equal urinary sodium losses up to an intake of 3 to 4 g. Adequacy of sodium intake can be monitored by carefully following body weight and blood pressure. Diets that are too restrictive increase the probability of noncompliance and inadequate nutrient intake, and may lead to sodium depletion in some patients, especially those on low protein diets.

Not all patients with renal disease need sodium restriction. In the early stages of pyelonephritis, medullary cystic disease, or bilateral hydronephrosis, excessive amounts of sodium are lost in the urine. Muscle cramps, convulsions, hypovolemia, and further deterioration of renal function occur if sodium needs are not met. Once the patient is stabilized on dialysis, the sodium allowance can be individualized using body weight and blood pressure as guides to adequacy of intake. Dietary sodium intake must be strictly limited in patients with severe oliguria when sodium excretion may cease. During nonoliguric renal failure or the diuretic phase, considerable sodium may be lost, and the dietary prescription must compensate for this.

POTASSIUM: Hyperkalemia, a common problem in renal failure, can lead to cardiac arrhythmias and eventual arrest. Although many renal patients require a low potassium diet to prevent hyperkalemia, such a restriction is usually not necessary under the following conditions: (a) when the urine output is greater than 1000 cc per day; (b) if the patient's serum potassium is normal (3.5 to 5.0 mg/dl) because intake and clearance are appropriate; or (c) in the absence of acidosis, catabolic stress, or hypoaldosteronism.

Factors to consider in restricting dietary potassium are urinary volume, medications used to control hyperkalemia, and the method of treatment for renal failure. A restriction to 40 to 60 mEq per day in the early stages will usually prevent problems, while a more liberal intake may be tolerated once dialysis is initiated. Since catabolism of body tissue can exacerbate hyperkalemia, an adequate caloric intake is essential.

Hypokalemia may result from the use of a potassium-losing diuretic or from peritoneal dialysis. In these instances, potassium-rich foods may need to be added to the diet until the condition is corrected. Careful monitoring of serum potassium is needed to maintain a normal level.

Potassium is widely distributed in foods. Meat, milk and dairy products, fruits, and vegetables are rich sources. Fresh and frozen fruits and vegetables contain more potassium than canned versions due to leaching of the mineral into the liquid. The potassium content of fresh fruits and vegetables can be reduced by soaking small pieces in tepid water for two hours, draining, and then cooking in large amounts of fresh water and draining again.

Because they are extremely concentrated sources of potassium, the use of potassium-containing salt substitutes is not recommended for patients with renal disease. (The salt substitute used at the University of Iowa Hospitals and Clinics contains 13.5 mEq potassium per packet.)

PHOSPHORUS: In moderate and severe renal failure, a reduced phosphorus intake is indicated because phosphate is excreted primarily in the urine. Hyperphosphatemia may trigger disturbances of calcium, vitamin D, and parathyroid hormone secretion, which in turn may cause hyperparathyroidism or renal osteodystrophy. Research is now suggesting that phosphorus be restricted to 600 to 1200 mg per day at the very early stages of renal failure to slow the progression of the disease.

The average American diet provides 1.5 to 2 g phosphorus per day. Meat and dairy products are especially rich sources, although it is present in nearly all foods. Restricting protein can result in a 25 to 50% decrease in phosphorus intake, depending on the foods selected. When diet alone does not result in appropriate serum levels, a phosphate-binding agent may be prescribed in addition to the diet. Labels should be read carefully, since phosphates are currently added to a wide variety of processed foods, including carbonated beverages, meats, cheeses, salad dressings, and refrigerated bakery products.

FLUIDS: When the patient appears in an ideal state of hydration, fluid intake is determined by the 24-hour urine output, other measurable losses, plus 400 to 600 cc for insensible losses. It is important not to restrict fluids for the patient with normal urine output, as this could result in dehydration and further deterioration of renal function. In the predialysis or conservative stage, most patients will be in balance with a fluid intake of 1000 to 3000 cc per day. Excessive fluid intake in patients with renal disease can lead to edema, hypertension, and congestive heart failure. Patients maintained on hemodialysis should not gain more than 0.5 to 1.0 kg per day for feasible removal of excess water weight. (One liter excess fluid weighs approximately 1 kg.) The fluid needs of patients utilizing peritoneal dialysis vary with the efficiency of ultrafiltration, and they seldom require restrictions of less than 1.5 liters per day.

79

The fluid content of solid foods is not routinely calculated in renal diets. However, it should be recognized that nonliquid foods do contain substantial amounts of water. The table below shows the average fluid content of common foods. Another factor to consider is the water produced from the metabolism of food: 0.60 cc/g carbohydrate, 0.41 cc/g protein, and 1.07 cc/g fat.

AVERAGE FLUID CONTENT OF COMMON FOODS

Cooked cereal (1/2 cup)	100 cc
Vegetables, fresh or drained (1/2 cup)	90 cc
Potato, boiled (1/2 cup)	95 cc
Potato, mashed (1/2 cup)	85 cc
Fruits, fresh or drained (1/2 cup)	80 cc
Lettuce (1/8 head)	70 cc
Spaghetti, rice, noodles, macaroni (1/2 cup)	55 cc
Egg (1)	40 cc
Meat (1 oz)	15 cc
Bread (1 slice)	10 cc
Jelly (1 tbsp)	5 cc
Butter (1 tsp)	1 cc
Hard candy	0 cc

Note: Calculated from USDA Handbook 456.

ADEQUACY: The adequacy of the diet depends on the number and severity of the restrictions. Diets restricted to less than 50 g of protein or 50 mEq potassium typically do not meet the Recommended Dietary Allowances for calcium, iron, niacin, riboflavin, thiamin, folic acid, and vitamins B_6, B_{12}, C, and D. Routine supplementation of these nutrients is advised, not only because of inadequate levels provided in the restricted diet and the altered metabolic utilization of nutrients, but also because water soluble nutrients are partially removed by dialysis.

RECOMMENDED DIETARY INTAKES FOR PATIENTS WITH RENAL FAILURE

Nutrient	Predialysis/ Conservative	METHOD OF TREATMENT Hemodialysis Adult Patient	Pediatric Patient	Peritoneal Dialysis
Protein	0.8 gm/kg Minimum 40 gm for men Minimum 35 gm for women and small men	1 gm/kg	1.5-2.0 gm/kg	1.2-1.5 gm/kg
Calories	25-30 kcal/kg	25-30 kcal/kg	Infants 100-120 kcal/kg Children 50-100 kcal/kg	25-30 kcal/kg
Sodium	Individualized (1-3 gm)	Individualized (2-3 gm)	Individualized (1-2 gm)	Individualized (3-4 gm)
Potassium	Urine volume >1000cc/day No restriction Urine volume ≤1000cc/day 40-60 mEq/day	Individualized (60-70 mEq)	Individualized (40-70 mEq)	Individualized (Usually no restriction)
Phosphorus	Individualized (600-1200 mg)	Individualized (1.0-1.2 gm)	Individualized (1.0-1.2 gm)	Individualized (1.2-1.5 gm)
Fluid	Equal to urine output plus insensible loss	Individualized (750-1500 cc)	Individualized (750-1500 cc)	Individualized (1000-1500 cc)
Supplements	Individualized General multivitamin-mineral supplement may be advisable	General multi-vitamin-mineral supplement Pyridoxine 10 mg Ascorbic Acid 100 mg Folic Acid 1 mg $FeSO_4$ 300 mg-3X/day	General multi-vitamin-mineral supplement Pyridoxine 10 mg Ascorbic Acid 100 mg Folic Acid 1 mg $FeSO_4$ 300 mg-3X/day	Prenatal vitamin supplement Pyridoxine 10 mg Ascorbic Acid 100 mg Folic Acid 1 mg $FeSO_4$ 300 mg-3X/day

PROTEIN, SODIUM, POTASSIUM, PHOSPHORUS, AND FLUID VALUES
FOR RENAL DIET EXCHANGES
(average figures)

Food Group	Protein (g)	Sodium (mg)	Potassium (mg)	Phosphorus (mg)	Fluid (cc)
Meat and Meat Substitutes					15
Low sodium	8	25	130	70	
Moderate sodium	8	75	130	70	
High sodium	8	300	130	70	
Very high sodium	8	600	130	70	
Dairy Products	4	60	170	120	120
Bread and Bread Substitutes					5-100
Low sodium	2	10	50	40	
Moderate sodium	2	150	50	40	
Vegetables					90
(Low sodium/Regular)					
Very low potassium	trace	trace	50	5	
List A	1	10/200	100	30	
List B	2	15/250	200	50	
Fruits					80
List A	--	--	100	15	
List B	--	--	200	20	
Fruits Juices					Varies with amount
List A	--	--	100	15	
List B	--	--	200	20	
Fats					1
Low sodium	--	--	--	trace	
Moderate sodium	--	50	--	trace	
Other Potassium- containing					Varies with amount
Beverages	--	--	90	5	

SAMPLE PROCEDURE FOR CALCULATING A RENAL DIET:

Diet Prescription

Protein	60	g
Potassium	60	mEq
Sodium	43	mEq
Phosphorus	60	mEq
Fluid	1000	ml

1. Convert the milliequivalents of Na, K, and P in the prescription to milligrams (multiply the number of milliequivalents by the atomic weight ÷ valence, see page 36).

2. Determine the amount of high biological value protein the patient should have, between 50 and 75% of the amount prescribed. (The lower the protein restriction, the higher the percentage of high biological value protein.)

3. Divide the high biological value protein between dairy exchanges and meat and meat substitute exchanges.

4. Divide the remaining protein between bread exchanges and vegetable exchanges.

5. Total the amount of potassium (K) in these exchanges. Subtract this amount from the total amount of potassium allowed.

6. Divide the remaining potassium among the fruits, juices, and other beverages.

7. Calculate the sodium level.

8. Calculate the phosphorus level.

9. Calculate the fluid level in ml or cc.

Example	Amount	Protein (g)	K (mg)

Step 1: 60 mEq K x 39 = 2340 mg K
43 mEq Na x 23 = 989 mg Na
60 mEq P x 31 ÷ 2 = 930 mg P

Step 2: Protein, 60 g x 50% = 30 g
60 g x 75% = 45 g
30-45 g high biological value protein

	Amount	Protein (g)	K (mg)
Step 3: Dairy products exchanges	1	4	170
Meat and meat substitute exchanges	5	40	650
Total protein from dairy and meat		44	

Step 4: 60 g protein in prescription
- 44 g protein from dairy and meat
16 g protein for bread and vegetables

	Amount	Protein (g)	K (mg)
Bread exchanges	6	12	300
Vegetable exchanges			
List A	2	2	200
List B	1	2	200
Total protein		60	

	Amount	Protein (g)	K (mg)
Step 5: Total potassium from sources other than fruit			1520

2340 mg potassium in prescription
- 1520 mg potassium from sources other than fruit and beverages
820 mg potassium for fruit and beverages

	Amount	Protein (g)	K (mg)
Step 6: Fruit exchanges			
List A	2	0	200
List B	1	0	200
Fruit juices			
List A	1	0	100
List B	1	0	200
Other beverages	1	0	90
Total potassium			2310

Example (continued):

Step 7: Calculate the sodium (average figures)

Sodium from 1 egg	75 mg
Sodium from 4 oz meat, low sodium	100 mg
Sodium from 1/2 cup milk	60 mg
Sodium from 3 unsalted breads	30 mg
and 3 regular breads	360 mg
Sodium from unsalted vegetables	35 mg
Sodium from 7 tsp salted	
(regular) butter or margarine	350 mg
Total sodium	1010 mg

Step 8: Calculate the phosphorus (average figures)

Phosphorus from 5 meats	350 mg
Phosphorus from 1/2 c milk	120 mg
Phosphorus from 6 breads	240 mg
Phosphorus from 2 "A" vegetables	60 mg
Phosphorus from 1 "B" vegetable	50 mg
Phosphorus from 2 "A" fruits and	
1 "A" fruit juice	45 mg
Phosphorus from 1 "B" fruit and	
1 "B" fruit juice	40 mg
Phosphorus from 1 "other" beverage	5 mg
Total phosphorus	910 mg

Step 9: Calculate the fluid

1/3 cup orange juice	80 ml
1 cup instant coffee	240 ml
1/2 cup milk	120 ml
1 1/2 cups Kool-Aid	360 ml
1/3 cup pineapple juice	80 ml
1/2 cup 7-Up	120 ml
Total fluid	1000 ml (or cc)

APPROXIMATE COMPOSITION OF SAMPLE MENU:

Calories	2113
Protein, g	69
Fat, g	63
Carbohydrate, g	323
Sodium, mg	969
Potassium, mg	2043
Phosphorus, mg	879

SAMPLE MENU FOR A RENAL DIET (60 g protein, 60 mEq potassium, 1000 mg sodium, 60 mEq phosphorus, 1000 cc fluid):

Breakfast	Luncheon	Dinner
1/3 cup orange juice	2 oz (60 g) chicken, unsalted	1/3 cup pineapple juice
1/2 cup unsalted farina	1/2 cup rice, unsalted	2 oz (60 g) roast beef, unsalted
1 slice toast, white enriched (regular)	1/2 cup green beans, unsalted	1/3 cup cubed white potatoes, unsalted
1 egg, soft cooked	1 slice bread, white enriched (regular)	1/3 cup carrots, unsalted
1 tsp butter or margarine (regular)	2 halves canned peaches, drained	1/2 cup lettuce salad
2 tsp grape jelly	3 tbsp cranberry sauce	1 slice bread, white enriched (regular)
2 tsp sugar	2 tsp butter or margarine (regular)	1 tbsp low sodium french dressing
1 cup instant coffee	1 cup Kool-Aid	3 tsp butter or margarine (regular)
1/2 cup whole milk		1/2 cup Kool-Aid

Midmorning Nourishment	Midafternoon Nourishment	Evening Nourishment
1 small apple	2 low sodium sugar cookies	2 halves canned pears, drained
	15 jelly beans	1/2 cup 7-Up

FOOD EXCHANGE LISTS FOR RENAL DIETS:

Meat and Meat Substitute Exchange List: Each exchange contains approximately 8 g protein, 130 mg potassium, and 70 mg phosphorus. Because the sodium content varies, the type of food allowed will depend on the patient's restriction. Portion sizes of meat, poultry, and fish refer to cooked weights without bone.

Low Sodium Content: Each exchange contains approximately 25 mg sodium.

Cheese[1], low sodium	1 oz (30 g)
Cottage cheese, low sodium	1/4 cup
Crab, fish, lobster, scallops, shrimp	1 oz (30 g)
Meat	
Beef, fresh unprocessed ham (not cured), lamb, liver[1], pork, poultry, wild game	1 oz (30 g)
Peanut butter[2], low sodium[1]	2 tbsp
Tuna or salmon, low sodium, water-pack	1/4 cup

---

[1]Limit on phosphorus restricted diet because of higher phosphorus content.

[2]Use only occasionally because of higher potassium content.

Moderate Sodium Content: Each exchange contains approximately 75 mg sodium.

Cottage cheese, regular, creamed[1,2]	1/4 cup
Egg, large[1]	1
Oysters	1 oz (30 g)

High Sodium Content: Each exchange contains approximately 300 mg sodium.

Canadian bacon	1 oz (30 g)
Cheese[1], natural (cheddar, parmesan)	1 oz (30 g)
Corned beef	1 oz (30 g)
Ham, processed (cured)	1 oz (30 g)
Luncheon meat	1 oz (30 g)
Meat or fish, canned with salt	1 oz (30 g)
Peanut butter[1,3], regular	2 tbsp
Pork link sausages	1 1/2 links (30 g)
Pork sausage	1 oz (30 g)

Very High Sodium Content: Each exchange contains approximately 600 mg sodium.

Bacon	4 slices (30 g)
Frankfurter	1 oz (30 g)

The following are high in sodium and should be avoided:

Chipped beef
Smoked fish, meat, or poultry

Dairy Products Exchange List: Each exchange contains approximately 4 g protein, 170 mg potassium, 60 mg sodium, and 120 mg phosphorus.

Milk	
Chocolate (commercial)[1]	1/2 cup
Evaporated	1/4 cup
Instant nonfat dry	2 1/2 tbsp
Sweetened condensed	3 tbsp
Whole, 2%, or skim	1/2 cup
Cream	
Half-and-half	1/2 cup
Heavy (whipping),	
before whipping	3/4 cup

---

[1]Limit on phosphorus restricted diet because of higher phosphorus content. Egg yolk is high in phosphorus, but egg whites are low and may be used (egg yolk = 85 mg phosphorus, egg white = 5 mg phosphorus).

[2]Use only occasionally because of higher sodium content.

[3]Use only occasionally because of higher potassium content.

Desserts

Custard, made without salt	1/4 cup
Ice cream or ice milk, any flavor (no nuts or fruit)	3/4 cup
Pudding[1], boxed or canned	1/2 cup
Pudding, cornstarch made without salt	1/2 cup
Yogurt, plain or vanilla flavored	1/2 cup

The following are high in sodium or potassium (indicated in parentheses) and should be avoided.

Buttermilk (Na)
Fruit flavored yogurt (K)
Low sodium milk (K)

Bread Exchange List: Each exchange contains approximately 2 g protein, 50 mg potassium, and 40 mg phosphorus. Because sodium content varies, the type of food allowed, low sodium or regular, will depend on the patient's restriction.

Low Sodium Content: Each serving contains approximately 10 mg sodium.

Breads and Crackers	
Bread, low sodium	1 slice
Crackers, low sodium	6
Melba toast, low sodium	4
Oyster crackers, low sodium	30
Pretzels, low sodium	4
Rice wafers	10
Rusk	1
Tortilla, plain or corn	1
Cereals, cooked (prepared without salt)	
Cream of Rice, Cream of Wheat, cornmeal, farina hominy grits, Malt-O-Meal, oatmeal[2], rolled wheat[2]	1/2 cup
Cereals, dry (processed without salt)	
Frosted Mini Wheats	4 biscuits
Low sodium cornflakes, low sodium toasted rice	1/2 cup
Puffed rice, puffed wheat, Puffa Puffa Rice, Sugar Smacks, Sugar Puffs, Sugar Crisp	1 cup
Shredded wheat, biscuit	1 large

---

[1]Limit to 1 serving each day due to higher sodium content. Use chocolate pudding only occasionally because of higher potassium content.

[2]Limit on phosphorus restricted diet because of higher phosphorus content.

Desserts
  Ladyfingers   1 large or 2 small
  Marshmallows   10 large
  Pie crust, double,
    made without salt   1/8 of 9-in. crust
  Sherbet   1/2 cup
  Shortbread cookies   4
Grains
  Cornmeal, dry   2 1/2 tbsp
  Flour   2 1/2 tbsp
  Masa harina, uncooked   3 tbsp
  Pearl barley, cooked   3 tbsp
Pasta and Rice (cooked without salt)
  Egg noodles, cooked   1/3 cup
  Macaroni, cooked   1/2 cup
  Rice, white, cooked   1/2 cup
  Spaghetti, cooked   1/2 cup
Miscellaneous
  Popcorn, unsalted   1 1/2 cups
    (average kernel)   popped

The following are high in sodium, potassium, or protein (indicated in parentheses) and should be avoided:

Bakery items containing low sodium baking powder (K)
Bran cereals (K)
Breads, crackers, and cereals of moderate sodium content (Na)
Cereals processed with fruit or nuts (K and protein)
High protein or protein fortified cereals (protein)
Instant cereals (Na)
Wheat germ (K and protein)

Moderate Sodium Content: Each serving contains approximately 150 mg sodium.

Bread and Crackers
  Bagel, medium   1/2
  Baking powder biscuit (2 in. diameter)   1
  Bread, regular white, vienna, french, rye,
    italian, whole wheat[1], raisin   1 slice
  Coffee cake[1]   2 in. square
  Cornbread[1] (1 1/2 in. cube)   1
  Crackers with unsalted tops   6 squares
  Dinner roll (2 in. diam)   1
  Doughnut, cake or yeast (3 in. diam)   1 or 1 oz
  English muffin, medium   1/2
  Graham crackers   2 squares
  Hotdog or hamburger bun   1 (12/pkg); or
                                            1/2 (8/pkg)
  Muffin[1], plain, homemade (3 x 2 x 1 1/2 in.)   1
  Pancake[1] (3 in. diam)   1
  Sweet roll or danish pastry, medium   1/2 or 1 oz
  Zwieback   2 pieces

---

[1]Limit on phosphorus restricted diet because of higher phosphorus content.

Cereals, cooked	
(lightly salted in preparation)	1/2 cup
Cream of Rice, Cream of Wheat,	
cornmeal, farina, hominy grits,	
Malt-O-Meal, oatmeal[1], rolled wheat[1]	
Cereals, dry[2]	
(processed with salt, without fruits or nuts)	3/4 cup

Desserts	
Angel food or sponge cake (1 1/2 in. wedge)	1
Animal crackers	8
Arrowroot cookies	5
Brownie (2 x 2 x 1 in.)	1
Cake, plain or frosted (3 x 2 x 1 in.)	1 slice
Gelatin	1/2 cup
Lemon pudding	1/2 cup
Oatmeal cookies (3 in. diam)	2
Pie crust, single (made with salt)	1/8 of 9-in. crust
Pound cake (3 x 3 x 1 in.)	1 slice
Rice Krispie bar (3 x 2 x 1 in.)	1
Sugar cookies (3 in. diam)	2
Sugar wafers, small	8
Vanilla wafers	10

The following are high in sodium, potassium, or protein, and should be avoided:

Cereals containing fruits or nuts (K and protein)
High protein or protein fortified cereals such as Life, Post Oat Flakes,
    Quaker Wheat Flakes (protein)
Pumpernickel bread (K)
Wheaties (Na)

Vegetable Exchange Lists: Very Low Potassium Content: The following vegetables contain approximately 50 mg potassium, 5 mg phosphorus, and negligible amounts of sodium and protein. One serving from this group may be used each day in addition to the other servings of vegetables.

Chicory, fresh	1/4 cup
Cabbage, chinese	1/4 cup
Chives, fresh chopped	2 tbsp
Cucumber, fresh pared	1/4 medium
Escarole, fresh	1/4 cup
Green pepper	1/4 medium shell
Lettuce, chopped	1/2 cup
Lettuce leaf (5 x 5 in.)	1
Onion, fresh chopped	3 tbsp
Parsley, fresh chopped	1 tbsp
Parsley sprig	1 large
Radish, fresh	1
Watercress	5 sprigs

---

[1]Limit on phosphorus restricted diet because of higher phosphorus content.

[2]Limit Cheerios on phosphorus restricted diet because of higher phosphorus content.

List A. Low Potassium Content: Each exchange contains approximately 1 g protein, 100 mg potassium, 30 mg phosphorus, and 10 mg sodium for fresh, frozen, or low sodium canned and 200 mg sodium for regular canned. The starred items are naturally higher in sodium, averaging 35 mg per serving.

Bean sprouts, fresh or fresh cooked	1/2 cup
Beets*, fresh cooked or canned	1/3 cup
Cabbage, fresh or fresh cooked	1/2 cup
Carrots*, canned	1/2 cup
Carrots*, fresh (1/4 x 3 in.)	6-8 sticks
Carrots*, fresh or frozen cooked	1/3 cup
Cauliflower, fresh, fresh or frozen cooked	1/3 cup
Celery*, fresh (6 x 1/2 in.)	1 stalk
Celery*, fresh chopped or cooked	1/4 cup
Corn-on-the-cob (4 x 2 in.)	1 ear
Corn, fresh or frozen cooked	1/3 cup
Corn, canned	1/2 cup
Corn, cream style	1/3 cup
Cucumber	1/2 medium or 1/2 cup
Eggplant, fresh or fresh cooked	1/3 cup
Endive	2/3 cup
Escarole	1/2 cup
Green beans, fresh, frozen, or canned	1/2 cup
Green pepper	1/2 medium
Green pepper, chopped	1/3 cup
Kale, fresh or frozen cooked	1/3 cup
Lettuce, chopped	2/3 cup
Mixed vegetables*, frozen cooked	1/3 cup
Okra, fresh or frozen cooked	1/3 cup or 5 pods
Onions, fresh	1/3 cup
Onions, fresh cooked	1/2 cup
Onions, green (5 x 1/2 in.)	2
Parsley, fresh chopped	4 tbsp
Peas, canned, fresh or frozen cooked	1/4 cup
Radishes (1 in. diam)	3
Summer squash, fresh or frozen cooked	1/3 cup
Watercress	10 sprigs
Watercress, chopped	1/3 cup
Wax beans, fresh, frozen or canned	1/2 cup
Zucchini, fresh or frozen cooked	1/3 cup

List B. Moderate Potassium Content: Each exchange contains approximately 2 g protein, 200 mg potassium, 50 mg phosphorus, and 15 mg sodium for fresh, frozen, or low sodium cooked and 250 mg sodium for regular canned. The starred items are naturally higher in sodium, averaging 35 mg per serving.

Asparagus, fresh or fresh cooked	2/3 cup
Asparagus, canned or frozen	1/2 cup
Beet greens*, fresh or cooked	1/2 cup
Broccoli, fresh, or fresh or frozen cooked	3 in. stalk
Broccoli, chopped, fresh or frozen cooked	1/2 cup
Brussels sprouts, fresh or frozen cooked	1/2 cup
Chard, swiss, fresh cooked	1/3 cup
Collards, fresh, or fresh or frozen cooked	1/2 cup
Cress, garden	1/2 cup
Dandelion greens, fresh or cooked	1/2 cup
Kohlrabi, fresh	1/3 cup
Kohlrabi, cooked	1/2 cup
Mushrooms, fresh	2/3 cup
Mushrooms, canned	1/2 cup

Mustard greens, fresh	2/3 cup
Mustard greens, cooked	1/2 cup
Parsnips, fresh cooked	1/3 cup
Parsnips, mashed	1/4 cup
Potatoes, mashed or boiled without skin	1/3 cup
Potatoes, french fried (3 1/2 in. long)	5 strips
Pumpkin, canned	1/3 cup
Rutabaga, fresh or cooked	1/2 cup
Spinach*, fresh, chopped	2/3 cup
Spinach*, fresh cooked, or canned	1/3 cup
Spinach*, frozen cooked	1/4 cup
Squash, winter	1/3 cup
Sweet potato, baked	1/2 small
Sweet potatoes, mashed	1/4 cup
Sweet potatoes, canned	1/2 cup
Sweet potatoes, candied	2 halves
Tomato, fresh	1/2 medium
Tomatoes, fresh cooked	1/4 cup
Tomatoes, canned	1/3 cup
Tomato juice or vegetable juice cocktail	1/3 cup
Turnips, fresh or mashed	1/2 cup
Turnips, cooked	2/3 cup
Turnips, mashed	1/2 cup
Turnip greens, canned	1/3 cup
Turnip greens, fresh cooked	2/3 cup

The following foods are high in sodium, potassium, or protein (indicated in parentheses) and should be avoided.

Artichoke (K)
Avocado (K)
Beans:
   Dry (K, protein)
   Lima (K, protein)
   Kidney (K, protein)
   Pork and beans (Na, K, protein)
   Soy (K, protein)
Lentils (K, protein)
Pickled vegetables (Na)
Potato, baked (K)
Sauerkraut (Na)
Split peas (K, protein)
Tomato puree (K)

Fruit Exchange Lists

List A. Low Potassium Content: Each exchange contains approximately 100 mg potassium, 15 mg phosphorus, and negligible protein and sodium.

Apple, fresh	1 small (2 1/2 in. diam)
Apple, fresh sliced	1 cup
Apple, dried	1/4 cup
Apple, frozen sliced	3/4 cup
Applesauce, fresh or canned	1/3 cup
Blackberries, fresh, canned, or frozen	1/2 cup
Blueberries, fresh, canned, or frozen	1 cup
Boysenberries, fresh, canned, or frozen	2/3 cup
Cherries, red sour, canned or frozen	1/3 cup

Cherries, sweet, canned or fresh	1/3 cup
Crabapple, fresh	1 small
Cranberry sauce	1 cup
Dates, fresh or dried	2 medium
Elderberries, fresh	1/4 cup
Fig, fresh or dried	1 medium
Figs, canned	2 medium
Gooseberries, fresh or canned	1/2 cup
Grapes, fresh	12 or 1/2 cup
Grapes, canned	1/3 cup
Lemon, fresh	1/2 medium
Lime, fresh	1/2 medium
Mandarin oranges, canned	1/2 cup
Mango, fresh	1/3 cup
Pears, canned	2 small halves
Pears, fresh sliced	1/2 cup
Persimmon (native)	1 medium
Pineapple, fresh (3 1/2 x 3/4 in.)	1 slice
Pineapple, fresh, canned, or frozen	1/2 cup
Plum, fresh	1 medium
Plums, canned	2 small
Raisins	1 tbsp
Raspberries (black or red), fresh, canned, or frozen	1/2 cup
Tangerine, fresh	1 small

List B. Moderate Potassium Content: Each exchange contains approximately 200 mg potassium, 20 mg phosphorus, and negligible protein and sodium.

Apricots, fresh	2 medium
Apricots, canned	3 halves
Apricots, dried	4 halves
Banana	1/2 small
Cantaloupe, cubed	1/2 cup
Cantaloupe (5 in. diam)	1/6 melon
Currants, fresh	1/3 cup
Fruit cocktail, fresh, frozen, or canned	1/2 cup
Grapefruit, fresh (4 in. diam)	1/2
Grapefruit sections, fresh or canned	1/2 cup
Honeydew, cubed	1/2 cup
Honeydew (5 in. diam)	1/4 melon
Mulberries, fresh	3/4 cup
Nectarine, fresh (2 1/2 in. diam)	1/2
Orange, fresh	1 small (2 in. diam)
Papaya, cubed	1/2 cup
Peaches, canned	2 halves
Peaches, sliced, canned, or frozen	2/3 cup
Peach, fresh	1 medium
Pear, fresh	1 medium
Pear, fresh sliced	1 cup
Persimmon, japanese (2 1/2 in. diam)	1/2
Pomegranate, fresh (3 1/2 in. diam)	1/2
Prunes	2 large or 3 medium
Rhubarb, fresh or frozen cooked	1/3 cup
Strawberries, fresh whole	3/4 cup or 10 large
Strawberries, canned or frozen	2/3 cup
Watermelon, cubed	1 cup
Watermelon wedge (5 in. diam, 1 in. thick)	1

Fruit Juice Exchange Lists

List A. Each exchange contains approximately 100 mg potassium, 15 mg phosphorus, and negligible protein and sodium.

Apple juice	1/3 cup
Awake imitation orange juice	1 1/3 cups
Cranapple juice	1/2 cup
Grape juice drink	1 1/4 cups
Grape juice, frozen and diluted	1 1/4 cups
Grape juice, bottled or canned	1/3 cup
Hawaiian punch	1 1/2 cups
Hi-C peach drink	1/3 cup
Hi-C strawberry drink	1/2 cup
Peach nectar	1/2 cup
Pear nectar	1 cup
Pineapple juice	1/3 cup
Tang[1], regular, all flavors	1 1/2 cups

List B. Each exchange contains approximately 200 mg potassium, 20 mg phosphorus, and negligible protein and sodium.

Apricot nectar	1/2 cup
Grapefruit juice	1/2 cup
Grapefruit-orange juice	1/2 cup
Hi-C fruit punch	1/2 cup
Orange juice	1/3 cup
Prune juice	1/3 cup

Other Beverages (containing potassium): Each exchange contains approximately 90 mg potassium, 5 mg phosphorus, and negligible protein and sodium.

Coffee, decaffeinated, instant	1 tsp powder
Coffee, instant	1 tsp powder
Tea, brewed	1 cup
Tea, instant	1 tsp powder
Poly Rich[2], nondairy creamer	1/2 cup
Gin, whiskey, rum	1 1/2 oz
Sherry, port tokay, aperitifs	3 oz
Apple or muscatel wine	1 1/2 oz
Table wine (burgundy, champagne, claret, Chianti, rosé, sauterne)	3 oz

---

[1]Limit on phosphorus restricted diet due to higher phosphorus content (1 1/2 cups Tang = 100 mg K and 42 mg P).

[2]Avoid on phosphorus restricted diet because of higher phosphorus content. (Poly Rich contains 43 mg per 4 oz.)

The following are high in potassium, sodium, or protein (indicated in parentheses) and should be avoided:

Flavored coffee (Na)
Gatorade (Na)
Instant hot cocoa and chocolate mixes (Na, protein, K)
Postum (K)
Kava (K)
Percolated and drip coffee (K)

Fat Exchange List: These foods increase calories without adding significant sodium, potassium, or phosphorus and should be used liberally to help maintain normal weight. Butter or margarine should be added to cooked cereals, breads, potatoes, and vegetables.

Low Sodium Content: These fats contain negligible amounts of protein, sodium, potassium, and phosphorus and may be used freely.

Butter or margarine, low sodium
Lard
Mayonnaise, very low sodium
Oil
Salad dressings, very low sodium, made without eggs or cheese
Vegetable shortening

Moderate Sodium Content: These fats contain 50 mg sodium and negligible amounts of protein, potassium, and phosphorus.

Butter or margarine, salted	1 tsp
Mayonnaise-type salad dressing	2 tsp
Mayonnaise	2 tsp
Sour cream[1]	2 tbsp

Avoid bacon drippings because of high sodium content.

Soup Exchange List

Each exchange is 1/2 cup and may be used within the fluid allowance. Soups are ready-to-serve or prepared according to package directions.

Bernard[2]

Dietetic chicken broth	1 serving/day (free)
Dietetic cream of celery	1 A vegetable
Dietetic cream of mushroom	1 B vegetable
Dietetic cream of potato soup mix	1 B vegetable
Dietetic cream of tomato	1 A vegetable
Dietetic vegetable beef	1 A vegetable

[1]Avoid on phosphorus restricted diet because of higher phosphorus content. (Cultured sour cream contains 20 mg per 2 tbsp.)

[2]Bernard Food Industries, Inc., P.O. Box 1497, Evanston, IL 60204.

Campbell[1]
  Low sodium chicken noodle   1/2 bread
  Low sodium cream of mushroom   1 A vegetable
  Low sodium green pea   2 bread
  Low sodium tomato   1 B vegetable
  Low sodium turkey noodle   1/2 bread
  Low sodium vegetable   1 A vegetable
  Low sodium vegetable beef   1 A vegetable

Featherweight[2]
  Low sodium chicken noodle   1 A vegetable
  Low sodium tomato   1 B vegetable
  Low sodium vegetable beef   1 B vegetable

Additional Foods List

The following foods are low in protein, sodium, potassium, and phosphorus and most add calories to the diet.

List A. Free (Any amount may be eaten each day.)

All purpose salad dressing, dietetic[3]	Jelly beans
Butterballs	Kool-Aid powder
Chewing gum	Light corn syrup
Cool Whip	Lollipops, unfilled
Cornstarch	Mints
Cotton candy	Popsicle (count as fluid)
Creme de menthe	Rich's Whip Topping
Dream Whip	Sugar, confectioners
Fondants	Sugar, granulated
French dressing, dietetic[3]	Tapioca, granulated
Gumdrops	Twist powdered soft drink mix
Italian dressing, low sodium[4]	

List B. Limit to 3 servings each day. One serving contains approximately 10 mg potassium.

Blue cheese style dressing, dietetic[5]	2 tbsp
Chili sauce, low sodium[4]	1 tsp
Coffee-mate	1/2 tsp
Cranberries, fresh	3 tbsp
Cranberry relish	3 tbsp
Cranberry sauce	3 tbsp
French dressing, low sodium[4]	1 tbsp

---

[1] Campbell Soup Company, Campbell Place, Camden, NJ 08101.

[2] Sandoz Nutrition, 5320 W. 23rd St., P.O. Box 370, Minneapolis, MN 55440.

[3] Bernard Food Industries, Inc., P.O. Box 1497, Evanston, IL 60204.

[4] Geoghegan's Dietetic, Low Calorie, and Special Diet Foods, Geoghegan Brothers Company, 8835 South Greenwood Ave., Chicago, IL 60619.

[5] William J. Elwood, Inc., 3 North Oak St., Copiague, NY 11726.

Honey	1 tbsp
Jam, jelly, marmalade	1 tbsp
Mayonnaise, low sodium[1,2]	2 tbsp
Mustard, low sodium[2,3,4]	1 tsp
Seafood cocktail sauce, low sodium[2]	1 tbsp
Soyamaise salad dressing[5]	1 tsp
Zero dressing[3]	2 tbsp
Zero style salad dressing[4]	2 tbsp

List C. Limit to one serving each day. One serving contains 30 to 100 mg potassium.

Barbecue sauce, low sodium[5]	1 tbsp
Brown sugar	2 tbsp
Catsup, low sodium[4,5]	1 tbsp
Chocolate syrup	2 tbsp
Creamy caesar salad dressing[5]	1 tbsp
Creamy cucumber salad dressing, low sodium[4]	1 tbsp
Creamy cucumber/onion salad dressing, low sodium[5]	1 tbsp
Coffee Rich	1/2 cup
French dressing, low sodium[3,5]	1 tbsp
French style dressing, low sodium[4]	1 tbsp
Herb salad dressing, low sodium[5]	1 tbsp
Maple syrup	2 tbsp
Pickle, low sodium[2,5]	1 oz
Red wine vinegar salad dressing, low sodium[4]	1 tbsp
Russian dressing, low sodium[2]	1 tbsp
2 Calorie Salad Dressing, low sodium[5]	1 tbsp

Free Juices and Beverages

These juices and beverages are very low in potassium and phosphorus and may be used as desired within the daily fluid allowance.

Cranberry juice cocktail
Hi-C fruit drinks:
    Apple
    Apple-cranberry
    Candy apple cooler
    Cherry
    Grape
    Lemonade
    Wildberry
Kool-Aid, all flavors
Lemonade, frozen and diluted

---

[1] Bernard Food Industries, Inc., P.O. Box 1497, Evanston, IL 60204.

[2] Geoghegan's Dietetic, Low Calorie, and Special Diet Foods, Geoghegan Brothers Company, 8835 South Greenwood Ave., Chicago, IL 60619.

[3] William J. Elwood, Inc., 3 North Oak St., Copiague, NY 11726.

[4] Estee Company, 169 Lackawanna Avenue, Parsippany, NJ 07054.

[5] Sandoz Nutrition, 5320 W. 23rd St., P.O. Box 370, Minneapolis, MN 55440.

Limeade, frozen and diluted
Minute Maid fruit punch
Twist (instant soft drink mix)

Soft Drinks

The kind of diet soda pop allowed depends on the levels of sodium, potassium, and phosphorus restriction. Soda pops in List A contain ≤ 2.9 mg Na, 1.67 mg K, and 1.0 mg P per oz, while those in List B contain more. The sodium and phosphorus content of the bottler's water supply is not included in the values reported. The amount of sodium and phosphorus varies depending on the water supply, season, and treatment. Special water treatment methods are used to produce beverages labeled "sodium free," containing 5 mg Na or less per 6 oz serving as per FDA regulations. Complete information was not available from all companies. Unless manufacturer's information or laboratory analyses indicate otherwise, soft drinks not listed should be avoided because of their higher sodium, potassium, or phosphorus content.

List A. These soft drinks may be used freely within the fluid allowance.

Barq's:
  Barq's Root Beer
Canada Dry:
  Barrelhead Root Beer
  Birch Beer
  Bitter Lemon
  Cactus Cooler
  California Strawberry
  Collins Mixer
  Concord Grape
  Golden Ginger Ale
  Half and Half
  Island Lime
  Pineapple
  Purple Passion
  Rooti
  Sunripe Orange
  Tahitian Treat
  Tonic Water
  Vanilla Cream
  Whiskey Sour
  Wild Cherry
  Wink
Coca-Cola:
  Fanta Ginger Ale
  Fanta Grape
  Fanta Orange
  Fanta Root Beer
  Mello Yello
  Ramblin' Root Beer
Pepsi-Cola:
  Mountain Dew
7-Up:
  7-Up, regular and diet
Shasta:
  Chocolate (NutraSweet-saccharin blend)
  Citrus Mist
  Creme
  Fruit Punch
  Ginger Ale (regular and NutraSweet-saccharin blend)
  Grape

Iced Tea
Orange
Tonic Water

List B. These soft drinks are limited to 1 12-oz serving per day due to their higher sodium, potassium, and/or phosphorus content.

A & W:
  A & W Root Beer, regular and very low sodium sugar-free
Canada Dry:
  Club Soda
  Diet Barrelhead Root Beer
  Diet Cola
  Diet Ginger Ale
  Diet Orange
  Diet Tonic Water
  Golden Ginger Ale
  Hi-spot
  Jamaica Cola
Canfield's (all are diet):
  Cherry-ola Cola
  Chocolate Fudge
  Cola
  50/50
  Ginger Ale
  Lemon Lime
  Orange
  Red Pop
  Root Beer
  Swiss Creme
  Club Soda Sparkling Water
  Quinine Tonic
  Seltzer
  Seltzer with lime
Coca-Cola:
  Cherry Coke
  Coca-Cola, regular and caffeine-free, diet, and caffeine-free diet Coke
  Fanta Diet Orange
  Fresca
  Mr. Pibb, regular and sugar-free
  Sprite, regular and diet
  Sugar-free Ramblin' Root Beer
  Tab, caffeine-free Tab
Dr. Pepper:
  Diet Dr. Pepper
  Dr. Pepper
  99% caffeine-free Dr. Pepper
  Sugar-free, Pepper-free Dr. Pepper
Pepsi-Cola:
  Diet Pepsi
  Diet Pepsi-Free
  Diet Slice
  Pepsi Cola
  Pepsi-Free
  Pepsi Light
  Slice
RC Cola:
  Cherry RC Cola

Diet Cherry RC
Diet Rite
Diet RC Cola, caffeine-free
RC Cola
7-Up:
Cherry 7-Up
Diet Cherry 7-Up
Like Cola, regular and diet
Shasta:
Birch Beer (NutraSweet-saccharin blend)
Black Cherry (regular, NutraSweet-saccharin blend)
Cherry Cola (regular, NutraSweet-saccharin blend)
Chocolate (100% NutraSweet)
Club Soda
Cola (regular, NutraSweet-saccharin blend, 100% NutraSweet)
Creme (NutraSweet-saccharin blend, 100% NutraSweet)
Dr. Diablo
Frolic (NutraSweet-saccharin blend)
Ginger Ale (100% NutraSweet)
Grape (NutraSweet-saccharin blend)
Grapefruit (NutraSweet-saccharin blend, 100% NutraSweet)
Lemonade
Lemon-lime (regular, NutraSweet-saccharin blend, 100% NutraSweet)
Orange (NutraSweet-saccharin blend, 100% NutraSweet)
Red Pop (regular, NutraSweet-saccharin blend)
Root Beer (regular, NutraSweet-saccharin blend, 100% NutraSweet)
Shasta-free Cola (regular, NutraSweet-saccharin blend)
Strawberry (regular, NutraSweet-saccharin blend)
Welch's:
Root Beer
Sparkling Apple
Sparkling Grape
Sparkling Orange
Sparkling Strawberry

D. RENAL DIABETIC DIET

DESCRIPTION: Renal failure is a common long-term complication of diabetes mellitus, especially in insulin-dependent patients. The purpose of the renal diabetic diet is to minimize complications associated with the metabolic changes of chronic kidney disease, as well as to control serum glucose and lipid levels. This diet incorporates the principles of the diabetic (see pages 141-44) and renal (see pages 78-80) diets. The guide on page 80 can be used for diabetic and nondiabetic patients, since their nutritional requirements are similar.

The distribution of calories in the usual diabetic diet is 55 to 60% from carbohydrate, 20 to 30% from fat, and 10 to 25% from protein. In the Renal Diabetic Diet, the percentage of calories from protein will be less, necessitating a higher proportion from carbohydrate and/or fat. Because of the increased risk of cardiovascular disease due to diabetes and renal failure, it is generally recommended that fat not exceed 40% of the calories. Most of the fat should be in the form of polyunsaturated fatty acids. When the protein is severely restricted, some carbohydrate may need to be supplied in the form of simple sugars. This form of dietary carbohydrate rarely presents problems with blood glucose regulation.

Diabetes control is typically more difficult in renal failure. The amount, type, and timing of food intake and insulin must be very carefully regulated to provide adequate nutrition without wide fluctuations in blood glucose levels. Although insulin requirements are often reduced as patients become progressively uremic, more insulin is often needed after starting dialysis.

Dietary compliance is difficult due to multiple restrictions. Making the diet as liberal and individualized as possible within necessary modifications is important for achieving optimal nutritional status. When a renal diabetic diet is ordered, the dietitian will develop a pattern using the renal diabetic exchange lists. The foods are categorized according to their composition of carbohydrate, protein, fat, calories, sodium, phosphorus, and potassium (see page 100). Because the composition of manufactured products is subject to change, labels and company literature should be checked periodically.

ADEQUACY: The adequacy of the diet depends on the number and severity of the restrictions. Diets restricted to less than 50 g protein or 50 mEq potassium typically do not meet the Recommended Dietary Allowances for calcium, iron, niacin, riboflavin, thiamin, folic acid, and vitamins B_6, B_{12}, C, and D. Routine supplementation of these nutrients is advised, not only because of inadequate levels provided in the restricted diet and the altered metabolic utilization of nutrients, but also because water soluble nutrients are partially removed by dialysis.

PROTEIN, SODIUM, POTASSIUM, PHOSPHORUS, CARBOHYDRATE, FAT, CALORIES, AND FLUID VALUES FOR RENAL DIABETIC EXCHANGES
(average figures)

Food Group	Calories (kcal)	Protein (g)	Fat (g)	Carbohydrate (g)	Sodium (mg)	Potassium (mg)	Phosphorus (mg)	Fluids (cc or ml)
Meat and Meat Substitutes								15
Low sodium	60	8	3	--	25	130	70	
Moderate sodium	60	8	3	--	75	130	70	
High sodium	60	8	3	--	300	130	70	
Very high sodium	60	8	3	--	600	130	70	
Dairy Products	85	4	5	6	60	170	120	120
Bread and Bread Substitutes								5-100
Low sodium	70	2	--	15	10	50	40	
Moderate sodium	70	2	--	15	150	50	40	
Vegetables								90
Low potassium	--	--	--	--	trace	50	5	
Group A - low carbohydrate	25	1	--	5	10/200	100	30	
Group A - high carbohydrate	70	1	--	15	10/200	100	30	
Group B - low carbohydrate	25	2	--	5	15/250	200	50	
Group B - high carbohydrate	70	2	--	25	15/250	200	50	
Fruits								80
Group A - low carbohydrate	40	--	--	10	--	100	15	
Group A - high carbohydrate	80	--	--	20	--	100	15	
Group B - low carbohydrate	40	--	--	10	--	200	20	
Group B - high carbohydrate	80	--	--	20	--	200	20	
Fruit Juices								Varies with amount
Low potassium	40	--	--	10	--	20	10	
Group A	40	--	--	10	--	100	15	
Group B	40	--	--	10	--	200	20	
Fats								1
Low sodium	45	--	5	--	0	--	trace	
Moderate sodium	45	--	5	--	50	--	trace	
Other Potassium-containing Beverages	--	--	--	--	--	90	5	Varies with amount

SAMPLE PROCEDURE FOR CALCULATING A RENAL DIABETIC DIET:

Diet Prescription

Calories	2000 kcal
Protein	60 g
Potassium	60 mEq
Sodium	43 mEq
Phosphorus	65 mEq
Fluid	1000 ml

1. Convert the milliequivalents of K, Na, and P in the prescription to milligrams (multiply the number of milliequivalents by the atomic weight ÷ valence, see page 36).

2. Determine the amount of protein of high biological value the patient should have, between 50 and 75% of the amount prescribed. (The lower the protein restriction, the higher the percentage of high biological value protein.)

3. Divide the high biological value protein between dairy exchanges and meat and meat substitute exchanges.

4. Divide the remaining protein between bread exchanges and vegetable exchanges.

5. Total the amount of carbohydrate and fat used in these exchanges and calculate the amount of calories supplied. Subtract this amount from the total number of calories prescribed to determine the calories remaining for fruit, juice, and fat exchanges.

6. Total the amount of potassium in the dairy, meat, bread, and vegetable exchanges. Subtract this from the total potassium allowed.

7. Divide the remaining potassium among the fruits, juices, and other beverages. Adjust calories with low and high carbohydrate fruit. (Vegetables may also be adjusted to low and high carbohydrate lists.)

8. Total the carbohydrate and calculate calories supplied. Subtract this amount from the total number of calories supplied to determine the calories remaining for fat and low protein products.

9. Divide remaining calories between fats and low protein products.

10. Calculate the sodium level.

11. Calculate the phosphorus level.

12. Calculate the fluid level in ml or cc.

13. Distribute the exchanges among meals and snacks.

Example	Amount	CHO (g)	Protein (g)	Fat (g)	K (mg)
Step 1: 60 mEq K x 39 = 2340 mg K					
43 mEq Na x 23 = 989 mg Na					
65 mEq P x (31 ÷ 2) = 1008 mg P					
Step 2: Protein, 60 g x 50% = 30 g					
60 g x 75% = 45 g					
30-45 g high biological value protein					
Step 3: Dairy product exchanges	1	6	4	4	170
Meat and meat substitute exchanges	4	--	32	12	520
Total protein from dairy and meat exchanges			36 g		
Step 4: 60 g protein in prescription					
-36 g protein from dairy and meat					
24 g protein remaining for bread and vegetables					
Bread exchanges	10	150	20	--	500
Vegetable exchanges					
List A, Low carbohydrate	2	10	2	--	200
List B, High carbohydrate	1	15	2	--	200
			60 g		
Step 5: Total amount of carbohydrate and fat		181 g		16 g	

Total calories - carbohydrate 181 x 4 = 724 kcal
protein   60 x 4 = 240 kcal
fat   16 x 9 = 144 kcal
Total   1108 kcal

2000 kcal in diet prescription
-1108 kcal from dairy, meat, bread, and vegetables
 892 kcal remaining for fruit, fruit juice, and fat exchanges

| Step 6: Total amount of potassium in dairy, meat, bread, and vegetable exchanges | | | | | 1590 mg |

2340 mg potassium in prescription
-1590 mg from dairy, meat, bread and vegetables
 750 mg potassium remaining for fruit and beverages

Step 7: Fruit exchanges					
List A, High carbohydrate	2	40	--	--	200
List B, High carbohydrate	2	40	--	--	400
Fruit juice exchanges					
Low potassium	2	20	--	--	40
Other beverages	1	--	--	--	90
Total potassium					2320 mg

Example (continued):	Amount	CHO (g)	Protein (g)	Fat (g)	K (mg)
Step 8: Total carbohydrate	281 g				

Total calories - carbohydrate 281 x 4 = 1124 kcal
                 protein   60 x 4 = 240 kcal
                 fat   16 x 9 = 144 kcal
                 Total   1508 kcal
       2000 kcal in diet prescription
      -1508 kcal from all exchanges except fat and low protein products
       492 kcal remaining

Step 9: 492 kcal ÷ 9 = 55 g fat

55 ÷ 5 = 11 fat exchanges					
Fat exchanges	11	--	--	55	--
No low protein products needed					

Summary:

Total carbohydrate, protein, fat		281 g	60 g	71 g	

Total calories - carbohydrate 281 x 4 = 1124 kcal
                 protein   60 x 4 = 240 kcal
                 fat   71 x 9 = 639 kcal
                                      2003 kcal

Step 10: Calculate the sodium (average figures, see page 100)

Sodium from 1 egg	75 mg
Sodium from 3 oz meat, low sodium	75 mg
Sodium from 1/2 cup milk	60 mg
Sodium from 6 low sodium breads	60 mg
and 4 regular breads	600 mg
Sodium from 3 unsalted vegetables	35 mg
Sodium from 2 tsp regular (salted) butter or margarine	100 mg
Total sodium	1005 mg

Step 11: Calculate the phosphorus (average figures, see page 100)

Phosphorus from 4 meats	280 mg
Phosphorus from 1/2 cup milk	120 mg
Phosphorus from 10 breads	400 mg
Phosphorus from 2 "A" vegetables	60 mg
Phosphorus from 1 "B" vegetable	50 mg
Phosphorus from 2 "A" fruits	30 mg
Phosphorus from 2 "B" fruits	40 mg
Phosphorus from 2 "Low Potassium" juices	20 mg
Phosphorus from 1 "other" beverage	5 mg
Total phosphorus	1005 mg

Example (continued):

Step 12: Calculate the fluid

1/2 cup milk	120 ml
3/4 cup cranberry juice, unsweetened	180 ml
1/3 cup Hi-C drink	80 ml
1 cup instant coffee	240 ml
1 cup lemonade, unsweetened	240 ml
1/2 cup Kool-Aid, unsweetened	120 ml
	980 ml (or cc)

Step 13: Distribute the exchanges among meals and snacks.

Exchange	Breakfast	AM Snack	Lunch	PM Snack	Dinner	HS Snack
Meat	1	--	1	--	1	1
Dairy	1	--	--	--	--	--
Bread						
Low sodium	2	--	2	--	2	--
Moderate sodium	--	1	--	1	--	2
Vegetables, low sodium						
A, low carbohydrate	--	--	1	--	1	--
B, high carbohydrate	--	--	--	--	1	--
Fruits						
A, low carbohydrate	--	1	--	1	--	--
B, high carbohydrate	--	--	1	--	1	--
Fruit juice						
Low potassium	1	--	--	--	--	1
Fats						
Low sodium	--	--	3	--	4	2
Moderate sodium	2	--	--	--	--	--
Other beverage	1	--	--	--	--	--

APPROXIMATE COMPOSITION OF SAMPLE MENU:

Calories	2116
Protein, g	59
Fat, g	74
Carbohydrate, g	284
Sodium, mg	1330
Potassium, mg	2012
Phosphorus, mg	805

SAMPLE MENU FOR A RENAL DIABETIC DIET (2000 calories, 60 g protein, 60 mEq (2340 mg) potassium, 43 mEq (989 mg) sodium, 65 mEq (1008 mg) phosphorus, and 1000 ml fluid):

Breakfast

3/4 cup cranberry juice, unsweetened
1 egg, soft cooked
2 slices toast, white enriched, unsalted
2 tsp margarine (regular)
1/2 cup whole milk
Artificial sweetener
1 cup instant coffee

Luncheon

1 oz (30 g) sliced chicken, unsalted
1/2 cup rice, unsalted
1/2 cup green beans, unsalted
1 slice bread, white enriched, unsalted
2 halves sweetened canned peaches, drained
3 tsp margarine, unsalted
1/2 cup Kool-Aid, artificially sweetened

Dinner

1 oz (30 g) roast beef, unsalted
1/3 cup cubed white potato, unsalted
1/3 cup carrots, unsalted
1/2 cup sweetened canned fruit cocktail, drained
1/2 cup lettuce salad
2 tbsp low sodium french dressing
2 slices bread, white enriched, unsalted
2 tsp margarine, unsalted
1/2 cup lemonade, artificially sweetened

Midmorning Nourishment

1/2 cup sweetened applesauce
2 graham crackers

Midafternoon Nourishment

6 vanilla wafers
1/3 cup sweetened canned cherries, drained
1/2 cup lemonade, artificially sweetened

Evening Nourishment

Sandwich:
2 slices bread, white enriched (regular)
1 oz (30 g) turkey, unsalted
2 tsp margarine, unsalted
1/3 cup Hi-C grape drink

FOOD EXCHANGES FOR RENAL DIABETIC DIETS:

<u>Meat and Meat Substitute Exchange List</u>: Each exchange contains approximately 8 g protein, 3 g fat, 130 mg potassium, 70 mg phosphorus, and 60 calories. Because the sodium content varies, the type of food allowed will depend on the patient's restriction. Portion sizes of meat, poultry, and fish refer to cooked weights without bone.

Low Sodium Content: Each exchange contains approximately 25 mg sodium.

Cheese[1], low sodium	1 oz (30 g)
Cottage cheese, low sodium	1/4 cup
Crab, fish, lobster, scallops, shrimp	1 oz (30 g)
Meat	
Beef, fresh unprocessed ham (not cured), lamb, liver[1], pork, poultry, wild game	1 oz (30 g)
Peanut butter[1,2], low sodium	2 tbsp
Tuna or salmon, low sodium, water-pack	1/4 cup

Moderate Sodium Content: Each exchange contains approximately 75 mg sodium.

Cottage cheese, regular, creamed[1,3]	1/4 cup
Egg, large[1]	1
Oysters	1 oz (30 g)

High Sodium Content: Each exchange contains approximately 300 mg sodium.

Canadian bacon	1 oz (30 g)
Cheese[1], natural (cheddar, parmesan)	1 oz (30 g)
Corned beef	1 oz (30 g)
Ham, processed (cured)	1 oz (30 g)
Luncheon meat	1 oz (30 g)
Meat or fish, canned with salt	1 oz (30 g)
Peanut butter[1,2], regular	2 tbsp
Pork link sausages	1 1/2 links (30 g)
Pork sausage	1 oz (30 g)

Very High Sodium Content: Each exchange contains approximately 600 mg sodium.

Bacon	4 slices (30 g)
Frankfurter	1 oz (30 g)

The following are high in sodium and should be avoided:

Chipped beef
Smoked fish, meat, or poultry

---

[1]Limit on phosphorus restricted diet because of higher phosphorus content. Egg yolk is high in phosphorus, but egg whites are low and may be used (egg yolk = 85 mg phosphorus, egg white = 5 phosphorus).

[2]Use only occasionally because of higher potassium content.

[3]Use only occasionally because of higher sodium content.

Dairy Products Exchange List: Each exchange contains approximately: 4 g protein, 5 g fat, 6 g carbohydrate, 60 mg sodium, 170 mg potassium, 120 mg phosphorus, and 85 calories.

Milk
  Evaporated, skim (add 1
    fat exchange) . . . . 1/4 cup
  Evaporated, whole . . . . 1/4 cup
  Instant nonfat dry milk
    (add 1 fat exchange) . . . . 2 1/2 tbsp
  Skim (add 1 fat exchange) . . . . 1/2 cup
  2% (add 1/2 fat exchange) . . . . 1/2 cup
  Whole . . . . 1/2 cup

Cream
  Half-and-half (omit 2
    fat exchanges) . . . . 1/2 cup

Desserts
  Custard, made with whole milk,
    artificially sweetened . . . . 1/4 cup
  D-Zerta pudding, made with
    whole milk . . . . 1/4 cup
  Ice cream, any flavor
    (no nuts or fruit) . . . . 1/2 cup
    (omit 1 low potassium fruit
    juice plus 1 fat exchange)

The following are high in sodium, potassium, or sucrose (indicated in parentheses) and should be avoided.

  Buttermilk (Na)
  Chocolate milk (CHO)
  Fruit flavored yogurt (CHO and K)
  Low sodium milk (K)
  Sweetened condensed milk (CHO)

Bread Exchange List: Each exchange contains approximately 2 g protein, 15 g carbohydrate, 50 mg potassium, 40 mg phosphorus, and 70 calories. Because sodium content varies, the type of food allowed, low sodium or regular, will depend on the patient's restriction.

Low Sodium Content: Each serving contains approximately 10 mg sodium.

Breads and Crackers
  Bread, low sodium . . . . 1 slice
  Crackers, low sodium . . . . 6 squares
  Melba toast, low sodium . . . . 4 slices
  Oyster crackers, low sodium 20
  Pretzels, low sodium 4
  Rice wafers 10
  Rusk 1
  Tortilla, plain or corn 1

Cereals, cooked	
(prepared without salt)	
Cream of Rice, Cream of	
Wheat, cornmeal, farina,	
hominy grits, Malt-O-Meal,	
oatmeal[1], rolled wheat[1]	1/2 cup
Cereals, dry	
(processed without salt)	
Puffed rice, puffed wheat,	
Puffa Puffa Rice, low sodium	
cornflakes, low sodium	
toasted rice	3/4 cup
Shredded wheat, biscuit	1 large
Desserts	
Marshmallows	3 large
Pie crust, single	
made without salt	1/8 of 9 in.
(omit 1 fat)	crust
Sherbet	1/4 cup
Grains	
Cornmeal, dry	2 1/2 tbsp
Flour	2 1/2 tbsp
Masa harina, uncooked	3 tbsp
Pearl barley, cooked	1/3 cup
Pasta and Rice	
(cooked without salt)	
Egg noodles, cooked	1/3 cup
Macaroni, cooked	1/2 cup
Rice, white, cooked	1/2 cup
Spaghetti, cooked	1/2 cup
Miscellaneous	
Popcorn, unsalted	
(average kernel)	1 1/2 cups
	popped

The following are high in sodium, potassium, or protein (indicated in parentheses) and should be avoided:

Bakery items containing low sodium baking powder (K)
Bran cereals (K)
Breads, crackers, and cereals of moderate sodium content (Na)
Cereals processed with fruit or nuts (K and protein)
High protein or protein fortified cereals (protein)
Instant cereals (Na)
Wheat germ (K and protein)

Moderate Sodium Content: Each serving contains approximately 150 mg sodium.

Breads and Crackers	1/2
Bagel, medium	1/2
Baking powder biscuit (2 in. diameter)	
(omit 1 fat exchange)	1
Bread, regular white, vienna, french, rye,	
italian, whole wheat, raisin	1 slice
Cornbread[1] (1 1/2 in. cube) (omit 1 fat exchange)	1

---

[1]Limit on phosphorus restricted diet because of higher phosphorus content.

Crackers with unsalted tops	6 squares
Dinner roll (2 in. diameter)	1
English muffin, medium	1/2
Graham crackers	2 squares
Hotdog or hamburger bun	1/2 (8 per pkg); or 1 (12 per pkg)
Muffin[1], plain, homemade (3 x 2 x 1 1/2 in.) (omit 1 fat exchange)	1
Pancake[1] (3 in. diameter) (omit 1 fat exchange)	1
Zwieback	2 pieces

Cereals, cooked
(lightly salted in preparation)

Cream of Rice, Cream of Wheat, cornmeal, farina, hominy grits, Malt-O-Meal, oatmeal[1], rolled wheat[1]	1/2 cup

Cereals, dry
(processed with salt, without sugar,
 fruits, or nuts)

Cornflakes, Rice Krispies, Product 19, Cheerios[1], Kix, Rice Chex	3/4 cup

Desserts

Angel food cake (unfrosted) (1 1/2 in. cube or 1/12 of 10-in. cake)	1 slice
Animal crackers	8
Arrowroot cookies	3
Cake, plain (2 x 2 x 2 in.) (omit 2 regular fat exchanges)	1 slice
Doughnut, plain, cake or yeast (3 in. diam) (omit 1 fat exchange)	1 or 1 oz
Gelatin, regular sweetened	1/3 cup
Marshmallows	3 large
Pie crust, single (made with salt) (omit 1 fat exchange)	1/8 of 9 in. crust
Sherbet	1/4 cup
Sponge cake	1 1/2 in. wedge
Vanilla wafers	6

The following are high in sodium, potassium, protein or carbohydrate (indicated in parentheses) and should be avoided:

Cereals containing fruit, nuts, or sugars (CHO, K, and protein)
High protein or protein-fortified cereals such as Life, Post Oat Flakes,
   Quaker Wheat Flakes (protein)
Pumpernickel bread (K)
Wheaties (Na)

---

[1]Limit on phosphorus restricted diet because of higher phosphorus content.

Vegetable Exchange Lists

Very Low Potassium Content: The following vegetables contain 50 mg potassium, 5 mg phosphorus, and negligible amounts of carbohydrate, sodium, and protein. One serving from this group may be used each day in addition to the other servings of vegetables.

Chicory, fresh	1/4 cup
Cabbage, chinese	1/4 cup
Chives, fresh chopped	2 tbsp
Cucumber, fresh pared	1/4 medium
Escarole, fresh	1/4 cup
Green pepper	1/4 medium
Lettuce, chopped	1/2 cup
Lettuce, leaf (5 x 5 in.)	1 leaf
Onion, fresh chopped	3 tbsp
Parsley, fresh chopped	1 tbsp
Parsley, sprig	1 large
Radish, fresh	1
Watercress	5 sprigs

List A. Each exchange of high or low carbohydrate vegetable contains approximately 1 g protein, 100 mg potassium, 30 mg phosphorus, and 10 mg sodium for fresh, frozen, or low sodium canned and 200 mg sodium for regular canned. The starred items are naturally higher in sodium, averaging 35 mg per serving. List A low carbohydrate vegetables contain approximately 5 g carbohydrate and 25 calories. List A high carbohydrate vegetables contain approximately 15 g carbohydrate and 70 calories.

List A. Low Carbohydrate Content:

Bean sprouts, fresh or fresh cooked	1/2 cup
Beets*, fresh cooked or canned	1/3 cup
Cabbage, fresh or fresh cooked	1/2 cup
Carrots*, canned	1/2 cup
Carrots*, fresh (1/4 x 3 in.)	6-8 sticks
Carrots*, fresh or frozen cooked	1/3 cup
Cauliflower, fresh, fresh or frozen cooked	1/3 cup
Celery*, fresh (6 x 1/2 in.)	1 stalk
Celery*, fresh chopped or cooked	1/4 cup
Cucumber	1/2 medium or 1/2 cup
Eggplant, fresh or fresh cooked	1/3 cup
Endive	2/3 cup
Escarole	1/2 cup
Green beans, fresh, frozen, or canned	1/2 cup
Green pepper	1/2 medium
Green pepper, chopped	1/3 cup
Kale, fresh or frozen cooked	1/3 cup
Lettuce, chopped	2/3 cup
Mixed vegetables*, frozen cooked	1/3 cup
Okra, fresh or frozen cooked	1/3 cup or 5 pods
Onions, fresh	1/3 cup
Onions, fresh cooked	1/2 cup
Onions, green (5 x 1/2 in.)	2
Parsley, fresh chopped	4 tbsp
Peas, canned, fresh or frozen cooked	1/4 cup
Radishes (1 in. diam)	3
Rutabaga, fresh or cooked	1/3 cup
Summer squash, fresh or frozen cooked	1/3 cup
Watercress	10 sprigs
Watercress, chopped	1/3 cup

| Wax beans, fresh, frozen, or canned | 1/2 cup |
| Zucchini, fresh or frozen cooked | 1/3 cup |

List A. High Carbohydrate Content:

| Corn-on-the-cob (4 x 2 in.) | 1 ear |
| Corn, fresh or frozen cooked, whole kernel or cream style canned | 1/3 cup |

List B. Each exchange of high or low carbohydrate vegetable contains approximately 2 g protein, 200 mg potassium, 50 mg phosphorus, and 15 mg sodium for fresh, frozen, or low sodium canned and 250 mg sodium for regular canned. The starred items are naturally higher in sodium, averaging 35 mg per serving. List B low carbohydrate vegetables contain approximately 5 g carbohydrate and 25 calories. List B high carbohydrate vegetables contain approximately 15 g carbohydrate and 70 calories.

List B. Low Carbohydrate Content:

Asparagus, fresh or fresh cooked	2/3 cup
Asparagus, canned or cooked	1/2 cup
Beet greens*, fresh or cooked	1/2 cup
Broccoli, fresh, fresh or frozen cooked	3 in. stalk
Broccoli, chopped, fresh or frozen cooked	1/2 cup
Brussels sprouts, fresh or frozen cooked	1/2 cup
Chard, swiss, fresh cooked	1/3 cup
Collards, fresh, fresh or frozen cooked	1/2 cup
Cress, garden	1/2 cup
Dandelion greens, fresh or cooked	1/2 cup
Kohlrabi, fresh	1/3 cup
Kohlrabi, cooked	1/2 cup
Mushrooms, fresh	2/3 cup
Mushrooms, canned	1/2 cup
Mustard greens, fresh	2/3 cup
Mustard greens, cooked	1/2 cup
Spinach*, fresh, chopped	2/3 cup
Spinach*, fresh cooked or canned	1/3 cup
Spinach*, frozen cooked	1/4 cup
Tomato, fresh	1/2 medium
Tomatoes, fresh cooked	1/4 cup
Tomatoes, canned	1/3 cup
Tomato juice or vegetable juice cocktail	1/3 cup
Turnips, fresh or mashed	1/2 cup
Turnips, cooked	2/3 cup
Turnips, mashed	1/2 cup
Turnip greens, canned	1/3 cup
Turnip greens, fresh cooked	2/3 cup

List B. High Carbohydrate Content:

Parsnips, fresh cooked	1/3 cup
Parsnips, mashed	1/4 cup
Potatoes, boiled without skin or mashed	1/3 cup
Potatoes, french fried (3 1/2 in. long) (omit 1 fat)	5 strips
Pumpkin, canned	1/3 cup
Squash, winter	1/3 cup
Sweet potato, baked	1/2 small
Sweet potatoes, mashed	1/4 cup
Sweet potatoes, canned	1/3 cup

The following are high in sodium, potassium, or protein (indicated in parentheses) and should be avoided.

Artichoke (K)
Avocado (K)
Beans:
   Dry (K, protein)
   Lima (K, protein)
   Kidney (K, protein)
   Pork and beans (Na, K, protein)
   Soy (K, protein)
Lentils (K, protein)
Pickled vegetables (Na)
Potato, baked (K)
Sauerkraut (Na)
Split peas (K, protein)
Tomato puree (K)

Fruit Exchange Lists

List A. Low Carbohydrate, Low Potassium Content: Each exchange contains approximately 100 mg potassium, 15 mg phosphorus, 10 g carbohydrate, and 40 calories for fruits that are fresh, frozen, or canned without sugar.

Apple, fresh (2 1/2 in. diam)	1 small
Apple, fresh sliced	1 cup
Apple, dried	1/4 cup
Applesauce	1/2 cup
Blackberries	1/2 cup
Blueberries	1/2 cup
Boysenberries	1/2 cup
Cherries, red sour	1/3 cup
Cherries, sweet	1/3 cup
Crabapple, fresh	1 small
Dates, fresh or dried	2 medium
Fig, fresh or dried	1 medium
Figs, canned	2 medium
Grapes, fresh	12 or 1/2 cup
Grapes, canned	1/3 cup
Mandarin oranges, canned	1/2 cup
Mango, fresh	1/3 cup
Pears, canned	2 small halves
Persimmon (native)	1 medium
Pineapple, fresh, canned, or frozen	1/2 cup
Plum, fresh	1 medium
Plums, canned	2 small
Raisins	1 tbsp
Raspberries (black or red), fresh or frozen	1/2 cup
Raspberries, canned	1/3 cup
Tangerine, fresh	1 medium

List A. High Carbohydrate, Low Potassium Content: Each exchange contains approximately 100 mg potassium, 15 mg phosphorus, 20 g carbohydrate, and 80 calories for fruits that are frozen or canned with sugar added.

Apple, frozen, sliced	1/3 cup
Applesauce	1/3 cup
Blackberries, canned or frozen	1/2 cup
Blueberries, canned or frozen	1/3 cup
Boysenberries, canned or frozen	2/3 cup
Cherries, red sour, canned or frozen	1/3 cup

Cherries, sweet, canned	1/3 cup
Figs, canned	2 medium
Grapes, canned	1/3 cup
Pears, canned	2 small halves
Pineapple, canned	1/2 cup
Pineapple, frozen	1/3 cup
Plums, canned	2 small
Raspberries (black or red), frozen	1/2 cup
Raspberries, canned	1/3 cup
Rhubarb, cooked, sweetened	1/4 cup

List B. Low Carbohydrate, High Potassium Content: Each exchange contains approximately 200 mg potassium, 20 mg phosphorus, 10 g carbohydrate, and 40 calories for fruits that are fresh, frozen, or canned without sugar.

Apricots, fresh	2 medium
Apricots, canned	3 halves
Apricots, dried	4 halves
Banana	1/2 small
Cantaloupe, cubed	1/2 cup
Cantaloupe, (5 in. diam)	1/6 melon
Currants, fresh	2/3 cup
Elderberries, raw	1/2 cup
Fruit cocktail, fresh, frozen, or canned	1/2 cup
Gooseberries, fresh or canned	3/4 cup
Grapefruit, fresh (4 in. diam)	1/2
Grapefruit, fresh, sections	1/2 cup
Grapefruit, canned, water-pack	1/2 cup
Honeydew melon, cubed	1/2 cup
Honeydew (5 in. diam)	1/4 melon
Mulberries, fresh	1/2 cup
Nectarine, fresh (2 1/2 in. diam)	1/2
Orange, fresh (2 in. diam)	1 small
Papaya, cubed	1/2 cup
Peach, fresh (2 1/2 in. diam)	1
Peaches, canned	2 small halves
Peaches, fresh sliced	1/2 cup
Pear, fresh (2 1/2 in. diam)	1
Pears, fresh sliced	1 cup
Pomegranate, fresh (3 1/2 in. diam)	1/2
Prunes	2 large
Strawberries, fresh whole	3/4 cup or 10 large
Watermelon, cubed	1 cup
Watermelon wedge (5 in. diam, 1 in. thick)	1

List B. High Carbohydrate: Each exchange contains approximately 200 mg potassium, 20 mg phosphorus, 20 g carbohydrate, and 80 calories for fruits that are frozen or canned with sugar added.

Apricots, canned	3 halves
Fruit cocktail, canned	1/2 cup
Grapefruit, canned	1/2 cup
Melon balls, frozen (honeydew, cantaloupe)	1/2 cup
Peaches, halves, canned	2 small
Peaches, sliced, canned	1/2 cup
Persimmon, japanese (2 1/2 in. diam)	1/2
Prunes, dried	3 large or 4 medium
Prunes, cooked, unsweetened	1/4 cup
Strawberries, frozen	1/3 cup

Fruit Juice Exchange List

Low Potassium Content: Each exchange contains approximately 20 mg potassium, 10 mg phosphorus, 10 g carbohydrate, and 40 calories.

Awake imitation orange juice	1/3 cup
Cranberry juice cocktail, sweetened	1/4 cup
Cranberry juice cocktail, unsweetened	3/4 cup
Grape drink	1/4 cup
Hawaiian punch	1/3 cup
Hi-C fruit drinks:	1/3 cup
Apple	
Apple-cranberry	
Candy apple cooler	
Cherry	
Grape	
Lemonade	
Wildberry	
Kool-Aid, sweetened	1/3 cup
Lemonade, sweetened	1/3 cup
Limeade, sweetened	1/3 cup
Tang, regular, all flavors[1]	1/3 cup

List A. Each exchange contains approximately 100 mg potassium, 15 mg phosphorus, 10 g carbohydrate, and 40 calories.

Apple juice	1/3 cup
Apricot nectar	1/3 cup
Cranapple juice	1/3 cup
Grape juice	1/4 cup
Hi-C peach or strawberry drink	1/3 cup
Orange-apricot juice	1/3 cup
Peach nectar	1/3 cup
Pear nectar	1/3 cup
Pineapple juice	1/3 cup
Pineapple-orange juice	1/3 cup
Pineapple-grapefruit juice	1/3 cup

List B. Each exchange contains approximately 200 mg potassium, 20 mg phosphorus, 10 g carbohydrate, and 40 calories.

Grapefruit juice	1/2 cup
Grapefruit-orange juice	1/2 cup
Hi-C fruit drinks:	1/3 cup
Citrus cooler	
Fruit punch	
Hula cooler	
Orange	
Orange juice	1/3 cup
Prune juice	1/3 cup

---

[1]Limit on phosphorus restricted diet due to higher phosphorus content.

<u>Other Beverages</u> (containing potassium)

Each exchange contains approximately 90 mg potassium and 5 mg phosphorus.

Coffee, decaffeinated, instant	1 tsp powder
Coffee, instant	1 tsp powder
Tea, instant	1 tsp powder
Tea, brewed	1 cup

The following are high in potassium, sodium, or protein (indicated in parentheses) and should be avoided.

Coffee, flavored (Na)
Coffee, percolated and drip (K)
Gatorade (Na)
Instant hot cocoa and chocolate mixes (Na, K, protein)
Kava (K)
Postum (K)

<u>Fat Exchange List</u>

These foods contribute calories to the diet without adding significant protein, sodium, potassium, or phosphorus. Butter or margarine can be added to cooked cereals, breads, potatoes, or vegetables.

Low Sodium Content: Each exchange contains 5 g fat, 45 calories, and negligible amounts of protein, sodium, potassium, and phosphorus.

Butter or margarine, low sodium	1 tsp
French dressing, low sodium	1 tbsp
Lard	1 tsp
Mayonnaise, low sodium	1 tsp
Oil	1 tsp
Salad dressings, low sodium, made without eggs or cheese	1 tsp
Vegetable shortening	1 tsp

Moderate Sodium Content: Each exchange contains 5 g fat, 45 calories, 50 mg sodium, and negligible amounts of protein, sodium, potassium, and phosphorus.

Butter or margarine, salted	1 tsp
French dressing, regular	1 tbsp
Mayonnaise-salad dressing type	2 tsp
Mayonnaise	1 tsp
Sour cream[1]	2 tbsp

---

[1]Avoid on phosphorus restricted diet because of higher phosphorous content. Cultured sour cream contains 20 mg per 2 tbsp.

Low Protein Exchange List

Each exchange contains approximately 15 g carbohydrate, 2 g fat, 15 mg sodium, 10 mg potassium, 7 mg phosphorus, and 80 calories.

Low protein bread[1]	1 slice, 23 g
Low protein butter cookie[2] (omit 1 fat exchange)	1
Low protein frosted orange cookie[2]	1
Low protein ice cream[3] (omit 1 fat exchange)	1/2 cup

The following products[4] can also be included in the amounts indicated:

Low protein anellini[5] (ring macaroni), cooked	1/3 cup, 75 g
Low protein bread, ready-to-serve	1 slice, 30 g
Low protein porridge (semolina), cooked	1/2 cup, 100 g
Low protein rigatini (ribbed macaroni), cooked	1/2 cup, 65 g
Low protein rusk	2 slices, 20 g
Low protein tagliatelle (flat, long noodle), cooked	1/3 cup, 80 g

Soup Exchange List

Each exchange is 1/2 cup, unless otherwise specified, and may be used within the fluid allowance. Soups are ready-to-serve or prepared according to package directions.

Bernard[6]

Dietetic chicken broth	1 serving/day (free)
Dietetic cream of celery	1 A low carbohydrate vegetable
Dietetic cream of mushroom	1 B low carbohydrate vegetable
Dietetic cream of potato soup mix	1 B low carbohydrate vegetable
Dietetic cream of tomato	1 A low carbohydrate vegetable
Dietetic vegetable beef	1 A low carbohydrate vegetable

Campbell[7]

Low sodium chicken noodle	1/2 bread
Low sodium cream of mushroom	1 A low carbohydrate vegetable
Low sodium green pea	1 bread
Low sodium tomato	1 B high carbohydrate vegetable
Low sodium turkey noodle	1/2 bread
Low sodium vegetable	1 A low carbohydrate vegetable
Low sodium vegetable beef	1 A low carbohydrate vegetable

---

[1]Kingsmill Food Company Limited, 1399 Kennedy Road, Unit 17, Scarborough, Ontario, Canada, MIP 2L6.

[2]Recipe in Appendix J.

[3]Limit on phosphorus restricted diet because of higher phosphorus content.

[4]Available from Dietary Specialties, Inc., P.O. Box 227, Rochester, NY 14601.

[5]Also available from Ener-g Foods, Inc., 6901 Fox Avenue South, Box 24723, Seattle, WA 98124-0723.

[6]Bernard Food Industries, Inc., P.O. Box 1497, Evanston, IL 60204.

[7]Campbell Soup Company, Campbell Place, Camden, NJ 08101.

Featherweight[1]

Low sodium chicken noodle	1 A low carbohydrate vegetable
Low sodium tomato (1/3 cup)	1 B high carbohydrate vegetable
Low sodium vegetable beef	1 B high carbohydrate vegetable

Additional Foods List

The following foods are low in carbohydrate, protein, fat, sodium, potassium, and phosphorus.

List A. Free (any amount may be eaten each day).

Sugar-free (artificially sweetened) Kool-Aid powder, all flavors except
   sunshine punch
Sugar substitutes (artificial sweeteners)

List B. Limit to the amount shown each day.

Barbecue sauce, low sodium[1]	1 tsp
Catsup, low sodium[1,2]	1 tbsp
Chewing gum, sugar-free	4 sticks
Chili sauce, low sodium[3]	1 tbsp
Coffee-mate	1 tsp
Cranberries, fresh or artificially sweetened	3 tbsp
Jams or jellies, sugar-free[1,2,3,4]	3 tbsp
Diet salad dressings:	
All purpose dietetic dressing (dill flavored)[5]	2 tbsp
Blue cheese style dressing, dietetic[4]	2 tbsp
French, low sodium[1,3,4,5]	2 tbsp
French style, low sodium[3]	2 tbsp
Italian, low sodium[3,4]	2 tbsp
Russian, low sodium[3]	2 tbsp
Zero or zero style[2,3]	2 tbsp
Dill pickle, low sodium[1,3]	1 oz
Mustard, low sodium[2,3]	1 tsp
Seafood cocktail sauce, low sodium[3]	1 tsp
Whipped toppings:	
Cool Whip	1 tbsp
Dream Whip	2 tbsp
D-Zerta low calorie whipped topping	1 tbsp
Featherweight low calorie whipped topping[1]	1 tbsp

[1] Sandoz Nutrition, 5320 W. 23rd St., P.O. Box 370, Minneapolis, MN 55440.

[2] Estee Company, 169 Lackawanna Ave., Parsippany, NJ 07054.

[3] Geoghegan's Dietetic, Low Calorie, and Special Diet Foods, Geoghegan Brothers Company, 8835 South Greenwood Ave., Chicago, IL 60619.

[4] William J. Elwood, Inc., 3 North Oak St., Copiague, NY 11726.

[5] Bernard Food Industries, Inc., P.O. Box 1497, Evanston, IL 60204.

<u>Free Beverages</u>

These beverages are very low in carbohydrate, protein, fat, sodium, potassium, and phosphorus. They may be used as desired within the fluid allowances unless indicated otherwise.

> Kool-Aid (artificially sweetened):
>   all flavors except sugar-free sunshine punch
> Lemonade, artificially sweetened
> Limeade, artificially sweetened

<u>Soda Pop</u>

The kind of diet soda pop allowed depends on the levels of sodium, potassium, and phosphorus restriction. Soda pops in List A contain ≤ 2.9 mg Na, 1.67 mg K, and 1.0 mg P per oz, while those in List B contain more. The sodium and phosphorus content of the bottler's water supply is not included in the values reported. The amount of sodium and phosphorus varies depending on the water supply, season, and treatment. Special water treatment methods are used to produce beverages labeled "sodium free," containing 5 mg Na or less per 6 oz serving as per FDA regulations. Complete information was not available from all companies. Unless manufacturer's information or laboratory analyses indicate otherwise, soft drinks not listed should be avoided because of their higher sodium, potassium, or phosphorus content.

List A. These soft drinks may be used freely within the fluid allowance.

> 7-Up:
>   Diet 7-Up
> Shasta:
>   Chocolate (NutraSweet-saccharin blend)
>   Ginger Ale (NutraSweet-saccharin blend)

List B. These soft drinks are limited to 1 12 oz serving per day due to their higher sodium, potassium, and/or phosphorus content.

> A & W:
>   A & W very low sodium, sugar-free Root Beer
> Canada Dry (all are diet):
>   Barrelhead Root Beer
>   Cola
>   Ginger Ale
>   Orange
>   Tonic Water
> Canfield's (all are diet):
>   Cherry-ola Cola
>   Chocolate Fudge
>   Cola
>   50/50
>   Ginger Ale
>   Lemon Lime
>   Orange
>   Red Pop
>   Root Beer
>   Swiss Creme
>   Club Soda Sparkling Water
>   Quinine Tonic
>   Seltzer

Seltzer with lime
Coca-Cola:
    Diet Coke, caffeine-free diet Coke
    Fanta Diet Orange
    Fresca
    Sugar-free Mr. Pibb
    Sugar-free Ramblin' Root Beer
    Diet Sprite
    Tab, caffeine-free Tab
Dr. Pepper:
    Diet Dr. Pepper
    Sugar-free, Pepper-free Dr. Pepper
Pepsi-Cola:
    Diet Pepsi, Diet Pepsi-Free
    Diet Slice
RC Cola:
    Diet Cherry RC
    Diet Rite
    Diet RC Cola, caffeine-free
7-Up:
    Diet Cherry 7-Up
    Diet Like Cola
Shasta:
    NutraSweet-saccharin blend:
        Birch Beer
        Black Cherry
        Cherry Cola
        Cola, Shasta-free Cola
        Creme
        Frolic
        Grape
        Grapefruit
        Lemon-lime
        Orange
        Red Pop
        Root Beer
        Strawberry
    100% NutraSweet:
        Chocolate
        Cola
        Creme
        Ginger Ale
        Grapefruit
        Lemon-lime
        Orange
        Root Beer

SECTION 4

Modification of Fat

A. FAT RESTRICTED DIETS

DESCRIPTION: The total amount of fat is restricted by omitting foods high in fat. Foods that frequently cause gaseous distention are also excluded when used for the patient with gallbladder disease. Medium-chain triglycerides are not considered part of the total fat restriction and may be used as desired and tolerated when caloric restriction is not necessary.

1. 45-Gram Fat Diet

DESCRIPTION: This diet limits fat intake to approximately 40 to 50 g per day. It may be indicated in diseases of the liver, gallbladder, or pancreas if disturbances in digestion and absorption of fat occur. Patients with ileal resection or disease would also benefit from restricted fat.

FOODS ALLOWED AND FOODS TO AVOID:

Food Group	Foods Allowed	Foods to Avoid
Beverages	Skim milk, drinks made with skim milk, buttermilk, coffee, tea, decaffeinated coffee, cereal beverages, mild carbonated beverages, fruit drinks	All beverages made with cream, ice cream, ice milk, whole milk, 2% milk, or egg
Breads	Enriched white and whole grain breads, graham crackers, saltine crackers	Quick breads such as muffins, biscuits, popovers; breads containing excess fat such as dinner rolls, sweet rolls, party crackers
Cereals	Any except those to avoid	Granola; any containing nuts, coconut, or fat; unless well tolerated, omit 100% bran

FOODS ALLOWED AND FOODS TO AVOID (continued):

Food Group	Foods Allowed	Foods to Avoid
Desserts	Angel food cake, cookies with less than 2 g fat/serving (arrowroot, fig bar, ginger-snap, vanilla wafer), cookies made with fat as MCT oil, fruit whips, gelatin desserts, sherbet, desserts made with skim milk or egg white (if dessert containing whole egg is used, omit the 1 egg allowed)	Ice cream; ice milk; desserts prepared with cream, coconut, fat, nuts, chocolate, or milk other than skim; most commercial desserts
Eggs	Limit to 1 whole egg daily, including that used in cooking (additional egg white may be used); any preparation without added fat	Fried egg
Fats	Butter, margarine, vegetable shortening and oil, lard, mayonnaise, peanut butter, salad dressings (limit to 3 tsp daily, 1 tsp at each meal, including that used in cooking), MCT oil or spread	Gravy, fatty sauces, all fats used in excess of 3 tsp
Fruits, Fruit Juices	All fruit juices, all fruits except those listed to avoid	Avocado, other fruit if not tolerated
Meat, Fish, Poultry, Cheese	5 oz per day lean meat, fish, poultry (baked, broiled, roasted, or stewed); cottage cheese; skim milk cheese	Highly seasoned or fatty meats such as sausage, luncheon meats, duck or goose; oil-pack fish; all other cheese
Potatoes or Substitutes	White and sweet potatoes, spaghetti, macaroni, noodles, rice, hominy	Fried potatoes, potato chips, any prepared with highly seasoned sauces or cream sauces made with whole milk
Soups	Fat-free, broth-based soups; soups made with skim milk	Commercial soups; soups prepared with cream, fat, or whole milk
Sugar, Sweets	Sugar, honey, jam, jelly, syrup, molasses, plain sugar candies	Candy containing nuts, chocolate, fat, cream, or coconut

FOODS ALLOWED AND FOODS TO AVOID (continued):

Food Group	Foods Allowed	Foods to Avoid
Vegetables, Vegetable Juices	All that do not cause discomfort	Unless well tolerated, omit broccoli, brussels sprouts, cabbage, cauliflower, cucumber, garlic, legumes, onions, green pepper, rutabagas, sauerkraut, turnips
Miscellaneous	Salt, flavorings, spices in moderation, cocoa powder, fat-free butter flavoring, nonstick vegetable pan sprays	Nuts, olives, cream sauces, breakfast cocoa, popcorn, coconut

APPROXIMATE COMPOSITION OF SAMPLE MENU:

Calories	1961
Protein, g	107
Fat, g	36
Carbohydrate, g	305

SAMPLE MENU FOR 45-GRAM FAT DIET:

Breakfast

1/2 cup orange juice
1/2 cup farina
1 egg, soft cooked
1 slice toast, cracked wheat
1 tsp butter or margarine
1 tbsp grape jelly
1 cup skim milk
2 tsp sugar
Coffee or tea

Luncheon

2 oz sliced chicken
1/2 cup rice
1/2 cup green beans
1/2 sliced tomato on lettuce
1 slice bread, cracked wheat
1 tsp butter or margarine
1/2 cup canned peaches
1 slice angel food cake
1 cup skim milk
1 tsp sugar
Coffee or tea

Dinner

3 oz roast beef, lean, trimmed
1/2 cup cubed white potato
1/2 cup cooked carrots
3/4 cup lettuce salad
1 tbsp zero dressing[1]
1 slice bread, cracked wheat
1 tsp butter or margarine
1/2 cup sherbet
3 vanilla wafers
1 cup skim milk
1 tsp sugar
Coffee or tea

Evening Nourishment

1 cup skim milk
4 saltine crackers

---

[1]Recipe in Appendix J.

2. 20-Gram Fat Diet

DESCRIPTION: The 20-Gram Fat Diet is used for patients with an acute intolerance to fat. High carbohydrate, low fat foods are included in meals and snacks to provide additional calories.

FOODS ALLOWED AND FOODS TO AVOID: The list of foods allowed and foods to avoid for the 45-Gram Fat Diet is used with the following exceptions:

Food Group	Foods Allowed	Foods to Avoid
Eggs	Egg white only, any preparation without added fat	Egg yolk
Fats	MCT oil	All others
Desserts	Angel food cake, fruit whips, gelatin, meringue, sherbet, fruit or water ices, pudding made without egg yolk	Desserts prepared with egg yolk, cream, chocolate, coconut, fat, nuts, or milk other than skim

APPROXIMATE COMPOSITION OF SAMPLE MENU:

Calories	2050
Protein, g	103
Fat, g	20
Carbohydrate, g	367

SAMPLE MENU FOR 20-GRAM FAT DIET:

Breakfast	Luncheon	Dinner
1/2 cup orange juice	2 oz sliced chicken	3 oz roast beef, lean, trimmed
1 cup farina	1/2 cup rice	1/2 cup cubed white potato
1 slice toast, cracked wheat	1/2 cup green beans	1/2 cup cooked carrots
1 tbsp grape jelly	1/2 sliced tomato on lettuce	3/4 cup lettuce salad
1 cup skim milk	1 slice bread, cracked wheat	1 tbsp zero dressing[1]
2 tsp sugar	1 tbsp honey	1 slice bread, cracked wheat
Coffee or tea	1/2 cup canned peaches	1 tbsp apple jelly
	1 slice angel food cake	1/2 cup sherbet
	1 cup skim milk	3 vanilla wafers
	1 tsp sugar	1 cup skim milk
	Coffee or tea	1 tsp sugar
		Coffee or tea

Midafternoon Nourishment	Evening Nourishment
1/2 cup gelatin	1 cup skim milk
2 saltine crackers	4 graham crackers

---

[1]Recipe in Appendix J.

B. MEDIUM-CHAIN TRIGLYCERIDE DIET

DESCRIPTION: Medium-chain triglyceride (MCT) preparations have proven effective in the dietary treatment of a variety of malabsorption syndromes such as steatorrhea from chyluria, pancreatitis, cystic fibrosis, sprue, gastrectomy, and massive resection of the small intestine. These 8 to 10 carbon fats provide 8.3 calories per gram and are directly absorbed into the portal circulation, bypassing the lymphatic system. Most naturally occurring fats are long-chain triglycerides and should be kept to a minimum on this diet.

MCT oils should gradually be introduced into the diet in small amounts until the prescribed dose is reached. From 50 to 100 g per day are usually well tolerated and should be divided into at least 3 meals and 3 snacks. It is possible to use MCT oil in food preparation[1], but it should not be heated above 300 to 320 degrees Fahrenheit because of oxidation. Because of the unstable nature and high expense of MCT oil, commercial formulas containing it are often used in place of the oil itself. The new ones are quite palatable and can contribute substantially to nutrition.

The percentage of calories from fat and the proportion of fat as MCT in the formulas should be determined (see table below). Those very low in fat can also be used. (See Section 10, Enteral Formulas and Nutritional Supplements.)

FAT AND MCT CONTENT OF SELECTED FORMULAS

Formula (240 cc)	Total Fat (g)	Calories from Fat (%)	MCT (g)	Fat Calories from MCT (%)	Total Calories from MCT (%)
Portagen - prepared according to directions for 1 cal/cc	11.45	41	9.8	86	34
Travasorb prepared according to directions for 1 cal/cc	8.2	30	6.5	80	23
Peptamen	9.36	33	6.5	70	22
Jevity	0.8	30	4.6	50	15
Osmolite	9.1	31	4.6	50	15
Vital HN	2.6	9	1.5	45	4
Precision LR Diet - prepared according to directions for 1.1 calorie/cc	0.5	1	0	0	0

---

[1]See Appendix J for recipes.

124

FOODS ALLOWED AND FOODS TO AVOID:

Food Group	Foods Allowed	Foods to Avoid
Beverages	Skim milk; skim buttermilk; supplemental formulas containing minimal fat, *or* MCT oil as the major source of fat; coffee; tea; Ovaltine; Postum; carbonated beverages	Whole or 2% milk; whole buttermilk; light, heavy, or sour cream; breakfast cocoa
Breads	Refined and whole grain breads	Biscuits, muffins, crackers, or baked products containing eggs, whole milk, or fat
Cereals	All except those to avoid	Granola; any containing nuts, coconut, or fat
Desserts	Angel food cake, meringue, gelatin, fruit whips, fruit or water ices	Ice cream; baked products or puddings containing whole milk, egg yolk, or fats other than MCT oil
Eggs	Egg white only	Egg yolk
Fats	Recipes using MCT oil	Butter, margarine, or shortening containing vegetable or animal fat
Fruits, Fruit Juices	All fruit juices and fruits except avocado	Avocado
Meat, Fish, Poultry, Cheese	5 oz per day lean meat, fish or poultry; cottage cheese; skim milk cheese	Cheese made from whole milk; all meats, fish, or poultry cooked with added animal or vegetable fat
Potatoes or Substitutes	All potatoes or substitutes to which no fat except MCT oil is added	Any prepared with butter, cream, or cheese; potato or corn chips
Soups	Fat-free bouillon, consommé, broth	Cream soups
Sugar, Sweets	Sugar, plain sugar candy, jelly, jam	Chocolate; candies made with chocolate, butter, cream, coconut, or nuts
Vegetables, Vegetable Juices	All vegetables to which no fat except MCT oil or MCT cream sauce[1] is added	Creamed, fried, au gratin, or buttered vegetables

---

[1]Recipe in Appendix J.

FOODS ALLOWED AND FOODS TO AVOID (continued):

Food Group	Foods Allowed	Foods to Avoid
Miscellaneous	Popcorn, cocoa powder, special recipes in which MCT oil is substituted for long-chain fats	Olives, coconut, nuts, buttered popcorn, gravies, peanut butter

APPROXIMATE COMPOSITION OF SAMPLE MENU:

Calories	2501
Protein, g	120
Fat, g	69
Carbohydrate, g	356

SAMPLE MENU FOR MEDIUM-CHAIN TRIGLYCERIDE DIET:

Breakfast	Luncheon	Dinner
1/2 cup orange juice	2 oz sliced chicken	3 oz roast beef, lean
1/2 cup farina	1/2 cup rice	1/2 cup cubed white potato
1 slice toast, white enriched	1/2 cup green beans	1/2 cup cooked carrots
2 tsp MCT oil spread[1]	1/2 sliced tomato on lettuce	3/4 cup tossed lettuce salad
1 tbsp grape jelly	1 slice bread, white enriched	1 tbsp MCT french dressing[1]
1/2 cup skim milk	2 tsp MCT oil spread[1]	1 slice bread, white enriched
2 tsp sugar	1/2 cup canned peaches	1 tsp MCT oil spread[1]
Coffee or tea	1 slice angel food cake	1/2 cup sherbet
	1 cup skim milk	1 cup skim milk
	1 tsp sugar	1 tsp sugar
	Coffee or tea	Coffee or tea

Midmorning Nourishment	Midafternoon Nourishment	Evening Nourishment
1 cup MCT formula[2]	1 cup MCT formula[2]	1 cup MCT formula[2]

---

[1] Recipe in Appendix J.

[2] Travasorb MCT or Portagen prepared according to label directions for beverage.

C. LOW CHOLESTEROL, FAT CONTROLLED DIETS FOR HYPERLIPIDEMIA

DESCRIPTION: Diet therapy is recognized as the primary treatment for hyper-cholesterolemia. The National Cholesterol Education Program's Adult Treatment Panel, the American Heart Association, and the American Dietetic Association recommend the Step-One and Step-Two Diets for lowering blood cholesterol. These diets are designed to progressively lower the intake of saturated fat and cholesterol while maintaining adequate nutrition. (See page 128.) The components of the diet having an impact on lowering plasma cholesterol include the following (in order of effectiveness): reducing saturated fat, modestly increasing monounsaturated and polyunsaturated fat, and lowering cholesterol intake. Achieving normalization of lipids lowers the incidence of coronary heart disease.[1]

The Step-One Diet limits saturated fatty acid intake to less than 10% of calories and cholesterol intake to less than 300 mg per day. Effectiveness of the Step-One Diet is typically demonstrated within three months. A 10-15% decline in blood cholesterol can be expected. If therapeutic goals are not achieved within three months, choices for dietary treatment include intensified counseling on the Step-One Diet or progression to the Step-Two Diet. The Step-Two Diet limits saturated fatty acid intake to less than 7% of calories and cholesterol intake to less than 200 mg per day. Because individual responsiveness to lipid-lowering dietary changes is variable, a six-month trial of intensive nutrition intervention is recommended.

Monounsaturated fats, such as olive oil and peanut oil, have received increased attention in recent years. Epidemiological data from the Mediterranean region show a very low incidence of heart disease in populations consuming a diet containing 15-20% of calories from monounsaturated fat and 7% or less of total calories from saturated fat. Preliminary studies have shown that the low density lipoproteins decreased and high density lipoproteins increased when monounsaturated fats were substituted for saturated fats. (High density lipoproteins protect against the formation of atherosclerotic plaque.) More studies need to be done before the American Heart Association recommends increased intake of monounsaturated fats.

A new area of research is omega-3 fatty acids, another category of polyunsaturates, commonly found in fish. A preliminary study by Connor showed that these fatty acids will lower serum triglyceride and cholesterol levels; however, the number of subjects was small and the controlled diets were also low in cholesterol and total fat. Other physiological effects of fish oils are being investigated, including their mechanisms of action. Because the optimal amount of omega fatty acids in the diet is not known, the general recommendation is for the public to consume more fish rather than fish oils themselves. Fish oil capsules being promoted in pharmacies, health food stores, and by mail order are specifically not recommended, since further research is needed to indicate what types and amounts are beneficial.

---

[1]Lipid Research Clinics program: The Lipid Research Clinics Coronary Primary Prevention Trial Results. JAMA 25(3):351-74, 1984.

DIETARY THERAPY FOR HIGH BLOOD CHOLESTEROL[a]

Nutrient	Recommended Intake	
	Step-One Diet	Step-Two Diet
Total fat	Less than 30% of total calories	Less than 30% of total calories
Saturated fatty acids	Less than 10% of total calories	Less than 10% of total calories
Polyunsaturated fatty acids	Up to 10% of total calories	Up to 10% of total calories
Monounsaturated fatty acids	10 to 15% of total calories	10 to 15% of total calories
Carbohydrates	50 to 60% of total calories	50 to 60% of total calories
Protein	10 to 20% of total calories	10 to 20% of total calories
Cholesterol	Less than 300 mg/day	Less than 200 mg/day
Total calories	To achieve and maintain desirable weight	To achieve and maintain desirable weight

[a]Arch Intern Med 148:36-69, 1988.

Close adherence to a low cholesterol, fat controlled diet is necessary to achieve effective reduction of serum cholesterol. Following this diet represents a long-term or permanent modification in life-style for the patient; therefore, the diet should be individualized as much as possible. This involves the use of a diet history, with emphasis on foods containing cholesterol and fat. An example of a form that may be used for this purpose is given on page 303. This history allows the nutritionist not only to estimate present cholesterol and fat intake, but also to identify food preferences and preparation techniques so that alternates can be suggested when appropriate (see Guide to Cholesterol Free and Fat Modified Products, page 139). Experience has shown that several counseling sessions are required to assist the patient in a permanent modification of eating habits.

UIHC "STANDARD" DIETS: At the University of Iowa Hospitals and Clinics, if a "low cholesterol" order is received, the patient is served a 200 mg cholesterol diet with 25% of the calories from fat. Until a patient interview has been completed, the patient who is also restricted in calories will be served meals selected according to the "Low Cholesterol Menu Patterns Using Fat Controlled Exchange Lists" table (see page 136).

Cardiovascular surgery patients are often placed on a "moderate cholesterol" diet to encourage consumption of adequate calories for healing. This diet is less restrictive than the standard low cholesterol diet. Two percent milk may be selected, and 1 serving per day of the following high fat foods is allowed: sweet rolls, quick breads, cookies, cake, or ice cream.

ADEQUACY: These diets meet the Recommended Dietary Allowances for all nutrients except iron for women of childbearing age.

FOODS ALLOWED AND FOODS TO AVOID:

Food Group	Foods Allowed	Foods to Avoid
Beverages	Skim milk, buttermilk, 1% milk, coffee, tea, decaffeinated coffee, cereal beverages, cocoa made with skim milk, carbonated beverages	Whole or 2% milk, cream, half-and-half

FOODS ALLOWED AND FOODS TO AVOID (continued):

Food Group	Foods Allowed	Foods to Avoid
Breads	Enriched white and whole grain breads, breadsticks, english muffins, melba toast, rusk, syrian bread, tortillas, zwieback; hot breads, pancakes, and waffles made with egg substitute or egg white and allowed fats (count as part of daily fat allowance); crackers: graham, Meal Mate, matzo, Rye Krisp, saltine, soda	High fat dinner rolls; egg or cheese breads; commercial biscuits, muffins, quick breads, doughnuts, sweet rolls, biscuit or quick bread mixes; commercial pancakes or waffles; high fat party crackers
Cereals	All except those to avoid	Granola, cereals with coconut or high levels of fat
Cheese	Rinsed cottage cheese, sapsago, Count Down cheese, cheeses containing less than 5 grams fat per oz if substituted for allowed meat servings (see Meat Exchange List on page 135)	Whole or part skim milk cheese (some may be substituted for allowed meat servings; see Meat Exchange List on page 135), cream cheese, filled cheese
Desserts	Fruits, fruit whips made with egg white, gelatin, fruit ices, fudgsicles, popsicles, sherbet, Weight Watchers frozen dessert, ice milk, commercial angel food cake, arrowroot cookies, gingersnaps, vanilla wafers, animal crackers, sugar or waffle ice cream cones, canned fruit pie fillings, pudding mixes prepared with skim milk, nonfat or 1% fat yogurt The following are permitted if made with allowed ingredients and if fat is counted in daily allotment: cakes, pies, cookies, pastries	Most commercial cookies, cakes, pie, or pastries; ice cream; nondairy ice cream; desserts containing chocolate, butter, cocoa butter, or coconut; pudding made with egg or milk other than skim; cookie and cake mixes (except angel food cake); 2% or 4% fat yogurt
Eggs	Egg whites, cholesterol-free egg substitutes	Egg yolk, whole egg, egg substitutes containing cholesterol

FOODS ALLOWED AND FOODS TO AVOID (continued):

Food Group	Foods Allowed	Foods to Avoid
Fats	Margarine (P/S ≥2); vegetable oils: canola, corn, soy, cottonseed, olive, safflower, sunflower, peanut; salad dressings: commercial or homemade french, italian, western, vinegar and oil, mayonnaise-type, buttermilk and mayonnaise, thousand island; polyunsaturated fat coffee creamers; peanut butter; nuts; olives (limit fat according to table on page 134)	Butter; margarine containing animal fat or with a P/S ratio <1; hydrogenated shortening or oil; oils: coconut, palm, palm kernel, oils used for restaurant frying; lard; bacon fat; other animal fat; salad dressings: blue cheese, green goddess, others containing cheese, whole milk, or sour cream; creamers containing saturated fat; sour cream; cocoa butter
Fruits, Fruit Juices	All	None
Meat, Fish, Poultry	Lean (≤15% fat, see pages 132-33) beef, pork, veal, lamb; chicken and turkey with skin removed; fish, clams, scallops, oysters, shrimp, lobster, water-pack tuna (limit according to table on page 134). (All meat, fish, and poultry should be trimmed of visible fat before cooking, and baked, broiled, roasted, stewed, or steamed to eliminate excess fat.)	All meat with >15% fat; duck, goose; poultry skin; oil-pack fish, caviar; organ meats (liver, kidney gizzard, heart, sweetbreads creamed or commercially fried meat, fish, or poultry; meats canned in gravy or sauce
Potatoes or Substitutes	White and sweet potatoes, macaroni, spaghetti, rice, hominy, cornmeal, cholesterol-free egg noodles, homemade noodles if made with egg substitute or egg white	Egg noodles; potato chips, corn chips, or similar products
Soups	Broth-based canned or homemade soups, if made with allowed ingredients and fat is counted in daily fat allotment; tomato if made with skim milk or water	Commercial cream soups; chowder or other soups made with cream, whole milk, or butter
Sugar, Sweets	Sugar, hard candy, gum drops, marshmallows, syrups (including chocolate), honey, jam, jelly, marshmallow creme	Chocolate candy, white chocolate, commercial fudge or other high fat candies, chocolate or butterscotch sauce

FOODS ALLOWED AND FOODS TO AVOID (continued):

Food Group	Foods Allowed	Foods to Avoid
Vegetables, Vegetable Juices	All if prepared with allowed foods	All those prepared or packaged with foods to avoid
Miscellaneous	Mustard; catsup; steak sauces; gravy made with fat-free broth, skim milk, and margarine or made from dry mixes containing only allowed foods; cocoa powder	Conventional gravy, commercially prepared popcorn, whipped toppings

CHOLESTEROL CONTENT OF COMMONLY USED FOODS

Item	Amount	Cholesterol (mg)	Item	Amount	Cholesterol (mg)
Skim milk	8 oz	5	Cereals		0
1% milk	8 oz	10	Nuts		0
2% milk	8 oz	20	Beef, 6-15% fat	1 oz	26
Whole milk	8 oz	34	Beef, 20-30% fat	1 oz	26
Sherbet	1/2 cup	3	Beef fat	1 tsp	5
Ice cream, 10% fat	1/2 cup	30	Veal	1 oz	28
Ice milk	1/2 cup	19	Pork, 10-15% fat	1 oz	26
Heavy cream, 35% fat	1 tbsp	20	Lamb	1 oz	27
Half-and-half, 12% fat	1 tbsp	6	Poultry, light (no skin)	1 oz	22
Butter	1 tbsp	7	Poultry, dark (no skin)	1 oz	25
Mayonnaise	1 tbsp	8	Kidney, beef	1 oz	228
American cheese, cheddar, blue, or swiss, >20% fat	1 oz	28	Liver (beef, calf, pork)	1 oz	124
			Heart	1 oz	78
Mozzarella, part skim	1 oz	15	Brains	1 oz	724
Cheese food and spread	1 oz	17	Sweetbreads	1 oz	132
			Giblets	1 oz	111
Cheese, Parmesan grated, dry	1 tbsp	6	Tuna	1 oz	17
			Salmon, pink	1 oz	10
Cottage cheese, 1% fat	1/2 cup	5	Fish, 2-6% fat	1 oz	23
			Fish, 12% fat	1 oz	23
Cream cheese, 35% fat	1 tbsp	15	Shrimp	1 oz	43
Egg yolk	1 large	274	Crab	1 oz	28
Egg whites		0	Lobster	1 oz	44
Vegetable margarine		0	Oysters	1 oz	13
Vegetable oils		0	Scallops	1 oz	15
Peanut butter		0	Clams	1 oz	18
Fruits		0			
Vegetables		0			

Note: Adapted from Nutrition Coding Center, Elemental Items: Food Table Information Listing Primary Nutrients and Food Units (1987).

PERCENTAGE OF FAT IN MEAT PRODUCTS:[1]

Variety Meats

Recommended

(% Fat)
3.5	Cold cuts: lowfat, dried, or pressed meat or poultry (Buddig, Land O' Frost)
4.0	Venison, rabbit, squirrel, and other wild game
4.1	Horsemeat
5.2	Guinea hen or pheasant with or without skin; wild duck, squab, and other wild game without skin
14.0	Opossum, raccoon
15.0	Rich's turkey variety meats

Not Recommended

(% Fat)
16.0	Salami (kosher)
19.8	Vienna sausage
22.0	Headcheese
23.2	Sausage (knockwurst)
25.8	Polish sausage, bratwurst
27.2	Frankfurters (average, cooked)
27.4	Braunschweiger
27.5	Bologna, cooked salami, or similar cold cuts (nonkosher)
30.0	Frankfurters (cooked, all beef, kosher)
38.1	Salami (dried, hard), pepperoni
44.1	Sausage (link, cooked)
44.2	Sausage (patty, cooked)

Fresh Pork

Recommended

(% Fat)
10	Leg (fresh ham), trimmed: rump, center, or shank
10	Leg, trimmed: cube steak
15	Loin, trimmed: roast or chops (blade, rib, center, top loin, sirloin); tenderloin
15	Shoulder, trimmed: arm picnic, roast or steak; blade Boston, roast or steak

Not Recommended

(% Fat)
30	Leg (fresh ham), untrimmed: whole, rump, center, or shank
30	Loin, untrimmed: roast or chops (blade, rib, center, top loin, sirloin); tenderloin
30	Pork, ground
15	Shoulder, untrimmed: arm picnic, roast or steak; blade Boston, roast or steak
40	Spareribs
40	Loin back ribs, country style

---

[1]Meat fat percentages were developed for the Coronary Primary Prevention Trial by the Iowa Lipid Research Clinic, Nutrition Section.

PERCENTAGE OF FAT IN MEAT PRODUCTS (continued):

Beef

Recommended		Not Recommended	
(% Fat)		(% Fat)	
6	Beef, chipped or dried	20	Chuck, untrimmed: pot roast, steak, or ground
6	Flank steak, plain, cubed, or rolled	25	"Ground beef"
6	Round, trimmed: bottom round roast or steak	30	Brisket, fresh
6	Shank, center cut, trimmed	30	Corned beef brisket, canned corned beef
10	Chuck, trimmed: arm pot roast or steak	30	Pastrami
10	Loin, trimmed: porterhouse, sirloin, and T-bone steaks; tenderloin roast, steak, or tips	30	Regular hamburger
10	Loin, trimmed: top loin (K.C., club) and top sirloin steaks	30	Loin, untrimmed: porterhouse, sirloin, and T-bone steaks
10	Plate ribs, short ribs, spareribs, trimmed	30	Loin, untrimmed: tenderloin, roast, steak, or tips: top loin steak (K.C., club); top sirloin steak
10	Plate skirt steak, boneless, cubed, rolled, trimmed	30	Plate ribs, short ribs, spareribs, untrimmed
15	Ground round	30	Rib eye, untrimmed, roast or steak (Delmonico)
15	Round, untrimmed: bottom round roast or steak, corned beef	30	Rib roast or steak, untrimmed
15	Rib eye, trimmed: roast or steak (Delmonico)	30	Shank, center cut, untrimmed
15	Rib roast or steak, trimmed		

Pork, Smoked and Cured

Recommended		Not Recommended	
(% Fat)		(% Fat)	
10	Ham, trimmed: center slices, rump, shank	17	Canadian bacon, untrimmed
15	Canadian bacon, trimmed	20	Ham, untrimmed; center slices, rump, shank
15	Pickled pigs' feet	25	Shoulder picnic or roll, untrimmed
15	Loin, trimmed: roast or chops	30	Loin, untrimmed, roast or chops
15	Shoulder picnic or roll, trimmed	30	Ham, deviled, canned
		35	Ham, country style, dry cure, untrimmed
		35	Hock, jowl, neckbones
		40	Ribs, loin back or spareribs
		50	Bacon, regular, sliced
		70	Salt pork, cooked
		85	Salt pork, raw

The following is a guide to aid in designating meat and fat exchanges for low cholesterol, fat controlled diets. Total calories need not be emphasized in the formal instruction unless weight loss is necessary.

MAXIMUM MEAT AND FAT EXCHANGES FOR LOW CHOLESTEROL, FAT CONTROLLED DIETS

	200 mg cholesterol, 25% fat		200 mg cholesterol, 20% fat		100 mg cholesterol, 20% fat	
	Meat	Fat	Meat	Fat	Meat	Fat
1000 Calories	5	1	4	1/2	3	1
1200 Calories	5	2	5	1	3	1
1500 Calories	5	3	5	2	3	2
1800 Calories	6	4	5	3	3	3
2000 Calories	7	4	6	3	3	4
2200 Calories	7	5	7	3	3	5
2400 Calories	7	6	7	4	3	5
2600 Calories	7	7	7	4	4	6
2800 Calories	7	8	7	5	4	6

Note: One dairy product from the Meat Exchange List (page 135) may be used in place of 1 oz meat in all diets, but only 1 such substitution may be made daily.

Values used for 1 meat exchange are 7 g protein, 3 g fat, and 55 calories.

FOOD VALUES OF EXCHANGE LISTS FOR LOW CHOLESTEROL, FAT CONTROLLED DIETS

Exchange Group	Amount	CHO (g)	Protein (g)	Fat (g)	Cholesterol (mg)	Calories
Skim milk	1 cup	12	8	1	4	90
Vegetable	1/2 cup	5	2	0	0	28
Fruit	Varies	15	0	0	0	60
Bread	Varies	15	3	1	0	80
Lean meat	1 oz	0	7	3	20-25	55
Very lean meat[a]	1 oz	0	7	1	20-25	37
Fat	Varies	0	0	5	0	45

[a]The very lean meat exchanges are the only ones allowed on the 100 mg cholesterol, 10% fat diet.

LOW CHOLESTEROL, FAT CONTROLLED EXCHANGE LISTS:

Meat Exchange List: Use *lean* meat exchanges on page 148 and the following list. These foods are equivalent to 1 oz allowed meat in cholesterol and fat content (not in calories). These items contribute less than 20 mg cholesterol and less than 5 g fat in the amounts listed. Only 1 substitute may be used per day because of the slightly higher fat content of foods in this list.

2% milk	1 cup	Cottage cheese, 2% fat	1 cup
Yogurt, lowfat	1 cup	Cottage cheese, creamed, 4% fat	1/2 cup
Lowfat, low calorie processed cheese foods containing 5 grams or less fat/oz	1 oz	Mozzarella cheese, part skim milk	1 oz

Fat Exchange List: These foods count as 1 fat exchange. All items contribute approximately 5 g fat and negligible or no cholesterol in the amounts listed.

Margarine (brands with liquid oil as first ingredient are recommended)	1 tsp	Mayonnaise	1 tsp
		Low calorie mayonnaise	2 tsp
Vegetable oil	1 tsp	Creamer, liquid polyunsaturated fat	3 tbsp
Salad dressing: mayonnaise-type, french, western, italian, thousand island, vinegar and oil	2 tsp	Peanut butter	2 tsp
		Nuts, chopped	1 tbsp
		Peanuts	10 nuts
Olives	6 medium		

Bread Exchange List: Use list on pages 146-47. The starch foods prepared with fat should be made with skim milk, oils from allowed list, and egg white or egg substitute.

Milk Exchange List: Use skim (no fat) milk only. One cup skim milk = 1 exchange.

Vegetable Exchange List: See list on pages 149-50.

Fruit Exchange List: See list on page 150-51.

APPROXIMATE COMPOSITION OF SAMPLE MENU:

Calories	2000
Protein, g	119
Fat, g	40
Carbohydrate, g	289
Cholesterol, mg	194

SAMPLE MENU FOR 2000 CALORIE, 200 mg CHOLESTEROL, 25% FAT DIET:

Breakfast

1/2 cup orange juice
1/2 cup oatmeal
1 slice toast,
  whole wheat
1 tsp margarine
1 cup skim milk
Coffee or tea

Luncheon

1/2 cup apple juice
3 oz sliced chicken
1/3 cup rice
1/2 cup green beans
1/2 sliced tomato on lettuce
1 slice bread, whole wheat
1 tsp margarine
4 halves unsweetened peaches
1 cup skim milk
Coffee or tea

Dinner

3 oz roast beef, lean,
  trimmed
1 cup cubed white potato
1/2 cup cooked carrots
3/4 cup tossed salad
1 tbsp french dressing
2 slices bread, whole
  wheat
1 tsp margarine
Banana
1 cup skim milk
Coffee or tea

Evening Nourishment

1 oz roast turkey
1 slice bread, whole
  wheat

LOW CHOLESTEROL MENU PATTERNS USING FAT CONTROLLED EXCHANGE LISTS
(200 mg cholesterol, 25% fat)

Exchanges	1000 Calories	1200 Calories	1500 Calories	1800 Calories	2000 Calories	2200 Calories	2400 Calories	2600 Calories	2800 Calories
Milk, skim	2	3	3	3	3	3	3	3	3
Vegetable	2	2	2	3	3	3	4	4	4
Fruit	2	2	3	5	6	7	8	9	9
Bread	4	5	7	8	9	10	11	12	14
Meat	5	5	5	6	7	7	7	7	7
Fat	1	2	3	4	4	5	6	7	8
Total Calories	998	1213	1480	1809	2005	2191	2405	2591	2798
Carbohydrate, g	124	151	196	246	276	306	341	371	401
Protein, g	67	78	84	96	106	109	114	117	123
Fat, g	26	33	40	49	53	59	65	71	78
Fat, %	23	24	24	24	24	24	24	25	25

LOW CHOLESTEROL MENU PATTERNS USING FAT CONTROLLED EXCHANGE LISTS
(200 mg cholesterol, 20% fat)

Exchanges	1000 Calories	1200 Calories	1500 Calories	1800 Calories	2000 Calories	2200 Calories	2400 Calories	2600 Calories	2800 Calories
Milk, skim	2	3	3	3	3	3	3	3	3
Vegetable	2	2	3	4	4	4	4	4	4
Fruit	3	4	5	7	7	8	10	10	11
Bread	4	4	6	7	9	10	11	13	14
Meat	4	5	5	5	6	7	7	7	7
Fat	1/2	1	2	3	3	3	4	4	5
Total Calories	981	1207	1502	1776	1993	2189	2435	2597	2783
Carbohydrate, g	139	166	216	266	296	326	371	401	431
Protein, g	60	75	83	88	101	111	114	120	123
Fat, g	21	27	34	40	45	49	55	57	63
Fat, %	19	20	20	20	20	20	20	20	20

LOW CHOLESTEROL MENU PATTERNS USING FAT CONTROLLED EXCHANGE LISTS
(100 mg cholesterol, 20% fat)

Exchanges	1000 Calories	1200 Calories	1500 Calories	1800 Calories	2000 Calories	2200 Calories	2400 Calories	2600 Calories	2800 Calories
Milk, skim	2	3	3	3	3	3	3	3	3
Vegetable	2	2	3	3	3	4	4	4	4
Fruit	4	4	4	6	7	9	10	10	11
Bread	4	5	8	10	11	11	13	14	16
Meat	3	3	3	3	3	3	3	4	4
Fat	1	2	2	3	4	5	5	6	6
Total Calories	1008	1223	1494	1821	2007	2200	2422	2603	2825
Carbohydrate, g	154	181	231	291	321	356	401	416	461
Protein, g	53	64	75	81	84	86	92	102	108
Fat, g	20	27	30	37	43	48	50	59	61
Fat, %	18	20	18	18	19	20	19	20	19

137

Extremely Lowfat Diet (100 mg cholesterol, 10% fat)

DESCRIPTION: This 100 mg cholesterol, 10% fat diet is useful in the treatment of Type I hyperlipidemia. When dietary fat is reduced to a minimum, the fasting chylomicronemia will disappear. Although more fat may be tolerated by some patients, many will need the more severe 10% fat restriction to obtain optimum results. Calorie restriction to attain ideal weight is helpful in initiating control of Type V hyperlipidemia.

Food values for calculating this diet are the same as those for the fat controlled exchange lists on page 134 with the following exception. The values for meat are 7 g protein, 1 g fat, and 37 calories, which is the average composition of the meat, fish, and poultry from the *very* low meat exchange list given below.

ADEQUACY: This diet meets the Recommended Dietary Allowances for all nutrients except iron for women of childbearing age. Although only approximately 10% of the calories are from fat, the essential fatty acid requirements (1% of the total calories as linoleic acid) are met.

VERY LOWFAT MEAT EXCHANGES FOR 10% FAT DIET: Only the meat, fish, and poultry included in this list are to be used; no fat is to be added. All should be baked, broiled, stewed, or steamed. Each cooked ounce (exchange) contains approximately 7 g protein, 1 g fat, and 37 calories.

> Chicken (light meat), skin removed
> Turkey (light meat), skin removed
> Wild duck, skin removed
> Wild rabbit
> Venison
> Plain dried beef
> Lean fish: barracuda, bass, bluefish, buffalo fish, bullhead, butterfish (gulf water only), carp, catfish, clams, cod, crappie, croaker, flatfish, flounder, grouper, haddock, halibut, herring (Pacific only), kingfish, perch, pickerel, pike, pollock, porgy, rockfish, sand dab, scub, smelt (Harvard), snapper, sole, sturgeon, suckers, swordfish, brook trout, tuna (cooked or canned in brine or water), green turtle, whiting, lobster, crab, scallops, oysters

Suggested menu patterns for this diet are provided below. To enhance the palatability of the diet, a small quantity of medium-chain triglycerides (MCT) may be incorporated into the diet. The calories from MCT (approximately 115/tbsp) may replace some of those from bread and/or fruit exchanges on a calorie-for-calorie basis.

LOW CHOLESTEROL MENU PATTERNS USING FAT CONTROLLED EXCHANGE LISTS
(100 mg cholesterol, 10% fat)

Exchanges	1000 Calories	1200 Calories	1500 Calories	1800 Calories	2000 Calories	2200 Calories	2400 Calories	2600 Calories	2800 Calories
Milk, skim	1	2	2 1/2	3	3	3	3	3	3
Vegetable	2	2	4	4	4	4	4	4	4
Fruit	7	7	9	9	10	10	11	11	13
Bread	4	5	6	9	11	13	15	17	18
Meat[a]	3	3	3	3	3	3	3	4	4
Fat	1/2	1/2	1	1	1	1	1	1	1
Total Calories	1023	1213	1517	1804	2026	2188	2410	2609	2810
Carbohydrate, g	187	214	275	326	371	401	446	476	521
Protein, g	45	56	67	80	86	92	98	111	114
Fat, g	10.5	12.5	16.5	20	22	24	26	29	30
Fat, %	9.2	9.3	9.8	10	9.8	9.9	9.7	10	9.6

[a]Each exchange equals 7 g protein, 1 g fat, and 37 calories.

GUIDE TO LOW CHOLESTEROL AND FAT MODIFIED PRODUCTS: Low cholesterol and fat modified products are available. This listing must be periodically updated to include new products and to determine any alterations in ingredients used. If a patient is able to substitute alternate products in favorite family recipes, chances of successful adherence will be increased.

Butter and Lard

Margarine: Brands listing liquid oil as the first ingredient are recommended
Nonstick sprays for coating pans
  Mazola No-Stick
  Pam
  Pan Pal
Vegetable oil: corn, safflower, soy, cottonseed, peanut, sunflower
Vegetable shortening

Cheese

Cheezola -- Fisher Cheese Company
Count Down -- Fisher Cheese Company
Heidi's low fat cheddar -- Heidi's cheese products
Rinsed[1] or dry cottage cheese
Sapsago
Weight Watchers imitation cream cheese
Reduced calorie cheeses containing 5 g or less fat/oz

Chocolate

Carnation Instant Breakfast
Chocolate extract
Cocoa powder
Hershey's chocolate syrup
Hot cocoa mixes made with skim milk and without coconut or palm oil

Coconut

Coconut extract

Dairy Creams and Toppings

Alba Dairy-lite instant nonfat creamer
Evaporated skim milk
Poly Rich (liquid creamer) -- Rich's
Powdered pudding mixes made with skim milk
Vanilla flavored yogurt

Eggs (whole)

Egg Beaters -- Fleischmann's; Nabisco
Egg white, fresh (2 whites = 1 whole egg)
Egg white, powdered
Scramblers -- Morningstar Farms
Second Nature -- Avoset Food Corporation

---

[1]Place cottage cheese in a strainer and run water through it until cream has been removed.

Frozen Desserts

Alba 77 cocoa prepared with crushed ice
Fruit ices
Fudgsicles
Popsicles
Sherbet
Weight Watchers frozen desserts

Meat

Texturized vegetable protein
  Bac-O's (bacon flavor)
  Loma Linda (canned vegetable protein entrees)
  Morningstar Farms breakfast links and patties (sausage flavored), slices (ham
    flavored), and strips (bacon flavored)
  Worthington Foods (canned vegetable protein entrees)
Tofu

Milk

Evaporated skim milk
Fresh buttermilk made from skim milk
Fresh skim milk
Powdered buttermilk made from skim milk
Powdered skim milk

Noodles

Creamette macaroni ribbons
Homemade noodles made with egg substitute
No Yolk Noodles -- Foulds, Inc.

Sour Cream

Buttermilk made from skim milk
Lowfat yogurt
Rinsed[1] or dry cottage cheese, blended until smooth

---

[1]Place cottage cheese in a strainer and run water through it until cream has been removed.

SECTION 5

Diabetic Diets, Diets for Weight Loss, and Modification of Carbohydrates

A. DIABETIC DIETS

DESCRIPTION: The primary objectives of a diabetic diet are to facilitate control of glycemia and to minimize the known risk factors for atherosclerosis. In addition it is thought that optimal regulation of blood glucose levels will delay or prevent the complications of neuropathy, retinopathy, and nephropathy. Although it is now widely recognized that dietary recommendations should be individualized, good nutrition must be maintained. Optimal management of diabetes can be achieved only if the diet is carefully controlled.

A nutritionally adequate diet that meets the U.S. Dietary Guidelines is an important step in making optimal management a reality. Considerations requiring special emphasis are calories, carbohydrate, protein, fat, cholesterol, and fiber.

Calories. Calories should be set at a level to allow persons with diabetes to achieve and maintain desirable body weight. Age, sex, height, weight, and physical activity determine the caloric requirement. Of these, activity level is the most difficult to determine. A nomogram (see Appendix E) or the Harris and Benedict equation (see page 246) are standard reference tools.

Carbohydrate. The amount of carbohydrate in the diet should be increased to 55 to 60% of the total calories, individualized according to the blood glucose and lipid levels. However, the diets of those individuals who are achieving good control on lower carbohydrate percentages may not require change. Whenever acceptable to the person with diabetes, complex carbohydrate, high fiber food should be substituted for highly refined carbohydrates. In some individuals, small amounts of sucrose may be acceptable, contingent upon metabolic control and body weight.

Protein. The recommended protein intake for persons with diabetes is 0.8 g/kg ideal body weight, the same as the RDA. Modest increases in protein are indicated during pregnancy, lactation, and periods of rapid growth. The elderly may also need more than 0.8 g/kg.

Higher levels of protein were used in the past, but recent studies show that limiting protein intake may help prevent or delay nephropathy. The optimal level is not known, but some researchers are suggesting 0.6 g/kg. For the 50 kg woman, this calculates to only 30 g protein per day. Five to six ounces of meat in her diet plan would provide 40 to 48 g protein. It may be more important to include this amount of meat to promote compliance with the overall diet plan than to restrict it in order to delay or prevent nephropathy.

Fat and Cholesterol. Saturated fat and cholesterol should be reduced to delay the progression of vascular disease. Total fat should comprise less than 30% of total calories, and cholesterol should not exceed 300 mg per day. To provide adequate calories while improving blood lipids, complex carbohydrate and limited amounts of polyunsaturated fat should replace much of the saturated fat. Gradual dietary changes may be required to facilitate patient compliance.

Fiber. Research indicates that diets high in fiber contribute to lower, more stable blood sugars. The goal is a minimum of 25 g and a maximum of 50 g dietary fiber per day. Additional nutrition recommendations are specific to either Type I or Type II diabetes. (See table on page 143.)

Dietary Management Principles Specific to Type I Diabetes
(Insulin Dependent, Ketosis Prone)

In Type I diabetes, foods must be eaten at appropriate times and in the right amount to correlate with the effects of insulin. Most patients using only intermediate or long-acting insulin should have a bedtime snack. With a conventional NPH/regular split dose regimen, 3 meals with 3 snacks are generally indicated. However, there may be variability in the size, number and timing of snacks dependent on an individual's life-style. For example, someone taking a split dose of NPH and regular insulin who eats breakfast at 8:30 a.m. and lunch at 12:00 noon probably will not require a morning snack. By the same token, another person on the same type of insulin regimen who exercises between 5:00 p.m. and 6:00 p.m. may need a larger than average afternoon snack to prevent exercise-induced hypoglycemia.

Those persons on a multiple daily injection (MDI) regimen or an insulin pump normally do not require snacks as part of their meal plans. However, individualization is necessary. A small bedtime snack (e.g., approximately 15 g carbohydrate and 100 calories) may be needed to prevent nocturnal hypoglycemia. With the MDI or pump regimen, an extra bolus dose of insulin is usually necessary if large snacks are included.

Ordinarily the nutrient needs of an individual with Type I diabetes can be met without the use of special "dietetic" foods. The use of wholesome foods appropriate for the entire family is advocated. As much as the type of food, it is the amount and timing of foods consumed which must be closely monitored. Since consistency is crucial, a major part of diabetes diet teaching must include emphasis on controlling portion sizes and eating at appropriate times.

Dietary Management Principles Specific to Type II Diabetes
(Non-insulin Dependent, Ketosis Resistant)

Approximately 80% of the diabetic population has obesity related diabetes (Type II). For these patients caloric restriction is the overriding consideration. This is true regardless of therapy, whether it be diet alone, diet and oral hypoglycemic agents, or diet and insulin. The American Diabetes Association exchange system diet is often used to help persons moderate their caloric intake. In other instances, programs providing ongoing support such as Weight Watchers International may be the best weight management alternative. For the person who is unable to follow a structured meal plan, the following general guidelines may be applicable:

- Eat well-balanced meals at regular times
- Eat smaller portions
- Eliminate sweet desserts and regular soda pop
- Decrease use of high fat foods
- Include more fruits, vegetables, or other foods high in complex carbohydrate and fiber

Insulin resistance is a common characteristic of Type II diabetes. Therefore, hypoglycemia is not often a problem (even for those who take insulin), unless meals are skipped altogether.

For the smaller number of persons with Type II diabetes who are of normal weight, dietary management objectives more closely resemble those guidelines appropriate for Type I diabetes.

142

DIETARY MANAGEMENT OF DIABETES MELLITUS

	Dietary Management Objectives		Different Treatment Regimens	
Type of Diabetes	Major Dietary Management Objectives	Dietary Modifications Needed to Achieve Objectives	Treatment Regimen	Typical Pattern of Meals and Snacks
Type I Diabetes (insulin dependent)	Aim for normoglycemia by balancing food intake with activity pattern and insulin action	Adequate calories for growth and maintenance of ideal weight	NPH or lente insulin (1 injection per day)	3 meals and evening snacks
	Prevent hypo- and hyperglycemia	Day-to-day consistency in intake of calories, carbohydrate, protein, and fat	NPH/regular insulin (split dose)	3 meals and 3 snacks
	Prevent or delay onset of micro- and macro-vascular complications	Appropriate timing of meals and snacks	Multiple daily injections (ultra-lente/ regular) or Insulin pumps	3 meals with even distribution of carbohydrate Snacks included occasionally, depending on individual variation
		Low fat, high carbohydrate, high fiber diet		
Type II Diabetes (non-insulin dependent)	Aim for normoglycemia through hypocaloric diets and weight loss until ideal body weight is achieved	Low calorie, low fat, high fiber diet	Diet and sulfo-nylurea agent	3 meals Snacks not necessary
	Prevent or delay onset of micro- and macro-vascular complications	Some flexibility in timing of meals and snacks permitted	Diet and insulin	3 meals and HS snack Snacks at a.m. and p.m. often not included unless indicated, based on self-glucose-monitoring records
		Extra food usually not required to prevent hypoglycemia		

143

DESIGNING AN EXCHANGE SYSTEM MEAL PLAN: The Exchange Lists for Meal Planning (American Diabetes Association 1986) provides the most common system used to help persons with diabetes achieve consistency in timing and quantity of foods consumed. Meal plans are designed to optimize diabetes management with consideration for patient preference. Factors to consider when individualizing a meal plan include:

- Type of diabetes
- Insulin regimen
- Oral hypoglycemic agent
- Activity level/exercise pattern
- Caloric need
- Patient food preferences
- Diet history
- Nutritional adequacy of diet
- ADA recommendations for 55-60% CHO and ≤30% fat
- Self-blood-glucose-monitoring data
- Clinical laboratory values
- Medical and weight history
- Life-style with special attention to job situation, timing of meals, and methods of food preparation
- Economic status
- Attitude about nutrition and diabetes
- Knowledge/educational level
- Support system

The procedure for designing an exchange system meal plan follows a logical progression. First a dietary history is obtained and medical, nutritional, and educational needs are assessed. Next a determination is made of estimated caloric needs, using data obtained from the dietary history as well as calculations determined via a nomogram (see Appendix E) or the Harris and Benedict equation (see page 246). The third step is to formulate realistic goals for diabetes diet management which are acceptable to the patient, physician, and other health care team members. From this a meal plan is developed by distributing exchanges into meals and snacks. It is then recalculated, ascertaining that the calories, carbohydrate, protein, and fat are distributed appropriately.

After discussing both long- and short-term goals with the patient, adjustments may be made to assure patient compliance for optimal diabetes management. The goals may need to be modified to achieve a practical level of control.

Finally, learning strategies and experiences selected to meet the needs and abilities of the individual patient are implemented. Ongoing evaluation of the suitability of the meal plan and of the patient's educational progress is essential.

Documentation in the patient record of both the meal plan and the patient's nutritional goals will facilitate follow-up and reinforcement by other health team members.

NUTRIENT VALUES OF EXCHANGES

Exchange List	Carbohydrate (g)	Protein (g)	Fat (g)	Calories
Starch/Bread	15	3	trace[a]	80
Meat				
Lean	--	7	3	55
Medium fat[b]	--	7	5	75
High fat	--	7	8	100
Vegetable	5	2	--	25
Fruit	15	--	--	60
Milk				
Skim	12	8	trace[a]	90
Lowfat	12	8	5	120
Whole	12	8	8	150
Fat	--	--	5	45

[a]A value of 1 is used in calculations.

[b]Generally the values for medium fat meats are used in calculating meal patterns assuming an average for a variety of different types of meat.

EXAMPLES OF DISTRIBUTION PATTERNS USING ADA FOOD EXCHANGE LISTS

		1000 Calories	1200 Calories	1500 Calories	1800 Calories	2000 Calories	2200 Calories	2500 Calories
B	Bread	1	2	2	2	3	3	3
R E	Meat	0	0	0	1	1	1	1
A K	Fruit	1	1	1	1	1	2	2
F A S	Skim milk	1	1	1	1	1	1	1
T	Fat	1	1	1	2	2	2	2
L U	Bread	1	1	2/1	3/2	3/2	3	4
N C	Meat	2	2/3	2/3	2/3	3	3	3
H /	Vegetable	1/2	1/2	1/2	1/2	2	2	2
D I	Fruit	1/0	1	1	1/2	1/2	1/2	2
N N	Skim milk	1/2-1/2	1/2-1/2	1	1	1	1	1
E R	Fat	0/1	0/1	2/1	1/2	1/2	2	3
	Total Calories	1005	1220	1480	1820	2003	2185	2495
CHO, g		114	144	171	216	236	266	311
Pro, g		59	69	80	93	105	108	114
Fat, g		35	41	53	65	71	77	89
%CHO		45	47	46	48	47	48	50
%Pro		24	23	22	50	21	20	18
%Fat		31	30	32	32	32	32	32

Note: Until a patient interview has been completed, meals will be selected according to these patterns. The 1800-calorie pattern, including an evening snack, will be served to any patient who arrives at mealtime without a diet prescription. An appropriate diet order should be written by the physician before the next meal.

Exchanges	1000 Calories	1200 Calories	1500 Calories	1800 Calories	2000 Calories	2200 Calories	2500 Calories
Bread	3	4	5	7	8	9	11
Meat	4	5	5	6	7	7	7
Vegetable	3	3	3	3	4	4	4
Fruit	2	3	3	4	4	5	6
Skim milk	2	2	3	3	3	3	3
Fat	2	2	4	5	5	6	8
Total Calories	1007	1221	1481	1821	2003	2189	2501
CHO, g	114	144	171	216	236	266	311
Pro, g	59	69	80	93	105	108	114
Fat, g	35	41	53	65	71	77	89
%CHO	45	47	46	48	47	48	50
%Pro	24	23	22	20	21	20	18
%Fat	31	30	32	32	32	32	32

1. Starch/Bread List

Each exchange contains approximately 15 g carbohydrates, 3 g protein, a trace of fat, and 80 calories. Whole grain products average about 2 g fiber per serving. Those foods that contain 3 or more grams of fiber per serving are identified with the fiber symbol §.

Cereals/Grains/Pasta

§Bran cereals, concentrated	1/3 cup
§Bran cereals, flaked	1/2 cup
Bulgur, cooked	1/2 cup
Cooked cereals	1/2 cup
Cornmeal, dry	2 1/2 tbsp
Grapenuts	3 tbsp
Other ready-to-eat unsweetened cereals	3/4 cup
Pasta, cooked	1/2 cup
Puffed cereal	1 1/2 cups
Rice, white or brown, cooked	1/3 cup
Shredded wheat	1/2 cup
§Wheat germ	3 tbsp

Dried Beans/Peas/Lentils

§Beans and peas, cooked (such as kidney, white, split, black-eye)	1/3 cup
§Lentils, cooked	1/3 cup
§Baked beans	1/4 cup

Starchy Vegetables

§Corn	1/2 cup
§Corn-on-the-cob (6 in. long)	1
§Lima beans	1/2 cup
§Peas, canned or frozen	1/2 cup
§Plantain	1/2 cup
Potato, baked	1 small (3 oz)
Potato, mashed	1/2 cup
Squash, winter (acorn, butternut)	3/4 cup
Yam, sweet potato, plain	1/3 cup

Bread

Bagel	1/2 (1 oz)
Bread sticks, crisp (4 in. x 1/2 in.)	2 (2/3 oz)
Croutons, lowfat	1 cup
English muffin, medium	1/2
Hot dog or hamburger bun	1/2 (1 oz)
Pita (6 in. diam)	1/2
Plain roll, small	1 (1 oz)
Raisin, unfrosted	1 slice (1 oz)
§Rye, pumpernickel	1 slice (1 oz)
Tortilla (6 in. diam)	1
White, whole wheat, vienna, french, italian	1 slice (1 oz)

Crackers/Snacks

Animal crackers	8
Graham crackers (2 1/2 in. sq)	3
Matzoh	3/4 oz
Melba toast	5 slices
Oyster crackers	24
Popcorn (popped, large kernel, no fat added)	3 cups
Pretzels	3/4 oz
Rye Crisp (2 in. x 3 1/2 in.)	4
Saltine-type crackers	6
Whole wheat crackers, no fat added (crisp breads such as Finn, Kavli, Wasa)	2-4 slices (3/4 oz)

Starch Foods Prepared With Fat
   (Count as 1 starch/bread plus 1 fat)

Biscuit (2 1/2 in. diam)	1
Chow mein noodles	1/2 cup
Corn bread (2 in. cube)	1 (2 oz)
Cracker, round butter-type	6
French fried potatoes (2 to 3 1/2 in. long)	10 (1 1/2 oz)
Muffin, plain, small	1
Pancake (4 in. diam)	2
Stuffing, bread (prepared)	1/4 cup
Taco shell (6 in. diam)	2
Waffle (4 1/2 in. sq)	1
Whole wheat crackers, fat added (such as Triscuits)	4-6 (1 oz)

2. Meat List

Each exchange contains approximately 7 g protein. The list is divided into 3 parts based on the amount of fat and calories: lean meat, medium fat meat, and high fat meat. One ounce (1 meat exchange) contains:

	Carbohydrate (g)	Protein (g)	Fat (g)	Calories
Lean	0	7	3	55
Medium Fat	0	7	5	75
High Fat	0	7	8	100

Lean Meat and Substitutes

Beef	USDA good or choice grades of lean beef such as round, sirloin, and flank steak; tenderloin; and chipped beef	1 oz
Pork	Lean pork such as fresh ham; canned, cured, or boiled ham, canadian bacon, tenderloin	1 oz
Veal	All except veal cutlets (ground or cubed)	1 oz
Poultry	Chicken, turkey, cornish hen (without skin)	1 oz
Fish	All fresh and frozen fish	1 oz
	Crab, lobster, scallops, shrimp, clams (fresh or canned in water)	2 oz
	Oysters	6 medium
	Tuna (canned in water)	1/4 cup
	Herring (uncreamed or smoked)	1 oz
	Sardines (canned)	2 medium
Wild Game	Venison, rabbit, squirrel	1 oz
	Pheasant, duck, goose (without skin)	1 oz
Cheese	Any cottage cheese	1/4 cup
	Grated parmesan	2 tbsp
	Diet cheeses (with less than 55 calories per ounce)	1 oz
Other	95% fat-free luncheon meat	1 oz
	Egg whites	3
	Egg substitutes with less than 55 calories per 1/4 cup	1/4 cup

Medium Fat Meat and Substitutes

Beef	Most beef products such as ground beef, roast (rib, chuck rump), steak (cubed, porterhouse, T-bone), and meatloaf	1 oz
Pork	Most pork products such as chops, loin roast, boston butt, cutlets	1 oz
Lamb	Most lamb products such as chops, leg, and roast	1 oz
Poultry	Chicken (with skin), domestic duck or goose (well-drained of fat), ground turkey	1 oz

Fish	Tuna (canned in oil and drained)	1/4 cup
	Salmon (canned)	1/4 cup
Cheese	Skim or part-skim milk cheese such as:	
	Ricotta	1/4 cup
	Mozzarella	1 oz
	Diet cheeses (with 56-80 calories per ounce)	1 oz
Other	86% fat-free luncheon meat	1 oz
	Egg	1
	Egg substitutes with 56-80 calories per 1/4 cup	1/4 cup
	Tofu (2 1/2 in. x 2 3/4 in. x 1 in.)	4 oz
	Liver, heart, kidney, sweetbreads	1 oz

High Fat Meat and Substitutes

Beef	Most USDA prime cuts of beef such as ribs, corned beef	1 oz
Pork	Spareribs, ground pork, pork sausage (patty or link)	1 oz
Lamb	Patties (ground lamb)	1 oz
Fish	Any fried fish product	1 oz
Cheese	All regular cheeses, such as American, blue, cheddar, monterey, Swiss	1 oz
Other	Luncheon meat such as bologna, salami, pimento loaf	1 oz
	Sausage, such as polish, italian	1 oz
	Knockwurst, smoked	1 oz
	Bratwurst	1 oz
	Frankfurter (turkey or chicken)	1 frank (10/lb)
	Peanut butter	1 tbsp

One High Fat Meat Plus One Fat Exchange

| | Frankfurter (beef, pork, or combination) | 1 frank (10/lb) |

3. Vegetable List

Each exchange contains approximately 5 g carbohydrate, 2 g protein, 25 calories, and 2 to 3 g dietary fiber. Unless otherwise noted, one exchange is 1/2 cup cooked vegetables or vegetable juice *or* 1 cup raw vegetables.

Artichoke (1/2 medium)
Asparagus
Beans (green, wax, italian)
Bean sprouts
Beets
Broccoli
Brussels sprouts
Cabbage, cooked
Carrots

VEGETABLE LIST (continued):

      Cauliflower
      Eggplant
      Greens (collard, mustard, turnip)
      Kohlrabi
      Leeks
      Mushrooms, cooked
      Okra
      Onions
      Pea pods
      Peppers (green)
      Rutabaga
      Sauerkraut
      Spinach, cooked
      Summer squash (crookneck)
      Tomato (1 large)
      Tomato/vegetable juice
      Turnips
      Water chestnuts
      Zucchini, cooked

4. Fruit List

Each exchange contains approximately 15 g carbohydrate and 60 calories. Fresh, frozen, and dried fruits have about 2 g fiber per serving. Fruits that have 3 or more grams of fiber per serving are identified with the symbol §. Unless otherwise noted, 1 exchange is 1/2 cup fresh fruit or fruit juice *or* 1/4 cup dried fruit.

<u>Fresh, Frozen, and Unsweetened Canned Fruit</u>

Apple, fresh	1 small (2 1/2 in. diam)
Applesauce	1/2 cup
Apricots, fresh	2 medium
Apricots, canned	1/2 cup or 4 halves
Banana (9 in. long)	1/2
§Blackberries, fresh	3/4 cup
§Blueberries, fresh	3/4 cup
Cantaloupe (5 in. diam)	1/3 melon
Cantaloupe, cubed	1 cup
Cherries, large	12
Cherries, canned	1/2 cup
Figs, fresh (2 in. diam)	2
Fruit cocktail, canned	1/2 cup
Grapefruit, fresh (4 in. diam)	1/2
Grapefruit sections	3/4 cup
Grapes, small	15
Honeydew melon, medium	1/8 melon
Honeydew, cubed	1 cup
Kiwi, large	1
Mandarin oranges	3/4 cup
Mango, small	1/2
§Nectarine, fresh (1 1/2 in. diam)	1
Orange, fresh (2 1/2 in. diam)	1
Papaya, cubed	1 cup
Peach, fresh (2 3/4 in. diam)	1 or 3/4 cup
Peaches, canned	1/2 cup or 2 halves

Fresh, Frozen, and Unsweetened Canned Fruit (continued):

Pear, fresh	1/2 large or 1 small
Pears, canned	1/2 cup or 2 halves
Persimmon (native)	2 medium
Pineapple, fresh	3/4 cup
Pineapple, canned	1/3 cup
Plum, fresh (2 in. diam)	2
§Pomegranate, fresh (3 1/2 in. diam)	1/2
§Raspberries, fresh	1 cup
§Strawberries, fresh, whole	1 1/4 cup
Tangerine, fresh (2 1/2 in. diam)	2
Watermelon, cubed	1 1/4 cup

Dried Fruit

§Apples	4 rings
§Apricots	7 halves
Dates	2 1/2 medium
§Figs	1 1/2
§Prunes	3 medium
Raisins	2 tbsp

Fruit Juice

Apple juice/cider	1/2 cup
Cranberry juice cocktail	1/3 cup
Grapefruit juice	1/2 cup
Grape juice	1/3 cup
Orange juice	1/2 cup
Nectar	
Apricot	1/2 cup
Peach	1/2 cup
Pear	1/2 cup
Pineapple juice	1/2 cup
Prune juice	1/3 cup

5. Milk List

Each milk exchange contains approximately 12 g carbohydrate and 8 g protein. The list is divided into 3 parts based on the amount of fat and calories: skim/very lowfat milk, lowfat milk, and whole milk. One milk exchange contains:

	Carbohydrate (g)	Protein (g)	Fat (g)	Calories
Skim/Very Lowfat	12	8	trace	90
Lowfat	12	8	5	120
Whole	12	8	8	150

Skim and Very Lowfat Milk

Skim milk	1 cup
1/2% milk	1 cup
1% milk	1 cup
Lowfat buttermilk	1 cup
Evaporated skim milk	1/2 cup
Dry nonfat milk	1/3 cup

Plain nonfat yogurt	8 oz

Lowfat Milk

2% milk	1 cup
Plain lowfat yogurt (with added nonfat milk solids)	8 oz

Whole Milk

Whole milk	1 cup
Evaporated whole milk	1/2 cup
Whole plain yogurt	8 oz

6. Fat List

Each exchange contains approximately 5 g fat and 45 calories.

Unsaturated Fats

Avocado	1/8 medium
Margarine	1 tsp
Margarine, diet	1 tbsp
Mayonnaise	1 tsp
Mayonnaise, reduced-calorie	1 tbsp
Nuts and Seeds:	
Almonds, dry roasted	6 whole
Cashews, dry roasted	1 tbsp
Pecans	2 whole
Peanuts	20 small or 10 large
Walnuts	2 whole
Other nuts	1 tbsp
Seeds, pine nuts, sunflower (without shells)	1 tbsp
Pumpkin seeds	2 tsp
Oil (corn, cottonseed, safflower, soybean, sunflower, olive, peanut)	1 tsp
Olives	10 small or 5 large
Salad dressing, mayonnaise-type	2 tsp
Salad dressing, mayonnaise-type, reduced-calorie	1 tbsp
Salad dressing (most varieties)	1 tbsp
Salad dressing, reduced-calorie	2 tbsp

Saturated Fats

Butter	1 tsp
Bacon	1 slice
Chitterlings	1/2 oz
Coconut, shredded	2 tbsp
Coffee whitener, liquid	2 tbsp
Coffee whitener, powder	4 tsp
Cream (light, coffee, table)	2 tbsp
Cream, sour	2 tbsp
Cream (heavy, whipping)	1 tbsp
Cream cheese	1 tbsp
Salt pork	1/4 oz

Free Foods

A free food is any food or drink that contains less than 20 calories per serving. Two or three of those items with serving size specified are allowed per day.

Drinks

Bouillon or broth without fat
Bouillon, low sodium
Carbonated drinks, sugar-free
Carbonated water
Club soda
Cocoa powder, unsweetened (1 tbsp)
Coffee/tea
Drink mixes, sugar-free
Tonic water, sugar-free

Nonstick Pan Spray

Combination Foods

Average exchange values for combination foods which fit into more than one exchange list are as follows:

Food	Amount	Exchanges
Casseroles, homemade	1 cup (8 oz)	2 starch, 2 medium fat meat, 1 fat
Cheese pizza, thin crust	1/4 of 15 oz or 1/4 of 10 in. diam	2 starch, 1 medium fat meat, 1 fat
§Chili with beans (commercial)	1 cup (8 oz)	2 starch, 2 medium fat meat, 2 fat
Chow mein (without noodles or rice)	2 cups (16 oz)	1 starch, 2 vegetable, 2 lean meat
Macaroni and cheese	1 cup (8 oz)	2 starch, 1 medium fat meat, 2 fat
Soup		
§Bean	1 cup (8 oz)	1 starch, 1 vegetable, 1 lean meat
Chunky, all varieties	10 3/4 oz can	1 starch, 1 vegetable, 1 medium fat meat
Cream (made with water)	1 cup (8 oz)	1 starch, 1 fat
Vegetable or broth	1 cup (8 oz)	1 starch
Spaghetti and meatballs (canned)	1 cup (8 oz)	2 starch, 1 medium fat meat, 1 fat
Sugar-free pudding (made with skim milk)	1/2 cup	1 starch
If Beans Are Used as a Meat Substitute		
§Dried beans, peas, lentils	1 cup (cooked)	2 starch, 1 lean meat

§3 grams or more of fiber per serving.

Foods for Occasional Use

Foods containing high amounts of sugar and fat should be used no more than 2 to 3 times/week. Exchanges for these foods are as follows:

Food	Amount	Exchanges
Angel food cake	1/12 cake	2 starch
Cake, no icing	1/12 cake, or a 3-in. square	2 starch, 2 fat
Cookies	2 small (1 3/4 in. diam)	1 starch, 1 fat
Frozen fruit yogurt	1/3 cup	1 starch
Gingersnaps	3	1 starch
Granola	1/4 cup	1 starch, 1 fat
Granola bar	1 small	1 starch, 1 fat
Ice cream, any flavor	1/2 cup	1 starch, 2 fat
Ice milk, any flavor	1/2 cup	1 starch, 1 fat
Sherbet, any flavor	1/4 cup	1 starch
Snack chips, all varieties	1 oz	1 starch, 2 fat
Vanilla wafers	6 small	1 starch, 1 fat

The exchange lists are the basis of a meal planning system designed by a committee of the American Diabetes Association and the American Dietetic Association. While designed primarily for people with diabetes and others who must follow special diets, the exchange lists are based on principles of good nutrition that apply to everyone.

B. DIETS FOR WEIGHT LOSS

DESCRIPTION: When diets are prescribed for weight loss, calories are reduced below the level necessary for maintenance of present body weight. At the same time, the intake of protein, vitamins, and minerals remains at or above the levels recommended by the National Research Council. The aim is to provide a diet tailored to the needs of the individual that will promote utilization of stored body fat for energy without causing excessive loss of lean body mass.

An estimated 26% of the adult population in the United States is overweight or obese. Obesity is defined as a body fat content of 25% or more in the male and greater than 30% in the female. Overweight signifies a body weight above an arbitrary standard, usually defined in relation to height.

Obesity and overweight are associated with increased risk of hypertension, hyperlipidemia, cardiovascular disease, gout, diabetes, arthritis, and surgical complications. Many undesirable social and psychological consequences occur as well.

Ideal Body Weight. The concept of ideal body weight is derived from data in which relative weight has been correlated with mortality. The Metropolitan Life Insurance Company tables are commonly used to determine desirable weight for height. The body mass index (weight in kilograms divided by height in meters squared) is also a convenient determination of desirable weight for height, and can be calculated without the use of tables. The National Health and Nutrition Examination Survey II used the following definitions for desirable body weight, overweight, and severe overweight:

CORRELATION OF BODY MASS INDEX
WITH WEIGHT LEVELS
[Body Mass Index (kg/m^2)]

	Desirable Body Weight	20% Excess Weight	40% Excess Weight
Men	22.7	27.8	31.1
Women	21.1	27.3	32.3

Another method often used for estimating desirable body weight is:

Women

100 pounds for the first
  5 feet of height, plus
  5 pounds for each
  additional inch

Men

106 pounds for the first
  5 feet of height, plus
  6 pounds for each
  additional inch

Determining Caloric Need. Determination of caloric need is used to anticipate the rate of loss and assist in planning long-term goals. A calorie deficit of 500 to 1000 calories per day which allows for a weight loss of 1 to 2 pounds per week is recommended.

The best methods for determining caloric needs consider weight (usually ideal weight if it can be decided), height, age, sex, and activity. Another influential factor is individual metabolic rate. The nomogram (see Appendix E) and Harris and Benedict equation (see page 246) are preferable, as they consider most of the factors known to influence caloric need. The following formula can be used to quickly determine caloric need for adults:

Basal requirement + activity requirement = caloric need

Daily basal requirement = 1 cal x ___ kg ideal body weight x 24 hours

Activity requirement: 20% of basal if very sedentary
30% of basal if sedentary
40% of basal if moderately active
50% of basal if very active

The estimated caloric need for maintenance is then compared with the caloric intake calculated from a thorough diet history.

Selecting a Diet Plan. Several approaches are used at UIHC to attain a hypocaloric diet. In all instances, assessments are made to determine advisability of vitamin and mineral supplementation, particularly at levels of less than 1200 kcal/day.

Exchange System. A balanced exchange system meal plan is designed based on individual preferences for a predetermined number of calories. An advantage of this method is the presumed development of good eating habits. A disadvantage is the time necessary to learn the system. Refer to pages 144-54 for additional information on the exchange lists for meal planning.

Calorie Counting. This method works well for the patient/client who has established good eating habits. He or she can then keep a diet diary and calculate calories on a daily basis.

Semistarvation. A very low calorie diet (200 to 600 kcal/day) results in significant physiological and biochemical changes. It should be carried out only with proper management and careful medical supervision. This approach to weight reduction may be desirable initially to enhance motivation, or when extensive weight loss is critical for patients with serious medical problems.

Protein-Sparing-Modified Fast (solid food version). The rationale for this diet is that high quality protein will minimize the loss of lean muscle mass. Close medical supervision is required. The diet prescription is 1.0 to 1.5 g protein per kilogram ideal body weight, very low fat, and minimal carbohydrate. The only fat present in the diet is that found in fish, poultry, or other lowfat protein foods. Carbohydrate is obtained from 3 or more servings of low calorie vegetables, included to promote compliance.

Specific Changes in Eating Habits. In some cases a significant number of calories can be eliminated by making changes in eating habits, without a "diet" per se. For example, a person drinking 4 cans of regular soda pop per day could eliminate 600 calories by altering that one behavior alone. Specific changes of this type can become well-defined attainable goals for the motivated individual.

Exercise and Behavior Modification. Successful weight management programs are those which include exercise and behavior modification techniques as well as a hypocaloric diet. The incorporation of exercise must be individualized according to motivational level and physical health. Assistance in determining physical activities that will be satisfying can be helpful, since enjoyable exercise routines tend to promote compliance. Obviously, exercise is a more significant variable in the younger person with only mild to moderate obesity than with the older individual who has other physical ailments. In any case, exercise is an important variable which should be included in weight management programs.

Behavior modification is based on the premise that behavior is controlled by environmental events that act as cues or stimuli and reinforcement. In weight management the emphasis is on changing behavior in order to decrease caloric consumption and increase physical activity. Generally, the use of behavior modification involves four steps:

1. Identifying the behavior to be changed

2. Setting realistic goals for behavior change

3. Modifying the social and physical environment to support the behavior change

4. Reinforcing or rewarding the behavior change

In weight control programs, behaviors are identified by asking a patient to keep a diary. Information included in the diary varies from program to program but usually includes:

- Time of initiation of eating
- Time of termination of eating
- Place of eating
- Perceived mood
- Food selected
- Amount of food consumed by volume and often by calories

The information obtained is used to identify specific behaviors requiring change, as well as the stimuli and consequences controlling these behaviors. Self-monitoring does reveal patterns of behavior the patient may not have previously recognized, and frequently can produce behavior change in and of itself. For effectiveness, the recording should occur immediately after the behavior.

Appropriate goal setting involves these principles:

- Goals should be established with patient/client involvement.
- Goals should be set at a moderate level of difficulty.
- Goals should be achievable and short term.
- Goals should be written and/or publicly stated.

Behavior modification programs attempt to help people reduce environmental cues associated with inappropriate behavior. Examples related to weight loss are:

- Prepare small quantities of food and serve them on a small plate.
- Remove the refrigerator light.
- Rearrange cupboards to make problem foods difficult to see and reach.
- Establish one place in the house which is the only place to eat.
- Remove serving dishes from the table.

A goal of intervention programs is to develop immediate tangible rewards for new appropriate behaviors, since those that are positively reinforced will be repeated.

<u>Evaluating Commercial Weight Loss Programs</u>. The increasing prevalence of obesity in our country has made weight control a prime business venture. Many commercial weight loss promotions are based on unsound theories which can be detrimental to health if followed for long periods.

Satisfactory weight loss programs are those that:

1. Avoid promises of rapid weight loss (should not be substantially more than 1% of total body weight per week).

2. Provide all nutrients in adequate amounts using a balanced diet containing approximately 15% protein, 30% fat, and 55% carbohydrate.

3. Teach how to make wise choices from the conventional food supply, rather than creating dependency upon special products or supplements.

4. Do not promote diets which are extremely low in calories, unless under the supervision of competent medical experts.

5. Encourage permanent, realistic life-style changes which include regular exercise and avoid the use of food as a coping device.

6. Avoid misrepresenting salespeople as "counselors" qualified to make nutrition recommendations.

7. Do not promote unproven or spurious weight loss aids such as starch blockers, diuretics, sauna belts, body wraps, ear stapling, passive exercise, or amino acid supplements.

C. VERTICAL BANDED GASTROPLASTY (VBG) DIETS

DESCRIPTION: The VBG operation for morbid obesity limits the capacity of the stomach. Patients eat less because of this reduced capacity and because they feel "full" sooner. The feeling of satiety persists longer than it did prior to surgery.

There are three steps to the surgery. First, a circular window is made through the stomach a few inches below the esophagus. Second, a small vertical pouch is made by stapling from the window toward the esophagus. Third, a band is placed through the window, around the outlet, and fastened together. This band controls the size of the outlet into the rest of the stomach and keeps the outlet from stretching.

The surgery is performed on patients who meet the following criteria: (1) exogenous obesity at least twice ideal weight according to the 1983 Metropolitan Life Insurance Company tables; (2) age 20 to 50 years; (3) acceptable surgical risk; (4) unsuccessful previous attempts at weight loss, using a medically safe diet; and (5) motivated to lose weight and willing to make the necessary changes in eating habits.

Typically a VBG clear liquid diet is given for 1 to 2 days after surgery. Clear, nontart juices, broth, and high protein gelatin are provided at each meal. The patient is encouraged to drink fluids such as clear juice and Citrotein between meals. Total daily intake often consists of only 24 to 32 ounces.

Within 1 to 2 days after surgery, the diet is advanced to the VBG pureed which is followed for approximately 2 weeks. Pureed food is recommended because (1) it decreases the likelihood of obstruction of the stoma due to large food particles, (2) it helps to educate the patient about appropriate food consistency, since food must be chewed to that texture before swallowing, and (3) it encourages the patient to modify eating habits since a normal variety of food is consumed from the beginning. One-fourth cup cooked refined cereal and a soft cooked egg are offered at breakfast. One-fourth cup each of pureed meat or blended casserole, vegetables, and fruit are on the lunch and dinner menus. Solid food intake may not exceed 2 to 4 tablespoons per meal for several days, but larger servings are offered because of the difficulty of keeping smaller portions warm. Between-meal fluids such as skim milk, juice, and Citrotein are encouraged. Solid foods are not allowed between meals.

Daily quantities after discharge typically consist of 1 to 2 oz meat, one egg, 1/2 cup juice, 1/2 cup fruit and vegetable, 2 servings grains, and 2 cups skim milk. The texture of the diet is gradually advanced 2 weeks post discharge; however, the quantity of food consumed remains the same.

Before and after surgery the dietitian is involved in patient counseling regarding diet and eating behavior. A protein-rich (at least 25 to 30 g/day), nutrient-dense, well-balanced diet is advocated. The emphasis is on quantity and quality of food eaten, rather than calories.

Solid food should be consumed at mealtime only, 3 times a day. Liquids are specifically *not* recommended at meals or within 30 to 45 minutes before or after, because there is not space for both solid food and liquids. For hydration and a feeling of fullness without excess calories, the following fluids and amounts are recommended to be sipped between meals: 2 cups water, 2 cups skim milk, and 4 oz either fruit juice, broth, coffee, tea, or flat diet soda pop. Given the limited size of the stomach and stoma, the volume of food or fluid consumed should not exceed 30 cc/15 minutes. Patients are advised to eat slowly, chew foods well, and stop eating when full to avoid rupture of the staples, obstruction of the stoma, and/or vomiting. A 30 ml medicine cup (used as a food container) and a clock are important behavior modification aids. Foods which patients report difficulty in tolerating include tough meats; membranes of oranges or grapefruit; cores, seeds, or skins of fruits or vegetables; fibrous vegetables such as corn, celery, or sweet potatoes; bread; spicy or fried foods; popcorn or nuts; and milk.

During the first 6 weeks after surgery, weight loss averages 5 to 7 pounds per week, and continues at a rate of 1 to 2 pounds per week for several months. Energy expenditure decreases as weight loss occurs, i.e., fewer calories are burned due to a smaller body size. Caloric intake often increases due to improved tolerance of food over time and stretching of the pouch. The net result is weight maintenance, often somewhat above ideal, or in rare cases, weight gain. Counseling regarding diet and exercise is necessary to identify and correct problems in following the guidelines, so that an acceptable body weight is achieved safely.

ADEQUACY: This diet does not meet the Recommended Dietary Allowances for any nutrient. A liquid or chewable daily multiple vitamin-mineral supplement is routinely prescribed. Frank nutritional deficiencies have not occurred in patients who consume the prescribed diet and vitamin-mineral supplement. Theoretically, the diet, supplement, and patient's stores supply the nutrient requirements.

APPROXIMATE COMPOSITION OF SAMPLE MENU:

Calories	647
Protein, g	38
Fat, g	15
Carbohydrate, g	93

SAMPLE MENU FOR VERTICAL BANDED GASTROPLASTY DIET (food sent):

Breakfast	Luncheon	Dinner
1/2 cup farina	1/4 cup pureed chicken,	1/4 cup pureed beef,
1 egg, soft cooked	diluted with broth	diluted with broth
Artificial	1/4 cup pureed green beans	1/4 cup pureed carrots
sweetener	1/4 cup pureed peaches	1/4 cup pureed pears

Midmorning Nourishment	Midafternoon Nourishment	Evening Nourishment
1/2 cup skim milk	1/2 cup skim milk	1/2 cup skim milk
	1/2 cup grape juice	

DIAGRAM OF VERTICAL BANDED GASTROPLASTY

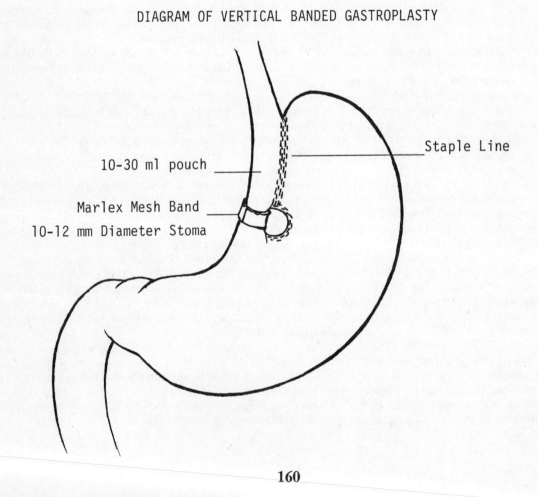

Staple Line

10-30 ml pouch

Marlex Mesh Band

10-12 mm Diameter Stoma

D. POSTGASTRECTOMY DIET

DESCRIPTION: A period of negative energy and protein balances immediately follows major gastric surgery due to postoperative catabolism and decreased oral intake. Parenteral nutrition may be advisable both before and after surgery for the patient who is nutritionally depleted. Severe nutritional depletion preoperatively is associated with increased postoperative mortality and morbidity rates. Even though healing occurs, an anastomotic site may become edematous and obstruct the lumen if protein malnutrition exists.

After an initial recovery period following surgery, oral feeding may be started. The postgastrectomy diet is designed to return the patient to an almost normal eating pattern as quickly as tolerated. Consideration is given to gastric size reduction, emptying alterations, reduction in acid secretion, and possible impairment in digestion and absorption of nutrients. The diet is individualized based on the patient's age, sex, activity level, initial disease, prior nutritional condition, and type of operation.

Dumping Syndrome. Dumping syndrome consists of fullness, nausea, sweating, flushing, rapid heart rate, diarrhea, and in rare cases, reactive hypoglycemia. The symptoms are caused by the physiological events resulting from the presence of undigested food in the jejunum. This undigested food is hypertonic, causing water to be drawn into the lumen to dilute the concentration. The extra fluid leads to intestinal distention, hyperperistalsis, and diarrhea. Hypoglycemia may occur 2 to 3 hours after eating. The rapid hydrolysis and absorption of carbohydrate cause a sudden, large increase in blood glucose. In an attempt to lower this, too much insulin may be secreted, resulting in hypoglycemia.

To decrease gastrointestinal transit time, patients are advised to eat small, low fiber meals of moderate temperature. Waiting 30 to 60 minutes after a meal to drink liquids also slows the rate at which food passes from the stomach to the intestine.

Carbohydrates, especially simple ones, are more rapidly hydrolyzed to osmotically active substances than are protein or fat. Thus the total carbohydrate in the diet should be restricted to approximately 40% of calories, primarily from complex sources. Fresh and unsweetened fruits and juices can provide 10 to 15% of total calories. The patient is advised to avoid concentrated sweets, especially in the form of sucrose, glucose, or dextrose. Protein and fat should supply approximately 20% and 40% of calories respectively. (In severe cases, carbohydrate may need to be restricted to 30% of total calories, with protein and fat supplying the other 70%.) The osmotic load is also reduced if each feeding contains sources of protein and fat as well as carbohydrate. These suggestions are consistent with the hyperinsulinism diet.

Small-Stomach Syndrome. Abdominal pain and vomiting may occur if too much food is consumed. The patient is advised to chew foods well and stop eating when full. In the first weeks after surgery, only small amounts can be taken at a time. The patient is encouraged to eat frequently, to gradually increase food quantity, and to sip liquids between meals. Within a few months, 3 meals with 2 or 3 snacks per day should be tolerated.

Postoperative Diarrhea. For a few days postsurgery, diarrhea is common. If it persists, it is important to determine and treat the cause which may be due to one or more of the following: dumping syndrome, steatorrhea, salmonella infection, gastrocolic fistula, anastomotic ulcer, blind loop syndrome with malabsorption, gluten enteropathy, and lactose intolerance. Broad spectrum antibiotics can allow overgrowth of the wrong type of intestinal flora. Yogurt or acidophilus milk may help to reestablish more compatible organisms.

Weight Loss. Many people lose weight immediately following surgery because of the reduction in stomach capacity. Eating 6 small meals per day increases caloric intake.

Two follow-up studies on patients 1 to 30 years postgastrectomy showed that continued weight loss was not significant, provided patients maintained caloric intake above the recommended daily allowance. Therefore, it is important to continually encourage patients to take frequent, small meals.

Vitamin B$_{12}$. Low serum vitamin B$_{12}$ is common after the twentieth postoperative month, but it may take as long as 3 years to deplete vitamin B$_{12}$ stores. Depending on the type and extent of surgery, lack of intrinsic factor (IF) may occur, and eventually vitamin B$_{12}$ supplementation will become necessary. The nutritional state of the patient before and after surgery will influence how soon supplementation should be started. In order to prevent pernicious anemia and serious neurological complications, vitamin B$_{12}$ injections may be required for a lifetime when IF is absent.

Iron. The major site of iron absorption is the duodenum. Although iron absorption can also occur in the ileum and jejunum, the decreased amount of gastric acid and the rapid passage of food through the small intestine often result in poor absorption. For some patients, serum iron levels may be low initially but return to normal within 6 months. Anemia responds readily to oral iron supplementation in most patients. Ascorbic acid, meat, and fish increase the absorption of non-heme iron; meat also enhances the absorption of heme iron.

Serum iron and iron-binding capacity should be studied in addition to hemoglobin level. Often iron deficiency is due to unrecognized bleeding from the gastrointestinal tract. Operative loss of blood may require temporary iron supplementation.

Vitamin A. Dietary fat is necessary for the metabolism and absorption of carotenoids and vitamin A in the intestine. Because steatorrhea is not uncommon in gastrectomized patients, vitamin A deficiency can and does occur. It can be resolved by treating the steatorrhea and providing supplemental vitamin A.

Vitamin D and Calcium. Postgastrectomy patients are at risk for calcium deficiency and eventual osteomalacia and osteoporosis for several reasons. Typical of many adults, a majority do not drink much milk. Lactose intolerance is a problem for some. Malabsorption of calcium and vitamin D also occurs. Some surgeries designed to treat morbid obesity bypass the duodenum and varying lengths of small bowel, thus predisposing the patient to depletion of bone mineral.

Several studies have been conducted to determine the calcium status of gastrectomized patients. Three to four years after surgery, no bone mineral loss or impaired calcium absorption is apparent. However, serum alkaline phosphatase and inorganic phosphorus levels are elevated, and urinary excretion of calcium is decreased. These are early signs of bone mineral depletion. Many patients manifest low bone mineral levels 10 years after surgery, but patients with total gastrectomies have low levels within 5 years. On the basis of these studies, most researchers recommend routine calcium and vitamin D supplementation for all postgastrectomy patients.

FOODS ALLOWED AND FOODS TO AVOID:

Food Group	Foods Allowed	Foods to Avoid
Beverages	Milk (3 cups); in moderation, artificially sweetened beverages, coffee, tea, decaffeinated coffee	Alcoholic beverages, sweetened carbonated beverages and drink mixes, large amounts of empty calorie fluids
Bread/Starch	Refined or whole grain, unsweetened breads, cereals, rice, pasta; potato; dried beans and peas	All others
Desserts	Custards, pudding, and gelatin sweetened with aspartame or saccharin	All others
Fats	All	None

FOODS ALLOWED AND FOODS TO AVOID (continued):

Food Group	Foods Allowed	Foods to Avoid
Fruits, Fruit Juices	(Limit to 10-15% of calories) All fresh or sweetened fruits and fruit juices	Fruits or fruit juices with added sugar
Meat, Fish, Poultry, Cheese, Eggs	All	None
Sugar, Sweets	Artificial sweeteners, aspartame	Candy, honey, jam, jelly, sugar, syrup, molasses
Vegetables, Vegetable Juices	All; the following should be counted as bread/starch exchanges: corn, lima beans, peas, potatoes, pumpkin, winter squash	None
Miscellaneous	All spices and herbs, unsweetened pickles, cocoa powder, nuts, mustard, sugar-free catsup	Sweetened pickles, catsup, gravy or cream sauces unless well tolerated

APPROXIMATE COMPOSITION OF SAMPLE MENU:

Calories	2135
Protein, g	117
Fat, g	86
Carbohydrate, g	218

SAMPLE MENU FOR POSTGASTRECTOMY DIET:

Breakfast

1/2 cup orange juice[1]
2 eggs, hard cooked
1 slice toast
1 tsp margarine

Luncheon

1/2 cup pineapple juice[1]
2 oz sliced chicken
1/2 cup rice
1/2 cup green beans
1 slice bread
1 tsp margarine

Dinner

2 oz roast beef
1/2 cup mashed potatoes
1/2 cup cooked carrots
1 tsp margarine
1/2 cup whole milk[1]

Midmorning Nourishment

1 oz cheddar cheese
6 saltine crackers
1/2 cup unsweetened applesauce
1/3 cup whole milk[1]

Midafternoon Nourishment

2 oz cold ham
2 slices bread
1 tsp mayonnaise
1/2 cup unsweetened pears
1/2 cup whole milk[1]

Evening Nourishment

1/4 cup cottage cheese
2 unsweetened peach halves
3 graham cracker squares
1/2 cup whole milk[1]

---

[1]If not tolerated with solids, fluids should be sipped slowly between meals and snacks.

E. DIET FOR HYPERINSULINISM (HYPOGLYCEMIA)

DESCRIPTION: The objective of dietary treatment of hyperinsulinism is to prevent overproduction of insulin. Since carbohydrate is the most potent stimulus to insulin secretion, sucrose and related sugars (glucose, dextrose) should be avoided. Moderate amounts of complex carbohydrates, comprising 40% of total calories, are recommended. Protein and fat should not exceed 20% and 40% of calories respectively. This distribution results in amelioration of symptoms, better compliance, and a balanced diet.

The diet should be divided into 6 small meals to allow gradual release of glucose into the blood stream. Each of the 6 feedings should contain sources of carbohydrate, protein, and fat. Since protein is also a stimulus to insulin secretion, the diet should not be excessively high in protein as was once thought advisable. In some cases, additional calories are needed from fat--preferably from polyunsaturated sources. Typically, the diabetic food exchange lists (pages 146-54) are used to help structure food choices.

ADEQUACY: This diet meets the Recommended Dietary Allowances for all nutrients, except iron for women of childbearing age.

FOODS ALLOWED AND FOODS TO AVOID:

Food Group	Foods Allowed	Foods to Avoid
Beverages	Milk (3 cups), artificially sweetened beverages, decaffeinated coffee	Alcoholic beverages, coffee, tea, sweetened carbonated beverages and drink mixes
Bread/Starch	Refined or whole grain, unsweetened breads, cereals, rice, pasta; potato; dried beans and peas	All others
Desserts	Custards, pudding, and gelatin sweetened with aspartame or saccharin	All others
Fats	All	None
Fruits, Fruit Juices	(Limit to 10-15% of calories) All fresh or unsweetened fruits and fruit juices	Fruits or fruit juices with added sugar
Meat, Fish, Poultry, Cheese, Eggs	All fresh, frozen, canned or dried meat, fish, poultry; eggs; all cheeses	Any meat, fish, or poultry with breading or sauces containing carbohydrate (unless calculated in the diet)
Sugar, Sweets	Artificial sweeteners, aspartame	Candy, honey, jam, jelly, sugar, syrup, molasses

FOODS ALLOWED AND FOODS TO AVOID (continued):

Food Group	Foods Allowed	Foods to Avoid
Vegetables, Vegetable Juices	All; the following should be counted as bread/starch exchanges: corn, lima beans, peas, potatoes, pumpkin, winter squash	None
Miscellaneous	All spices and herbs, unsweetened pickles, cocoa powder, nuts, mustard, sugar-free catsup	Sweetened pickles, catsup, gravy or cream sauces (unless calculated in the diet)

APPROXIMATE COMPOSITION OF SAMPLE MENU:

Calories	2025
Protein, g	117
Fat, g	79
Carbohydrate, g	212

SAMPLE MENU FOR HYPERINSULINISM:

Breakfast

1/2 cup orange
  juice
1/2 cup oatmeal
1 egg, soft cooked
1 slice toast,
  whole wheat
1 tsp margarine
1 cup 2% milk
Artificial
  sweetener
1 cup decaffeinated
  coffee

Luncheon

3 oz sliced chicken
1/2 cup rice
1/2 cup green beans
1 slice bread, whole wheat
1 tsp margarine
Fresh peach
1 cup 2% milk

Dinner

3 oz roast beef
1/2 cup mashed potatoes
1/2 cup cooked carrots
3/4 cup tossed lettuce salad
1 tbsp french dressing
1 slice bread, whole wheat
1 tsp margarine
1/2 cup unsweetened
  applesauce
1 cup 2% milk

Midmorning Nourishment

1/2 slice toast,
  whole wheat
1/2 oz cheese

Midafternoon Nourishment

6 saltine crackers
2 tsp peanut butter

Evening Nourishment

1 slice bread, whole wheat
1 oz ham
1 tsp margarine

F. LACTOSE RESTRICTED DIET

DESCRIPTION: This diet is designed for patients with an intolerance for lactose, the carbohydrate component of milk. The intolerance may be primary, a genetic predisposition to low levels of lactase; or secondary, a transient intolerance following diarrheal disease. Since the degree of intestinal lactase activity is highly variable, the diet should be individualized. Lactalbumin, lactate (lactic acid), and calcium compounds do not contain the disaccharide lactose and are not eliminated. All labels of food products and medication should be carefully read for addition of lactose, milk, or milk solids. Small amounts of lactose may be tolerated, especially if consumed at body temperature with other food and spaced throughout the day. The amounts of lactose in chewing gum and most commercial bakery products are not of sufficient quantity to produce symptoms. Milk in fermented form such as yogurt or cheese in which the lactose has been converted to lactic acid is sometimes tolerated. Acidophilus milk which has been treated with lactobacillus acidophilus, and milk treated with Lact-Aid[1] have been successfully used by many lactase-deficient persons.

For those patients with some degree of intolerance to small amounts of lactose, items which contain limited amounts of lactose are indicated in the center column. These foods may be used in addition to the lactose-free foods listed in the left-hand column.

ADEQUACY: This diet does not meet the Recommended Dietary Allowances for calcium, riboflavin, and vitamin D. A supplementary source of calcium, riboflavin, and vitamin D (for children) should be prescribed.

FOODS ALLOWED AND FOODS TO AVOID:

Food Group	Lactose-free Foods (allowed on all diets)	Foods Containing Lactose in Limited Amounts (allowed on some diets)	High Lactose-containing Foods (not allowed)
Beverages	Coffee, tea, carbonated beverages, nondairy creamers, soy milk substitutes and beverages	1/2 cup regular milk treated to reduce lactose[2], powdered or tableted soft drinks	Milk and milk drinks
Breads	Crackers, rusk, homemade bread without milk, french or vienna bread	Commercial bread and bread products containing milk or lactose (muffins, biscuits, pancakes)	
Cereals	All cereals except those containing milk or lactose	Instant Cream of Wheat, dry cereals containing milk or lactose	

---

[1] Sugarlo Company, Pleasantville, NJ.

[2] Examples are the sweet acidophilus milk and milk treated with Lact-Aid powder. Lact-Aid-treated milk has a greater reduction in lactose.

FOODS ALLOWED AND FOODS TO AVOID (continued):

Food Group	Lactose-free Foods (allowed on all diets)	Foods Containing Lactose in Limited Amounts (allowed on some diets)	High Lactose-containing Foods (not allowed)
Desserts	Cookies, fruit ices, fruit pies and crisps, angel food or sponge cake, gelatin desserts, homemade baked products without milk	Commercial cake mixes, sherbet, yogurt	Ice cream, custard, pudding, cream pies, cheese cake
Eggs	All except preparations containing milk	Eggs prepared with small amounts of milk	Creamed eggs
Fats	Butter, milk-free margarine, vegetable oils, lard, shortening, mayonnaise, peanut butter, bacon, milk-free salad dressings, nondairy whipped topping	Margarine, whipped cream	Salad dressing made with milk, sour cream spreads and dips, cream cheese
Fruits, Fruit Juices	All except those listed as not allowed		Fruit drinks containing lactose
Meat, Fish, Poultry, Cheese	Plain baked, broiled, roasted or stewed beef, fish, lamb, poultry, pork, or veal	Breaded foods	Creamed food, cheese and cheese products[1], cold cuts, wieners
Potatoes or Substitutes	White or sweet potato, hominy, macaroni, noodles, rice, spaghetti	Some commercial potato products	Any prepared with milk or cheese
Soups	Broth-based soups made with allowed foods		Cream soups, soups made with milk

---

[1]Certain persons are able to tolerate a limited quantity of cheese (1 oz).

FOODS ALLOWED AND FOODS TO AVOID (continued):

Food Group	Lactose-free Foods (allowed on all diets)	Foods Containing Lactose in Limited Amounts (allowed on some diets)	High Lactose-containing Foods (not allowed)
Sugars and Sweets	All except those listed as not allowed	Cream or chocolate candies, tableted candies, any commercial or homemade candies containing milk, lactose, or molasses	
Vegetables, Vegetable Juices	All except those listed as not allowed		Any prepared with milk or cheese
Miscellaneous	Popcorn, vinegar, catsup, mustard, pure flavorings, salt, pepper, herbs, and spices		Cocoa mixes with dry milk solids, cream sauce, nonfat dry milk

APPROXIMATE COMPOSITION OF SAMPLE MENU:

Calories	1992
Protein, g	70
Fat, g	54
Carbohydrate, g	309

SAMPLE MENU FOR LACTOSE-FREE DIET:

Breakfast	Luncheon	Dinner
1/2 cup orange juice	2 oz sliced chicken	3 oz roast beef
1/2 cup farina	1/2 cup rice	1/2 cup cubed white potato
1 egg, soft cooked	1/2 cup green beans	1/4 cup beef broth gravy
1 slice vienna bread toasted	1/2 sliced tomato on lettuce	1/2 cup cooked carrots
2 tsp milk-free margarine	2 tsp mayonnaise	3/4 cup tossed lettuce salad
1 tbsp grape jelly	1 slice vienna bread	1 tbsp french dressing
2 tsp sugar	2 tsp milk-free margarine	1 slice vienna bread
Coffee or tea	1/2 cup canned peaches	2 tsp milk-free margarine
	1 slice angel food cake	Small banana
	1 tsp sugar	1 tsp sugar
	Coffee or tea	Coffee or tea

	Midafternoon Nourishment	Evening Nourishment
	1 cup 7-Up	1 cup apricot nectar

SECTION 6

Other Restricted Diets

A. FOOD ALLERGIES

DESCRIPTION: In the management of allergies, food may be influential when (1) elimination diets are used as a tool for diagnosis and (2) dietary modification is necessary to remove the allergen(s) from the patient's environment.

One of four procedures for suspected food allergy is used at the University of Iowa Hospitals and Clinics, depending upon the individual patient:

1. The most common allergens are eliminated from the diet immediately such as nuts, seafoods, and metabisulfites.

2. An elimination test diet is used to determine the origin of the suspected allergen(s). The Animal Protein Test Diet is used first and then the Plant Protein Test Diet.

3. A more severe elimination diet consisting mainly of chicken and rice, or lamb is begun, adding a new food every 2 to 3 days.

4. The most rigid elimination diet is the elemental diet (e.g., Tolerex) which contains L-amino acids rather than proteins.

This manual includes the Animal Protein Test Diet, the Plant Protein Test Diet, the Chicken-Rice or Lamb Diet, the Wheat Test Diet (use the Gluten Restricted Diet on pages 179-81), and the Milk-free Test Diet (a modified Lactose Restricted Diet allowing lactose but not milk).

The widely published Rowe elimination diets exclude foods that most frequently cause food allergy. These diets are divided into four categories. The usual procedure is to eliminate foods from category one. If symptoms persist, the patient proceeds to the second category, and if necessary, to the third and fourth categories. The first category eliminates the use of beef, pork, poultry, milk and milk products, rye, corn, legumes, and potatoes. The second category eliminates beef, lamb, legumes, milk and milk products, rice, and potatoes. The third category eliminates lamb, poultry, corn, rice, rye, and milk and milk products. The fourth category consists of milk, tapioca, and cane sugar. Foods are generally added one by one to the fourth category until symptoms reappear and the allergen is identified.

An elemental formula (see pages 294-95) may be used for the patient suffering from severe food allergy symptoms or for whom the elimination diets fail to isolate the allergen(s). This diet regimen effectively eliminates all food allergens, which can then be more easily identified as they are reintroduced into the diet.

Upon diagnosis of a particular food allergy, the patient must learn to recognize products and labeling terms related to the allergen. Terms relating to common food allergens can be found in the chart on page 170. Composition of manufactured products is subject to change, requiring that labels be checked carefully. Because foods with a standard of identity may lack a label listing ingredients, a chart listing foods that may contain these common allergens is included on pages 170-71.

ADEQUACY: The nutritive adequacy depends upon the number and type of food sensitivities.

169

TERMS INDICATING THE PRESENCE OF COMMON ALLERGENS:

Common Allergen	Terms	Common Allergen	Terms

Milk	Casein
	Caseinate
	Casein hydrolysate
	DMS (dried milk solids)
	Lactalbumin
	Lactate solids
	Milk solid pastes
	Sweetened condensed milk
	Whey or whey solids
		Legume	Food gums from the legume family:
			  Acacia gum
			  Arabic gum
			  Carob
			  Haraya gum
			  Locust bean gum
			  Tragacanth
			Hydrolyzed vegetable protein
			Soy concentrate
			Soy protein
			Soya flour
			TVP (textured vegetable protein)
			Vegetable protein concentrate

Egg	Albumin Dried egg solids Globulin Ovomucin Vitellin		
Corn	Corn solids Cornstarch Corn syrup Vegetable starch		

STANDARDS OF IDENTITY: These Standard of Identity foods contain a particular ingredient that may cause an allergic reaction in certain individuals but may lack a label listing ingredients.

Food Group	Wheat ✓	Corn	Eggs ✓	Soybean ✓	Milk ✓
Beverages	Whiskey	Bourbon whiskey			Milk, cream
Breads	Raisin and whole wheat breads and rolls	White, raisin, and whole wheat breads and rolls	Raisin and whole wheat breads and rolls	Raisin and whole wheat breads and rolls	Raisin and whole wheat breads and rolls
Candies, sweets			Nougat, kisses, frappés, marshmallows	Nougat, kisses, frappés, marshmallows	Fudge, caramels, chocolates
Cereal Products	Farina	Grits			
Cheese					Standards allow some cheeses to be made from goat or cow milk
Dressings	Salad dressings	Salad dressings, mayonnaise	Salad dressings, mayonnaise		

170

Standards of Identity (continued):

Food Group	Wheat	Corn	Eggs	Soybean	Milk
Fish	Breaded	Breaded		Tuna packed in soy oil	
Flours	Phosphated wheat	Corn, cornmeal			
Fruits, Fruit Drinks		Canned with corn syrup			
Ice Creams, Sherbets		Includes corn syrup solids	French style creams, ice creams, sherbets		Ice creams, sherbets, ice milk
Jams		Jellies and jams using corn syrup			
Macaroni Products	Semolina		Noodles		Macaroni products
Sauces, Condiments		Catsup			
Spreads				Peanut butter, margarine	Margarine
Vegetables	Generic canned green beans, peas, corn			Canned green beans, peas, corn	Vegetables in sauces
Miscellaneous				Lecithin (may be found in frozen sauces containing milk or egg)	Chocolate products

1. Animal Protein Test Diet

DESCRIPTION: Foods in this diet contain protein from animal sources only. All foods containing protein from vegetable sources are omitted. Any food to which the patient has a known and definite sensitivity must of course be omitted.

FOODS ALLOWED AND FOODS TO AVOID:

Food Group	Foods Allowed	Foods to Avoid
Beverages	Coffee, tea, milk, cream	Fruit juices, cereal, beverages

FOODS ALLOWED AND FOODS TO AVOID (continued):

Food Group	Foods Allowed	Foods to Avoid
Breads	Arrowroot cookies	All others
Cereals	Arrowroot starch only	All others
Desserts	Arrowroot pudding (caramel), junket (vanilla, caramel), baked or stirred custard (butterscotch, caramel, vanilla), gelatins without added fruit or fruit juice	All others
Eggs	Baked, soft or hard cooked, poached, fried in animal fats only	Any prepared with vegetable fats
Fats	Lard, bacon fat, chicken fat, any meat fat	Vegetable fats or oils
Fruits, Fruit Juices	None	All
Meat, Fish, Poultry, Cheese	All plain meats, fish, poultry, and unprocessed cheese	Meat, fish, or poultry with breadings, batters, or containing cereal products; processed cheese containing vegetable gums
Potatoes or Substitutes	None	All
Sugar, Sweets	Refined sugar	All others
Soups	Meat soups thickened only with arrowroot	Any vegetable or cereal additions
Vegetables, Vegetable Juices	None	All
Miscellaneous	Salt, small amount of pepper	Nuts, peanut butter, chili sauce, catsup, spices (except small amount of pepper), herbs

APPROXIMATE COMPOSITION OF SAMPLE MENU:

Calories	2419
Protein, g	166
Fat, g	117
Carbohydrate, g	172

SAMPLE MENU FOR ANIMAL PROTEIN TEST DIET:

Breakfast	Luncheon	Dinner
1 egg, soft cooked	3 oz sliced chicken	2 oz roast beef
3 bacon strips	1/2 cup cottage cheese	1/2 cup beef broth
4 arrowroot cookies	4 arrowroot cookies	4 arrowroot cookies
1 tsp butter	1 tsp butter	1 tsp butter
1 cup milk	1 cup junket	1 cup flavored gelatin
1 tsp sugar	1 cup milk	cubes with
1 oz cream	1 tsp sugar	1/4 cup custard sauce
Coffee or tea	1 oz cream	1 cup milk
	Coffee or tea	1 tsp sugar
		1 oz cream
		Coffee or tea

2. Vegetable Protein Test Diet

DESCRIPTION: Foods in this diet contain protein from vegetable sources only. All foods containing protein from animal sources are omitted. Any food to which the patient has a known and definite sensitivity must, of course, be omitted.

FOODS ALLOWED AND FOODS TO AVOID:

Food Group	Foods Allowed	Foods to Avoid
Beverages	Tea, coffee, fruit juices, soybean milk	Milk or milk drinks
Breads	All breads, crackers, and hot breads that do not contain milk, eggs, or animal fats	All others containing milk, eggs, or animal fats
Cereals	All that do not contain animal protein	Dry cereals containing dried milk
Desserts	Fruit, puddings made with fruit and thickened with cornstarch or tapioca, fruit pies and baked goods made with vegetable shortening, fruit ices made without gelatin or egg whites	Any containing cream, eggs, animal fats, milk, or gelatin
Eggs	None	All
Fats	Vegetable fats and oils, margarine free of animal fat and protein	Butter, mixed margarine, any meat fat, mayonnaise or salad dressing containing egg or milk
Fruits, Fruit Juices	All fresh, frozen, canned, dried	None

FOODS ALLOWED AND FOODS TO AVOID (continued):

Food Group	Foods Allowed	Foods to Avoid
Meat, Fish, Poultry, Cheese	Soybean foods	All others
Potatoes or Substitutes	Baked, broiled, fried, and steamed potatoes	Noodles; all foods prepared with or containing milk, cheese, or animal fat
Sugar, Sweets	Sugar, jam, jelly, marmalade, honey, syrup	Those containing butter, gelatin, or egg
Soups	Vegetable soup made without meat stock	Meat, cream, egg, cheese, or noodle soups
Vegetables, Vegetable Juices	All fresh, frozen, canned, and dried	None
Miscellaneous	Peanut butter, nuts, salt, pepper, spices, herbs	Seasoned sauces containing animal products

APPROXIMATE COMPOSITION OF SAMPLE MENU:

Calories	1664
Protein, g	44
Fat, g	60
Carbohydrate, g	241

SAMPLE MENU FOR VEGETABLE PROTEIN TEST DIET:

Breakfast	Luncheon	Dinner
1/2 cup orange juice	2 tbsp peanut butter	3 oz soy "meat" analog
1/2 cup farina	1 baked potato	1/2 cup cubed white potato
1 slice vienna bread, toasted	1/2 cup green beans	1/2 cup cooked carrots
1 tsp milk-free margarine	1/2 sliced tomato on lettuce	3/4 cup tossed lettuce salad
1 tbsp grape jelly	1 slice vienna bread	1 tbsp french dressing
2 tsp sugar	2 tsp milk-free margarine	1 slice vienna bread
Coffee or tea	1/2 cup canned peaches	1 tsp milk-free margarine
	Puffed rice bar	1 tsp sugar
	1 tsp sugar	Coffee or tea
	Coffee or tea	

3. Chicken-Rice or Lamb Diet

DESCRIPTION: Allergies to cereals and/or fruits may be identified by either of these diets. The diet is followed for 1 to 2 weeks and consists *only* of the following foods:

Chicken-Rice	Lamb
Chicken	Lamb
Turkey	White potato
Rice	Pearl tapioca
Pearl tapioca	Carrots
Cottonseed oil	Peas

Chicken-Rice (continued:)	Lamb (continued:)
Sesame seed oil	Cottonseed oil
Salt	Sesame seed oil
Sugar	Salt
Water	Sugar
Soy-based formulas, if	Water
tolerated	Soy-based formulas, if
	tolerated

Allergies to chicken, rice, potato, and/or cottonseed may be suspected if the patient does not improve, and other sources of allergy have been ruled out. If symptoms subside, the diet is continued for 2 weeks. When the patient is symptom-free, peas and squash are added to the chicken-rice diet; potatoes and squash, to the lamb diet. Other fruits, vegetables, cereals, and milk are added (one at a time, several days apart), until symptoms reappear. The problematic food is then identified and retested at later intervals.

Other sources of potential allergens which should not be used during the elimination diets include flavored mouthwashes, toothpaste, denture fixatives, and chewing gum. The patient should also be cautioned against using over-the-counter medications during the trial diet period without consulting the physician.

4. Salicylate Restricted Diet (Tartrazine Restricted)

DESCRIPTION: In general, patients who are allergic to salicylates need eliminate only aspirin (acetyl salicylic acid) and tartrazine which are ordinarily responsible for such adverse reactions as urticaria and/or bronchospasms. The amount of sodium salicylates or other salicylates *naturally* found in foods is negligible, not enough to cause symptoms.

Tartrazine, also known as F.D. & C. yellow number 5, is a certified coloring dye used in foods, drugs, fabrics, and cosmetics to produce yellow, orange, green, or red tints. Although some controversy exists regarding the extent of cross-sensitivity of patients to aspirin and tartrazine, the consensus is that most patients who require salicylate restriction should also avoid tartrazine. Federal law now requires manufacturers to identify tartrazine on food labels. Because the composition of manufactured products is subject to change, brand names of commercial products containing salicylate and/or tartrazine are not listed here. Labels should be checked carefully. See the chart on page 176 for foods which may contain tartrazine.

The amount of salicylates used as *additives* in foods, beverages, flavorings, fragrances, cosmetics, drugs, and other products may be high enough to cause symptoms only in rare instances. A very small number of patients would need to avoid salicin, an additive which produces the wintergreen or mint flavor or fragrance in many foods, drugs, and cosmetics. Sources which may be overlooked are candles, liniments, lotions, and antimildew solutions. The chart below lists nonfood sources of salicylates.

NONFOOD PRODUCTS CONTAINING SALICYLATES

Drugs (all salicylate-tartrazine sensitive patients should avoid):

Acetine	Coricidin	Pepto-Bismol
Alka-Seltzer	Darvon compound	Persistin
Anacin	Dristan	Sal-Sayne
Anahist	Ecotrin	Stanback
ACP	Empirin compound	Theracin
Aspirin	Excedrin	Trigesic
BC	4-Way cold tablets	Aspergum headache
Bromo-quinine	Inhiston	powder
Bromo-seltzer	Liquiprin	Equagesic tablets
Bufferin	Midol	Sigmagen tablets
		Vanquish tablets

Acetyl salicylic acid
Aluminum acetyl
  salicylate
Ammonium salicylate
Arthropan
Calcium acetyl
  salicylate
Choline salicylate
Ethyl salicylate

Lithium salicylate
Methyl salicylate
Para amino salicylic acid
Phenyl salicylate
Procaine salicylate
Sal ethyl carbonate
Salicylamide

Salicylsalicylic
  acid
Santyl (santalyl
  salicylate)
Sodium salicylate
Strongcylate
Strontium salicylate

Plants Containing Salicylates (rarely need to be avoided):

(Any part of the plant--leaves, flowers, fruits, stem, bulbs, bark, root)

Acacia
Aspens
Birches
Camellia
Calcythemus

Hyacinth
Marigold
Milkwort
Poplars
Spiraea

Teaberry
Tulips
Violets
Willows

Foods Which May Contain Tartrazine (F.D. & C. Certified Food Color No. 5):

Beverages:
  Carbonated beverages
  Flavored drink mixes

Bread Products:
  Breaded foods such as
    fish sticks
  Quick bread mixes
  Refrigerated rolls and
    quick breads

Candy:
  Butterscotch chips
  Candy coatings
  Candy drops
  Chocolate chips
  Hard candies
  Marshmallows

Cereals

Desserts:
  Cake mixes
  Cake and cookie decorations
  Frostings
  Ice creams
  Gelatin desserts
  Pastries
  Pies and pie crust mixes
  Puddings
  Sherbets
  Whipped toppings

Extracts and flavorings

Pasta and Potato Products:
  Aproten low protein pasta
  Pasta mixes such as
    macaroni and cheese
  Potato mixes

Miscellaneous:
  Gravy mixes
  Pickles
  Salad dressings and toppings
  Sauces
  Seasonings
  Snack foods such as corn chips

5. Foods Containing Other Additives That May Cause Allergic Responses

DESCRIPTION: In addition to tartrazine, other food additives that may cause allergic reactions include metabisulfites, vegetable gums, benzoic acid, and cottonseed (but not cottonseed oil). Common vegetable gums are from the acacia, carob, guar, haraya, and tragacanth plants.

Metabisulfites are antioxidants commonly used in food preservation. They are also sometimes used as sanitizing agents for food containers. Sulfite sensitivity is most common in patients with asthma (the frequency is estimated to be between 5% and 10% of this population). The symptoms include flushing, difficulty in swallowing, gastric distress, dizziness, weakness, chest tightness, shortness of breath, wheezing, and hypotension. The FDA banned the use of sulfites on raw produce, effective August 8, 1986, but they are allowed in many packaged foods and some seafoods to retard spoilage. If used, the label must disclose the additive. Sulfites are *not* allowed on fresh meats, or foods that are a good source of thiamin such as enriched bread or flour, because of sulfite's adverse effects on the nutrient.

Clinical management of these food sensitivities focuses mainly on identifying and avoiding the offending additives. Careful reading of food labels is necessary. In addition, patients should inquire about ingredients (and the use of sulfiting agents in the case of metabisulfite sensitivity) when eating out. Patients should be advised that laws regarding sulfite use are different in other countries. Products that *may* contain these additives are listed in the chart on page 178.

FOODS THAT MAY CONTAIN ADDITIVES THAT CAUSE ALLERGIC RESPONSES

Cottonseed	Metabisulfites	Soybean Seed	Vegetable Gums
Brown cookies	Beverages:	Biscuits	Cheeses:
Dog food	Beer	Candies containing	Cheese spreads
Fig bars	Carbonated beverages	lecithin	Cream cheese
Fried cakes, rolls,	Cider	Crackers	Neufchatel cheese
and pastries	Cordials	Formulas	Cold pack cheese
Pan-greasing	Fruit drinks	Frankfurters	foods
products	Wine	Frozen desserts	Processed cheese
		Luncheon meats	
	Breads and Crackers:	Margarine	Desserts:
	Those containing	Meat sauces	Cake icing mixes
	dough conditioners	Pork links	Cake mixes
	or dried fruits and	Sausage	Candy fillings
	vegetables	Soy:	Frozen desserts
		Flakes	Ice cream
	Cheeses, processed	Milks	Ice milk
		Nuts	Whipped toppings
	Cakes, especially	Sauce	
	those containing		
	dried fruits or		Miscellaneous:
	vegetables		Chewing gum
			Prepared mustard
	Fish		Salad dressing
			Toothpaste
	Fruits:		
	Canned		
	Dried		
	Pickled		
	Gelatin		
	Potato, pasta, and		
	rice mixes		
	Salad dressings and		
	mixes		
	Seasonings, especially		
	those containing		
	dried vegetables		
	Starches used to		
	thicken food		
	Sugar (beet sugar)		
	Syrups, corn or pancake		
	Vegetables:		
	Canned		
	Dried		
	Pickled		
	Vinegars		

B. GLUTEN RESTRICTED DIET

DESCRIPTION: Wheat, rye, oats, barley, and products containing these grains are omitted from the diet in order to substantially reduce gluten intake. Because some patients are extremely sensitive to trace amounts of gluten, all potential sources (including "gluten-free wheat starch" and white vinegar) should be avoided.[1] Corn, rice, and products made from them may be used instead. Other substitutes include tapioca; and soybean, arrowroot, and potato flours.

A possible substitute is amaranth, a pseudo-cereal (not in the grass family), that has been advertised as containing little or no gluten. Because gluten does not appear in other members of the Amaranthaceae family, the chance that amaranth contains gluten is remote. The scientific studies and clinical trials to determine its presence had not been performed as of the press date (Saunders 1989).

This diet is used in the treatment of gluten-induced enteropathy. Many celiac patients have other malabsorption problems. Therefore, the diet should contain optimal calories, protein, vitamins, and minerals. Initially, some persons may require a lactose restriction until symptoms are resolved. Alcohol should be avoided in the recuperative stage, but may be consumed in moderation later.

NOTE: Because many processed foods contain wheat, rye, oats, barley, or flours from these grains, LABELS SHOULD BE READ CAREFULLY.

FOODS ALLOWED AND FOODS TO AVOID:

Food Group	Foods Allowed	Foods to Avoid
Beverages	Milk, carbonated beverages, coffee, tea, decaffeinated coffee, fruit-flavored beverages, rum, brandy, tequila, dry table wines, dessert wines	Cereal beverages; malted milk; ale; beer; beverages containing wheat, rye, oats, barley, or malt, including whiskeys (scotch, bourbon, gin) and vodka unless made from potatoes or grapes
Breads	Breads made from cornmeal; corn, potato, rice, soybean, tapioca, and arrowroot flours	All bread and crackers containing wheat, rye, oats, or barley; "gluten-free" wheat starch[2], triticale; millet and buckwheat[3]
Cereals	Cornmeal, rice, precooked rice cereal, dry cereals containing only rice or corn	All cooked and prepared cereals containing wheat, rye, oats, barley, malt, bran, or wheat germ

---

[1]The Celiac Sprue Association of the United States (CSA/USA) and the Gluten Intolerance Group of North America (GIG).

[2]The current recommendation is to avoid wheat starch since even "gluten-free" wheat starch may contain trace amounts of gluten.

[3]Although botanically different from other gliadin-containing grains, additional information is needed before these can be approved.

FOODS ALLOWED AND FOODS TO AVOID (continued):

Food Group	Foods Allowed	Foods to Avoid
Desserts	Custard; gelatin desserts; fruit ice; puddings, cakes, cookies, and other desserts made with allowed flours or starches	Cakes, cookies, pastries, or commercial pudding mixes containing restricted flours; ice cream cones; fruit sauces thickened with wheat flour; commercial ice cream or sherbet containing a wheat stabilizer
Eggs	Baked, poached, soft or hard cooked, scrambled, fried	Creamed eggs, soufflé, or fondue unless made with allowed flours
Fats	Butter, margarine, cream, vegetable oils and shortenings, lard, bacon, salad dressings thickened with allowed flours or starches	Salad dressings or gravies containing wheat, rye, oats, or barley
Fruits, Fruit Juices	All fresh, frozen, canned, and dried	None
Meat, Fish, Poultry, Cheese	Baked, broiled, roasted, or steamed beef, lamb, liver, pork, veal, poultry, fish; cottage cheese, cream cheese, nonprocessed cheeses	Meat, fish, poultry, or cheese products containing restricted cereals (the following foods frequently contain these cereals: meatloaf; meat patties; breaded meat, fish, or poultry; canned meat products; cold cuts unless guaranteed all meat; cheese spreads)
Potatoes or Substitutes	White and sweet potatoes, rice, hominy, potato chips	Creamed or scalloped potatoes unless made with allowed flours, macaroni, noodles, spaghetti
Soups	Broth-based and cream soups made from allowed foods	Soups containing wheat, rye, oats, barley, or products made from these grains; soups thickened with wheat flour
Sugar, Sweets	Sugar, syrup, honey, jelly, molasses, candy, chocolate, chewing gum	Commercial candies containing wheat, rye, oats, barley, or malt
Vegetables, Vegetable Juices	All fresh, frozen, and canned	None

FOODS ALLOWED AND FOODS TO AVOID (continued):

Food Group	Foods Allowed	Foods to Avoid
Miscellaneous	Salt, flavorings, spices, cider vinegar, peanut butter, coconut, popcorn, olives, pickles, catsup, mustard, chocolate, cocoa powder, gravy or cream sauce if thickened with allowed flours or starches	Pretzels, distilled white vinegar[1], gravy thickened with flours or starches other than allowed

APPROXIMATE COMPOSITION OF SAMPLE MENU:

Calories	2221
Protein, g	98
Fat, g	76
Carbohydrate, g	296

SAMPLE MENU FOR GLUTEN RESTRICTED DIET:

Breakfast	Luncheon	Dinner
1/2 cup orange juice	2 oz sliced chicken	3 oz roast beef
1/2 cup cream of rice cereal	1/2 cup rice	1/2 cup cubed white potato
1 egg, soft cooked	1/2 cup green beans	1/2 cup cooked carrots
Cornmeal muffin	1/2 sliced tomato on lettuce	3/4 cup tossed lettuce salad
1 tsp butter or margarine	Rice muffin	1 tbsp french dressing
1 tbsp grape jelly	1 tsp butter or margarine	Rice muffin
1 cup 2% milk	1/2 cup canned peaches	2 tsp butter or margarine
2 tsp sugar	Puffed rice bar	1 cup 2% milk
Coffee or tea	1 cup 2% milk	Coffee or tea
	Coffee or tea	

---

[1]Because grain is used as a starting material for white vinegar, it is possible that trace amounts of gluten may appear in the distillate.

C. LOW OXALATE, RESTRICTED ASCORBIC ACID DIET

DESCRIPTION: This diet may be helpful in preventing renal calculi for patients with hyperoxaluria caused by small bowel dysfunction or high intakes of oxalate rich foods.

The most common type of hyperoxaluria is associated with ileal bypass procedures for obesity, ileitis, and ileal resection. A lowfat, low oxalate diet may be needed. This is based on the theory that calcium binding by excess fecal fat due to fat malabsorption leaves dietary oxalates unbound; their increased absorption by the colon results in oxaluria and oxalate stones.

Data are not well documented regarding hyperoxaluria due to ingestion of foods containing high amounts of oxalate. Oxalic acid is found in certain fruits, vegetables, beverages, and nuts. Animal products contain negligible amounts. Considerable variation in the oxalate content of plants can occur depending on the season, species, variety, age, maturity, and part of the plant, as well as soil conditions during growth. There is also considerable variation in the amount and percentage of oxalate absorbed from different foods. The factors that affect absorption include the form of the oxalate, and the mineral, protein, and fiber content of the diet. In normal persons, oxalate is usually poorly absorbed.

Several different analysis techniques exist for determining the oxalate content of foods. The enzymatic method is the most reliable, although only a limited number of foods have been analyzed this way.

The following table lists foods containing more than 20 mg oxalate per serving, and fluids containing more that 10 mg per serving. (Instant coffee is shown for comparison purposes.) Most patients who require the diet need avoid only the extremely high sources, spinach and rhubarb.

A high magnesium intake is encouraged because it increases the solubility of oxalic acid in aqueous solutions. Calcium is also helpful, since it binds oxalate.

The main pathways of oxalate synthesis are from glyoxylate and ascorbic acid, the former representing the major source. Since about one-third of endogenous oxalate arises from the metabolism of ascorbic acid, the RDA for the vitamin should not be exceeded. In practical terms, this means avoiding foods fortified with ascorbic acid, and eating only 1 serving per day of vitamin C-rich food from the table on page 183.

On this diet it is especially important to consume 2 to 3 liters water daily, distributed throughout the day, to assure a constant output of dilute urine.

ADEQUACY: This diet meets the Recommended Dietary Allowances for all nutrients except iron for women of childbearing age.

FOODS CONTAINING OVER 10-20 MG OXALATE/SERVING

Food/Fluid	Amount	Oxalate Content (mg)
Food/Description		
Rhubarb, stewed	1/2 cup	312-536
Spinach, boiled	1/2 cup	320-702
Green beans, boiled	1/2 cup	5-40
Beets[a], boiled	1/2 cup	82-93[a]
Peanuts	1 oz	52
Parsley, fresh	2 tbsp	33
Chocolate	1 oz	16-35
Fluid/Description		
Cocoa (1 tbsp powder/cup milk)	1 cup	131
Tea, dried, brewed for 2-6 minutes	1 cup	12-33
Coffee, instant (2 tsp dry)	1 cup	0.7-7
Coffee, brewed (4 g/100 ml for 13 minutes)	1 cup	16
Ovaltine (4-5 heaping tsp or 21.3 g/cup)	1 cup	7-10

[a]Kasidas and Rose (1980) reported 425 mg/1/2 cup by the enzymatic method. Other confirmations of this extremely high level are needed before this value can be accepted.

PORTIONS OF FRUITS AND VEGETABLES PROVIDING 30-50 mg ASCORBIC ACID

Fruit	Vegetables
1/2 cup cantaloupe	1/4 cup broccoli
1/2 cup grapefruit	1/2 cup other cabbage family vegetables
1/4 cup grapefruit juice	
1/2 medium kiwi fruit	1 cup fresh or cooked greens (no spinach)
1 cup fresh or frozen mulberries	
1/4 cup orange juice	1/2 cup raw or fresh cooked edible pea pods
1/2 cup papaya	1/4 cup green or red pepper
1 cup fresh or frozen raspberries	1 medium fresh or fresh cooked tomato
1/4 cup strawberries	1 cup tomato juice

APPROXIMATE COMPOSITION OF SAMPLE MENU:

Calories	2036
Protein, g	105
Fat, g	65
Carbohydrate, g	269
Ascorbic acid, mg	60

SAMPLE MENU FOR LOW OXALATE-RESTRICTED ASCORBIC ACID DIET:

Breakfast

1/4 cup orange
  juice
1/2 cup farina
1 slice toast,
  cracked wheat
1 tsp butter or
  margarine
1 tbsp grape jelly
1 cup 2% milk
1 tsp sugar
Coffee

Luncheon

1/2 cup grape juice
3/4 cup creamed chicken on
1 biscuit
1/2 cup green beans
1 slice bread, cracked
  wheat
1 tsp butter or margarine
1/2 cup canned peaches
1 slice angel food cake
1 cup 2% milk
Coffee

Dinner

3 oz roast beef
1/2 cup mashed potatoes
1/2 cup cooked carrots
3/4 cup lettuce salad
1 tbsp french dressing
1 slice bread, cracked
  wheat
1 tsp butter or margarine
Banana
3 vanilla wafers
1 cup 2% milk
Coffee

Evening Nourishment

1 cup 2% milk

D. LOW PURINE DIET

DESCRIPTION: The low purine diet may be useful in the treatment of gout that does not respond to drug therapy.[1] Although exogenous sources of uric acid and its precursors account for half or less of serum uric acid, foods high in purines are restricted to avoid unnecessary metabolic stress (see table below).

Obesity is often associated with gout and may be a contributing factor in the onset of the disease. Gradual weight reduction is recommended for the obese patient, since fasting or drastic dieting will increase blood uric acid. Reduction in fat intake is indicated, since a high fat diet decreases urinary excretion of urates. A minimum of 2 quarts fluid intake per day is suggested to promote urinary excretion of uric acid.

Overconsumption of alcoholic beverages may precipitate attacks of gout. Excessive intake results in accumulation of lactic acid which inhibits renal secretion of urates. Complete abstinence is not necessary, but discretion and moderation are advised. The alcohol that is consumed should be diluted as in mixed drinks and taken with food.

The low purine diet is no longer recommended for the treatment of uric acid calculi, since studies show that it is ineffective. When stone formation is due to a persistently acid urine caused by a defect in ammonium excretion, treatment consists of alkalinizing the urine and increasing fluid intake to a minimum of 2 quarts per day.

ADEQUACY: If all meat, fish, and poultry are eliminated on a purine-free regimen, the diet is low in iron, thiamin, and niacin.

PURINE YIELDING FOODS PER 100 GRAMS

Group I (0-50 mg) Unlimited	Group II (50-150 mg) 1 Serving/Day	Group III (150-825 mg) Not Allowed
Vegetables (except Group II)	Meats	Sweetbreads
Fruits	Meat soups/broths	Anchovies
Milk	Whole grain breads and cereals	Herring
Cheese	Mackerel
Eggs	Wheat germ and bran	Scallops
Breads and cereals (except whole grain and oatmeal)	Fish	Sardines
	Seafoods	Liver
Sugar	Poultry	Kidney
Coffee	Beans, dry	Meat extracts
Tea	Peas, dry	Wild game
Carbonated beverages	Lentils	Goose
Gelatin	Asparagus	
Nuts	Cauliflower	
	Spinach	
	Peas	
	Mushrooms	

Note: Adapted from Turner, 1970, and Pennington and Church, 1985.

[1]The drug Allopurinol (Zyloprim™) interferes with uric acid synthesis by inhibiting the enzyme, xanthine oxidase.

E. TYRAMINE RESTRICTED DIET

DESCRIPTION: This diet restricts foods high in tyramine and levodopa for patients who are receiving monoamine oxidase (MAO)-inhibiting drugs. (Primarily used as antidepressants, the drugs act by inhibiting brain MAO, resulting in increased levels of certain neurotransmitters.)

Normally, the pressor amines in foods (vasoactive amines which influence blood pressure) are of no concern because monoamine oxidase and diamine oxidases inactivate them in the intestine, liver, or kidney. Ingested tyramine, for example, is converted to 4-hydroxyphenylacetic acid. However, when a patient is receiving MAO-inhibiting drugs, a high concentration of serum tyramine can occur, indirectly causing severe hypertension by releasing norepinephrine from stores in sympathetic nerve endings.

Many foods normally contain small amounts of tyramine and other pressor amines, but the formation of large quantities has been reported only in aged, fermented, or spoiled products. More than 60 different foods have been implicated for symptoms of acute hypertension, headache, palpitations, and flushing; however, scientific evidence is inconclusive in many cases. Foods allowed and foods to avoid are based on a critical review of the literature by McCabe (1986). The highly variable tyramine values reported are probably due to differences in processing, fermentation, ripening, incidental contamination, or degradation by bacteria. Foods which spoil quickly, especially milk, meat, fish, and poultry products, should be purchased, prepared, and stored under sanitary conditions. They should be used within 72 hours of purchase.

Distilled spirits contain tyramine, but the patient will not get too much tyramine from this source unless he or she drinks more than 4 oz/day. For other health reasons, the patient should not exceed 1 to 2 oz distilled spirits per day.

A diet history should be taken with emphasis on foods that are to be avoided or used in limited quantities. The patient should be warned about hidden sources of cheese and wine in cooking. Advising consumption of freshly prepared foods is important in order to avoid tyramine from bacterial degradation.

It is not uncommon for patients to try prohibited foods to test the diet. Adverse effects may not occur if the serum level of oxidases is not depleted, such as soon after the drug has been prescribed and/or if the food is not consistently high in tyramine. Monitoring by food recall after weekend passes, or by telephone or live interview after discharge, is recommended.

The diet should be followed for 2 weeks after the drug has been discontinued to allow for enzyme recovery.

FOODS ALLOWED AND FOODS TO AVOID:

Food Group	Foods Allowed	Foods to Avoid
Beverages	All except those to avoid; limit each of the following to one 4 oz serving per day: port and white wines, and yogurt and cream from unpasteurized[1] milk	Ale, beer, Chianti, and vermouth wines
Breads	All except those to avoid	Bread or crackers containing cheese

---

[1]Unpasteurized yogurt, cream, or milk is not recommended; however, small quantities do not contain sufficient tyramine to warrant exclusion on this basis.

FOODS ALLOWED AND FOODS TO AVOID (continued):

Food Group	Foods Allowed	Foods to Avoid
Cereals	All	None
Desserts	All	None
Eggs	All	None
Fats	All except salad dressings made with cheese other than cottage	None
Fruits, Fruit Juices	All; limit raspberries to 1/2 cup serving per day	None
Meat, Fish, Poultry, Cheese	Cottage cheese, cream cheese, ham, bacon, all other meats except those to avoid	Cheese (except cottage or cream cheese), smoked or pickled fish, liver, summer sausage, salami, meat extracts
Potatoes or Substitutes	All	None
Soups	Soups made with foods allowed	Soups containing foods to avoid
Sugar, Sweets	All except those to avoid; limit chocolate to 4 oz per day	Sweets containing foods to avoid
Vegetables, Vegetable Juices	All except those to avoid; limit avocado to 1/2 cup serving per day	Italian green beans (broad bean pods or fava broad beans), sauerkraut
Miscellaneous	Baked products raised with yeast; limit peanuts and soy sauce to 1/2 cup servings per day	Yeast vitamin supplements (brewer's yeast); meat extracts; gravies, soups, or sauces made from meat extracts

There is insufficient evidence to support exclusion of the following foods:

Beets	Curry powder	Pineapple
Coca Cola	Egg	Raisins
Cookies (English biscuits)	Figs	Salad dressings
Corn	Fish (fresh)	Tomato juice
Cucumber	Junket	Worcestershire sauce
	Mushrooms	Yeast bread

APPROXIMATE COMPOSITION OF SAMPLE MENU:

Calories	2023
Protein, g	97
Fat, g	62
Carbohydrate, g	282

SAMPLE MENU FOR TYRAMINE RESTRICTED DIET:

Breakfast	Luncheon	Dinner
1/2 cup orange juice	1/2 cup grape juice	3 oz roast beef
1/2 cup farina	3/4 cup creamed chicken on 1 biscuit	1/2 cup mashed potatoes
1 slice toast, cracked wheat	1/2 cup green beans	1/2 cup cooked carrots
1 tsp butter or margarine	1/2 sliced tomato on lettuce	3/4 cup tossed lettuce salad
1 tbsp grape jelly	1 slice bread, cracked wheat	1 tbsp french dressing
1 cup 2% milk	1 tsp butter or margarine	1 slice bread, cracked wheat
1 tsp sugar	1/2 cup canned peaches	1 tsp butter or margarine
Coffee or tea	1 slice angel food cake	Banana
	1 cup 2% milk	3 vanilla wafers
	Coffee or tea	1 cup 2% milk
		Coffee or tea

CURRENT MAO INHIBITOR DRUGS

Generic Name	Trademark and Producer	General Use
Tranylcypromine Sulfate	Parnate Smith, Kline & French Laboratories	Antidepressant
Phenelzine Sulfate	Nardil Warner-Chilcott Laboratories	Antidepressant
Nialamide	Niamid Pfizer Laboratories	Antidepressant
Isocarboxazid	Marplan Roche Laboratories	Antidepressant
Furazolidone	Furozone Eaton Laboratories	Antimicrobial
Procarbazine	Natulane Roche Laboratories	Antineoplasm
Pargyline HCl	Eutonyl Abbott Laboratories	Antihypertensive
Pargyline HCl and Hethylclothiazide	Eutron Abbott Laboratories	Antihypertensive

F. VEGETARIAN DIET

DESCRIPTION: A vegetarian diet is usually categorized into one of three types: Lacto-ovo (includes eggs and dairy products), lacto-vegetarian (includes dairy products), or strict vegetarian (no foods relative to an animal are used). However, some people who call themselves vegetarian may eat fish or poultry, but no meat of larger animals. The restrictions are individual and may be based upon religious, health, or environmental ideologies. The patient must be interviewed to determine individual food variations. Dietary modifications necessary for a medical condition(s) should be reviewed with the patient. A nutrient dense diet of a wide variety of foods is especially important for the vegetarian. The guidelines from the basic four food groups can be used, substituting eggs, meat analogues, legumes, nuts, and seeds for meat, poultry, and fish. Intake of low nutrient foods should be limited. If additional calories are needed, servings of whole grain breads or cereals and milk may be added. The diet should be planned using foods which have complementary amino acid patterns (see the complementary protein chart on page 190). The table on page 192 shows the calorie content and the portion size equivalent for 7 g protein.

Planning an adequate vegetarian diet involves understanding the concepts of limiting amino acid(s) and complementary protein foods. For protein synthesis to proceed, each of the 9 essential amino acids must be present simultaneously in the proper proportions. If a given amino acid is limited in amount, the utilization of the remaining amino acids is reduced by the same proportion. Various combinations of foods provide mixtures of proteins that are complementary; that is, foods low in 1 or more amino acids are combined with foods containing adequate amounts of 1 or more limiting amino acids. In general, cereals that are deficient in lysine are complemented by legumes that are deficient in methionine. The following food combinations work well together to provide complete proteins: grains with milk products, grains with legumes, seeds with legumes. See the table on page 190 to determine other combinations. Histidine (which does not appear in the table) is also an essential amino acid, but it is readily available in all foods containing protein.

In addition to supplying adequate protein, the vegetarian should consume adequate calories so that the protein consumed will be utilized for tissue growth and repair rather than for energy. Since many plant foods are low in calories, the large bulk of food necessary to meet caloric needs can become a problem for the strict vegetarian.

If oversupplementation of vitamins and/or minerals is a problem, appropriate levels should be recommended. Patients consuming toxic doses should be advised to discontinue them. If the supplementation is high, but not in the toxic range, a gradual reduction in dosage is recommended. The body may have adjusted to a higher intake and a sudden drop could result in a temporary deficiency state.

ADEQUACY: For lacto and lacto-ovo vegetarians, the Recommended Dietary Allowances can be met depending upon the foods and portions consumed. Very careful planning is necessary for the strict vegetarian diet to be adequate. The nutrients which are most often deficient are the minerals calcium, iron, iodine, and zinc; and the vitamins B_6, B_{12}, folic acid, riboflavin, and D. The chart on pages 195-97 lists rich nonmeat sources of these nutrients. Vitamin B_{12} is found almost exclusively in foods of animal origin, but it is possible for some vegetable foods to contain vitamin B_{12} due to the presence of microorganisms such as yeasts, molds, or bacteria that are often an intrinsic part of fermented foods. Thus vitamin B_{12} may be found in vegetable foods as a result of contamination. Since these foods are *not* dependable sources, a person following a strict vegetarian diet should use cereal or soy milk fortified with vitamin B_{12} or a vitamin preparation that includes it. The strict vegetarian is at risk for iron deficiency, megaloblastic and pernicious anemia, goiter, nervous disorders, and eventual osteoporosis.

COMPLEMENTARY AMINO ACID COMPOSITION OF SOME FOODS

Essential Amino Acids	Cheese Eggs Milk Meat	Corn	Cereal	Legumes	Whole Grains (with germ)	Nuts Seed Oils Soybeans	Sesame and Sunflower Seeds	Peanut Protein	Green Leafy Vegetable Leaf Protein	Gelatin[a]	Yeast
Cystine[b]			--	--			X				
Methionine			X	--	X	--	X	--	--	--	X
Isoleucine	X										
Leucine	X										
Lysine	X	--	--		X	X	X	--	--	--	
Phenylalanine											--
Threonine	X		--	--	X	--	X	--			X
Tryptophan			--	--			X			--	
Valine	X										

Source: Erhard (1971).

Note: X equals high amount of amino acid present; -- equals low amount of amino acid present; blank spaces indicate a generally good balance of amino acids present with respect to other amino acids in the food. (Be sure to complement a low amino acid with a food high in that amino acid at the same meal.)

[a]Not a good source of all essential amino acids.

[b]Not essential but added because it is hard to get in a vegetarian diet. Methionine and cystine can be compared as one.

VEGETARIAN FOOD USAGE:

Food Group	Foods Commonly Used	Foods Often Avoided
Beverages	Milk, cocoa, soybean milk, herbal teas[1]	
Breads	Whole grain breads, graham crackers	Saltine crackers
Cereals	Farina, oatmeal, bran cereals, brown rice, complementary grains	White bread, refined cereals other than farina
Desserts	Any (those high in calories and low in other nutrients should be consumed in very limited amounts if at all)	
Eggs	All	
Fats	Any, except bacon fat; limited amounts are recommended	Bacon fat, excessive amounts of other fats

[1]Some types can cause serious side effects, especially if taken in large amounts.

VEGETARIAN FOOD USAGE (continued):

Food Group	Foods Commonly Used	Foods Often Avoided
Fruits, Fruit Juices	All, especially fresh	
Meat, Fish, Poultry, and Substitutes	Cheese; fish for some; tofu (soybean curd); meat analogues; complementary protein foods (see chart on page 190)	Meat analogues
Potatoes or Substitutes	All	
Soups	Typically homemade without meat, fish, or poultry	Broth-based, fish chowder for some
Sugar, Sweets	Honey, brown sugar, molasses in limited amounts	White sugar
Vegetables, Vegetable Juices	Any	

PLANT PROTEIN EQUIVALENT CHART

Foods	Amounts Containing 7 g Protein	Caloric Content
Legumes (cooked)		
Beans:		
Black	1/2 cup	115
Fried (frijoles)	1/2 cup	110
Kidney	1/2 cup	110
Lima	1/2-3/4 cup	95-110
Navy	1/2 cup	110
Pinto	1/2 cup	115
Soy	1/3 cup	75
Peanuts	3 tbsp	155
Peas:		
Black-eyed (cow peas)	1/2 cup	90
Chick (garbanzos)	1 cup	110
Green	1 cup	110
Split	1/2 cup	115
Sprouts:		
Alfalfa	150 g	60
Mung	2 cups	56
Soy	1 cup	50
Lentils	1/2 cup	105
Cereals/Grains		
Bulgur	1 cup	225
Bread	2 1/2-3 slices	150
Corn	1 1/3 cups	175
Grits	2 1/2 cups	310
Rice	1 1/3 cups	310
Wheat, rolled	1 1/2 cups	225
Wheat germ	1/4 cup	90
Seeds/Nuts		
Almonds	1/3 cup	260
Brazil nuts	2 oz or 14 nuts	370
Cashews	1/3 cup	260
Filberts	1/2 cup	365
Pecans	3/4 cup	610
Pine nuts:		
Pignolias	1 oz	155
Pinon	2 oz	360
Pistachios	1 1/2 oz	250
Pumpkin seeds	3 tbsp	145
Sunflower seeds	3 tbsp	150
Walnuts:		
Black	1/4 cup	195
English	1/2 cup	390

COMPARISON OF SELECTED VEGETABLE PROTEIN AND ANIMAL PROTEIN TO AMINO ACID CONTENT

(Portions equivalent to approximately 7 g protein)	Amino Acids (mg)							
	Tryptophan	Phenylalanine	Leucine	Isoleucine	Lysine	Valine	Methionine	Threonine
Complete Protein								
Egg (1)	99	360	546	409	397	459	192	310
Milk (7 oz, 3.5% fat)	102	339	700	425	572	470	184	326
Legumes - Incomplete Protein								
Beans, kidney (1/2 cup)	429	51[a]	671	437	577	468	78[a]	335
Beans, lima (1/2 cup)	56[a]	366	515	360	415	391	99[a]	291
Peas, split (1/2 cup)	80	365	606	409	532	409	87[a]	285
Peanuts (3 tbsp)	150	690	831	561	486	678	120[a]	366
Cereals/Grains - Incomplete Protein								
Bread (3 slices wheat)	324	90[a]	288[a]	438	213[a]	339[a]	111[a]	216[a]
Rice, brown, cooked (1 1/3 cups)	55[a]	247[a]	425	233[a]	192[a]	345[a]	88[a]	192[a]
Corn (1 1/3 cups)	34[a]	320	629	210[a]	210[a]	35[a]	109[a]	234[a]
Nuts/Seeds - Incomplete Protein								
Brazil nuts (14)	98	325	507	267[a]	198[a]	369[a]	423	189[a]
Pumpkin seeds (3 tbsp)	130	271[a]	573	406	334	391[a]	138[a]	217
Walnuts, english (1 1/2 cup)	88	383	614	383	220[a]	487	153	295

Sources: Pennington and Church (1985); Adams (1975).
[a]Low (limiting amino acid).

SAMPLE MENUS FOR VEGETARIAN DIETS

APPROXIMATE COMPOSITION OF SAMPLE MENU (lacto-ovo vegetarian):

Calories	1942
Protein, g	73
Fat, g	75
Carbohydrate, g	259

Lacto-ovo vegetarian

Breakfast	Luncheon	Dinner
1/2 cup orange juice	1/2 cup cottage cheese	1/2 cup kidney beans
1/2 cup farina	1 cup green beans	1 baked potato
1 egg, soft cooked	1/2 cup sliced tomato on lettuce	3/4 cup tossed salad
1 slice toast, whole grain	2 tsp mayonnaise	2 tbsp french dressing
1 tsp butter	2 tbsp raisins	2 slices bread, whole wheat
1 tsp honey	1 slice rye bread	2 tsp butter
1 cup milk	1 tsp butter	1/2 grapefruit
1 cup tea	1 tsp honey	1/2 cup sherbet
	1 cup milk	1 cup milk

APPROXIMATE COMPOSITION OF SAMPLE MENU (strict vegetarian):

Calories	2142
Protein, g	77
Fat, g	101
Carbohydrate, g	269

Strict vegetarian

Breakfast	Luncheon	Dinner
1/2 cup orange juice	4 oz tofu	1/2 cup kidney beans
1/2 cup farina	1 cup green beans	1 baked potato
3 tbsp peanuts	1/2 cup sliced tomato on lettuce	3/4 cup tossed salad
1 slice toast, whole grain	2 tsp mayonnaise	2 tbsp french dressing
1 tsp honey	2 slices rye bread	2 slices bread, whole wheat
1 cup soybean milk	2 tsp margarine	2 tsp margarine
1 cup tea	2 tbsp raisins	1/2 grapefruit
	1 cup soybean milk	1/4 cup black walnuts
		1 tsp honey
		1 cup soybean milk

GOOD NONMEAT SOURCES OF NUTRIENTS THAT ARE OFTEN LOW IN VEGETARIAN DIETS

Food Group	Description	Portion Size	VITAMINS					MINERALS			
			Riboflavin (mg) Adult USRDA 1.7 mg	Vitamin B6 (mg) Adult USRDA 2 mg	Vitamin B12 (mcg) Adult USRDA 6 mcg	Folic Acid (mcg) Adult USRDA 400 mcg	Vitamin D (I.U.) Adult USRDA 400 I.U.	Calcium (mg) Adult USRDA 1000 mg	Iron (mg) Adult USRDA 18 mg	Iodine (mcg) Adult USRDA 150 mcg	Zinc (mg) Adult USRDA 15 mg
Bakery and Grain	Bread, whole wheat	1 slice	0.03	0.04	0			23	0.5	0-95	0.4
	Bulgur wheat, cooked	1/2 cup			0						1.4
	Carob flour	2 tbsp	unknown					62	0.9		0.6
	Egg noodles, cooked	1/2 cup							1.2		0.2-0.4
	English muffin	1 whole	0.04-0.40					48-112	0.7-1.4		
	Rolled oats, dry	1/2 cup	0.06	0.06				21	1.8		1.4
	Soy flour	2 tbsp				48			1.0		
	Wheat germ	1/4 cup	0.13-0.23			118			2.7		4.4
	Whole wheat flour	2 tbsp							0.5		
	Wild rice	1/2 cup	0.16	1.3		35			1.1		1.2
Eggs and Dairy Products	Cheese	1 oz	0.10-0.15		0.2-0.3		23-44[a]	150-200		5-44	0.2-0.9
	Cottage cheese	1/2 cup	0.17-0.21		0.8			63		18-71	0.4
	Egg	1 med	0.13	0.1	0.6		23	56	1.0	18	0.7
	Eggnog	1 cup	0.48		1.1		approx 100[a]	330		60-150	1.2
	Ice cream	1 cup	0.33-0.45		0.6		50[a]	176	0.5	26-70	1.4
	Kefir (cultured milk product)	1 cup	0.40		0.9						
	Milk	1 cup	0.34-0.40	0.1	0.9		100[a]	291		51-140	0.9
	Yogurt, lowfat	1 cup	0.49	0.1	1.3	25	100[a]	415		48-134	2.0
Fruits and Fruit Juices	Banana	1 avg		0.7	22			52			
	Orange	1 avg			40						
	Orange juice	1 cup			109						
	Prune juice	1/2 cup							1.5		
	Prunes	5							1.0		
	Raisins, packed	1/4 cup							0.9		

195

GOOD NONMEAT SOURCES OF NUTRIENTS THAT ARE OFTEN LOW IN VEGETARIAN DIETS (continued)

Food Group	Description	Portion Size	VITAMINS					MINERALS			
			Riboflavin (mg) Adult USRDA 1.7 mg	Vitamin B$_6$ (mg) Adult USRDA 2 mg	Vitamin B$_{12}$ (mcg) Adult USRDA 6 mcg	Folic Acid (mcg) Adult USRDA 400 mcg	Vitamin D (I.U.) Adult USRDA 400 I.U.	Calcium (mg) Adult USRDA 1000 mg	Iron (mg) Adult USRDA 18 mg	Iodine (mcg) Adult USRDA 150 mcg	Zinc (mg) Adult USRDA 15 mg
Legumes (all cooked from dry)	Black beans	1/2 cup	unknown	0.11		49		30	1.7		0.5
	Black-eyed peas	1/2 cup	0.07-0.17	0.07-0.10		120		19-28	1.7-2.1		0.9-1.5
	Garbanzo beans	1/2 cup	0.10	0.17		57		46	2.6		1.3
	Kidney beans	1/2 cup	0.06-0.10	0.14		34-58		27-48	1.7-3.0		0.9-1.0
	Lentils	1/2 cup	0.05-0.11	0.10-0.14		30		19-25	1.6-3.4		0.9-1.0
	Navy beans	1/2 cup	0.07-0.11	0.36		38-54		47-60	2.5-2.6		0.9-1.0
	Pinto beans	1/2 cup	0.07	0.17		73		47	2.9		1.3
	Soybeans	1/2 cup	0.08-1.0	0.17-0.25		38-58		66	2.4-2.7		1.1
	Split peas	1/2 cup	0.08-0.09	0.06		unknown		10-22	1.4-1.5		1.1
	Tofu	2 oz (1/4 cup)				58		8-160 (varies considerably)	1.1-2.1		0.5
Nuts and Seeds	Almonds, whole	1/4 cup	0.21-0.39			22-31		76-95	1.3-1.5		1.0-1.9
	Brazil nuts	1/4 cup	0.04	0.06-0.09				65-75	1.2		1.7-1.8
	Cashews	1/4 cup	0.06-0.09	0.08-0.1		23-46		13-16	1.3-2.1		1.5-1.9
	Filberts, chopped	1/4 cup	0.03-0.18	0.18		21-24		54-86	0.94-1.1		0.7-1.0
	Peanut butter	2 tbsp	0.03-0.04	0.10-0.12		26		11-22	0.58		0.9
	Peanuts, roasted	1/4 cup	0.04-0.05	0.13-0.14		19-38		13-31	0.8-1.5		1.1-1.2
	Pecans, chopped	1/4 cup	0.04	0.05-0.06		8-12		11-22	0.6-0.8		1.2-1.6
	Pistachios	1/4 cup	0.06-0.08	unknown		19		23-43	2.2-2.3		0.5
	Pumpkin squash kernels	1/4 cup	0.05-0.11			32		15-25	3.9-8.5		2.6-4.2
	Sunflower seeds	1/4 cup	0.08-0.09	0.40-0.48		42-85		19-92	2.3-2.7		1.8
	Walnuts, english	1/4 cup	0.03-0.04	0.16-0.18		19-20		25-28	0.73-0.8		0.6-0.8
Vegetables	Asparagus, green, cooked	1/2 cup	0.12-0.16	0.06-0.13		58-88		14-22	0.5-2.2		0.5-1.1
	Beet greens, cooked	1/2 cup	0.11-0.21	0.08-0.15		24		72-99	1.4-1.9		0.4-0.7
	Broccoli, cooked	1/2 cup	0.07-0.16	0.10-0.15		43-142		38-89	0.6-0.9		0.1-0.3
	Brussels sprouts, cooked	1/2 cup	0.07-0.11	0.09-0.16		28-125		16-28	0.6-0.9		0.3

Food	Serving									
Chinese cabbage, cooked	1/2 cup	0.05-0.07	0.11				26-79	0.2-0.9		
Lettuce, loose leaf	1/2 cup				30		19	0.4		
Lima beans, cooked	1/2 cup	0.04-0.08	0.08-0.16		20-90		22-33	1.2-2.3		0.4-0.8
Peas, green cooked	1/2 cup	0.05-0.12	0.05-0.17		10-72		14-22	0.8-1.5		0.6-1.0
Potato, baked	1 large (5 oz)	0.06-0.07	0.3-0.7		19-23		14-21	1.0-2.6		0.3-0.7
Spinach, cooked	1/2 cup	0.12-0.21	0.07-2.0		58-153		107-139	1.4-3.2		0.5-0.8
Sweet potato, cooked	1/2 cup	0.04-0.18	0.07-0.31		18-27		12-28	0.7-1.3		0.2-1.1
Turnip greens cooked	1/2 cup	0.03-0.18	0.06-0.13		33-85		99-137	0.6-1.3		0.1-0.3
Winter squash, cooked	1/2 cup	0.01-0.13	0.09-0.24		12-23		12-54	0.3-1.1		0.1-0.4
Miscellaneous										
Brewer's yeast	1 tbsp	0.34-0.43	0.20		313		17-21	1.4-1.7		0.63
Cod liver oil	1 tsp					400				
Iodized salt	1 tsp								400-570	
Margarine	1 tbsp					45[a]				
Soy milk, fortified	1 cup	0.02-0.08	0.28	unknown	unknown	unknown	55-150	3.0	unknown	0.4
Fish, Shellfish, Poultry										
Cod	3.5 oz	0.10	0.13	0.72			29-31	0.9	102	
Chicken, cooked	1 cup	0.16-0.26	0.46-0.84	0.3-0.5			18-20	1.4-1.7		1.6-2.9
Haddock	3.5 oz	0.07-0.08	0.11	1.2			13-40	0.5-1.1	122-1086	0.3
Oysters	3.5 oz	0.18-0.30	0.04	18			28-206	5.5-8.1	15-30	6-100
Perch	3 oz	0.10	0.14	0.9			32	1.2	18	
Salmon	3.5 oz	0.20	0.01-0.8	6.0-7.6	1-22	407-497	154-285	0.9-1.3		1.0
Tuna, canned	1/2 cup	0.08-0.10	0.34-0.6	1.8-3.4	200-212		6-14	1.4-1.5		0.9
Turkey, cooked	1 cup	0.26	0.68	0.54			28	2.5-2.8		4.2

Sources: Agricultural Research Service (1976-1988); Leveille et al. (1983); ESHA Research (1985).

Note: A blank does not mean that the nutrient is absent, only that it is not a significant source in quantities normally consumed by vegetarians.

[a] Fortified with vitamin D or made from vitamin D fortified milk.

197

SECTION 7

Infants' and Children's Diets

A. CHILDREN'S GENERAL DIET

DESCRIPTION: The Children's General Diet is designed for the child 2 to 16 years of age. There are no dietary restrictions. Individual intolerances may necessitate the exclusion of certain food items. Salt, pepper, and sugar are routinely added to the tray.

      The amounts served vary to meet the physical needs of children within a wide age range. Interval feedings are routinely offered.

APPROXIMATE COMPOSITION OF SAMPLE MENU:

Calories	2699
Protein, g	86
Fat, g	82
Carbohydrate, g	420

SAMPLE MENU FOR CHILDREN'S GENERAL DIET (11-year-old boy):

Breakfast

1/2 cup orange juice
1 cup dry cereal
1 slice toast,
  cracked wheat
1 tsp butter or
  margarine
1 tsp grape jelly
1 cup 2% milk

Luncheon

1/2 cup creamed chicken on
1 biscuit
1/2 cup green beans
1/2 sliced tomato on lettuce
1 tbsp mayonnaise
1 slice bread, cracked
  wheat
1 tsp butter or margarine
1/2 cup canned peaches
1 slice angel food cake
1 cup 2% milk

Midafternoon Nourishment

1 cup grape juice
Apple

Dinner

2 oz roast beef
1/2 cup mashed potatoes
1/2 cup cooked carrots
3/4 cup tossed lettuce
  salad
2 tbsp french dressing
1 slice bread, cracked
  wheat
2 tsp butter or margarine
1 cup sherbet
Oatmeal cookie
1 cup 2% milk

Evening Nourishment

1 cup apple juice
Banana

MODIFICATIONS OF THE CHILDREN'S GENERAL DIET:

1. Soft

DESCRIPTION: This diet is used for a variety of circumstances requiring a softer than normal diet. The age and illness of the child determine the consistency of food served. The food may vary in texture from that in a baby soft diet to that in an adult soft diet.

2. Sodium Restricted

DESCRIPTION: This diet is designed to reduce edema and maintain water balance. The sodium content of a mild sodium restricted diet varies with the food intake of the child. Soft or general food may be served. Milk is limited to 3 to 4 cups per day. There is no reduction in the sodium content of the baby soft foods: a child from 2 to 5 years of age would receive about 1.5 to 2 g sodium; a child from 6 to 16 years of age would receive about 2 to 4 g sodium on a "no-added-salt" diet. The approximate sodium content of selected foods is found on page 66.

The salt substitute used at the University of Iowa Hospitals and Clinics contains 13.5 mEq K+ per packet and is not given unless ordered by a physician.

See page 57 for foods allowed and foods to avoid.

B. ADVANCED BABY SOFT DIET

DESCRIPTION: This is a general diet for a child between 10 months and 1 1/2 years of age who can eat table and finger foods. Interval feedings are offered routinely. The pureed selective hospital menu is used for this type of diet. Meats are pureed, ground, or chopped. Vegetables, fruits, and desserts vary in consistency from pureed to tender pieces.

FOODS ALLOWED AND FOODS TO AVOID:

Food Group	Foods Allowed	Foods to Avoid
Beverages	Whole or 2% milk and milk drinks	Coffee, tea, skim or 1% milk
Breads	Enriched white and whole grain breads, plain and graham crackers, zwieback	Breads with seeds or nuts
Cereals	Cooked cereals; iron-fortified infant cereals; dry cereals of corn, oats, rice, wheat	Excessive amounts of 100% bran cereals
Desserts	Plain desserts, plain cakes and cookies, custards, puddings, ice cream, gelatin desserts, fruit whips	Desserts containing coconut, nuts, or seeds
Eggs	All	None
Fats	Butter, margarine, cream, bland salad dressings	Excessive amounts of fried foods
Fruits, Fruit Juices	All fruit juices; all ripe, canned, or frozen fruits that are soft and do not contain pits, coarse seeds, or tough skins	All others
Meat, Fish, Poultry, Cheese	Beef, lamb, veal, liver, pork, chicken, turkey, fish without bones (all should be pureed or finely ground or chopped); cottage cheese; natural or processed cheese	Tough pieces of meat

FOODS ALLOWED AND FOODS TO AVOID (continued):

Food Group	Foods Allowed	Foods to Avoid
Potatoes or Substitutes	White and sweet potatoes, spaghetti, hominy, macaroni, noodles, rice	None
Soups	Soups made from foods allowed	None
Sugar, Sweets	Sugar, syrup, jelly	Chocolate, nut candy, hard candy in small pieces, honey[1]
Vegetables, Vegetable Juices	All cooked or canned vegetables and juices	Raw vegetables
Miscellaneous	Salt, spices in moderation, smooth peanut butter, cream sauce, catsup, gravy in limited amounts	Horseradish, nuts, unpitted olives, popcorn, excessive spices

APPROXIMATE COMPOSITION OF SAMPLE MENU:

Calories	1353
Protein, g	61
Fat, g	48
Carbohydrate, g	171

SAMPLE MENU FOR ADVANCED BABY SOFT DIET:

Breakfast	Luncheon	Dinner
1/2 cup frozen orange juice	1/4 cup creamed chicken on	2 oz chopped roast beef
1/4 cup farina	1/4 cup rice	1/4 cup cubed white potato
1 egg, soft cooked	1/4 cup green beans	1/4 cup cooked carrots
1/2 slice toast, white enriched	1/2 slice bread, white enriched	1/2 slice bread, white enriched
1 tsp butter or margarine	1 tsp butter or margarine	1 tsp butter or margarine
1/2 cup milk	1/4 cup canned peaches	1/4 cup canned pears
1 tsp sugar	1/2 cup milk	1/2 cup milk

Midmorning Nourishment	Midafternoon Nourishment	Evening Nourishment
1/2 cup apricot nectar	1/2 cup sherbet	1 cup milk

---

[1]The intestinal tracts of some infants under 1 year of age are susceptible to infant botulism. Because the susceptibility of individual infants remains unknown, it is reasonable to avoid use of nutritionally nonessential foods such as honey in infant feedings (Arnon et al. 1979).

C. BABY SOFT DIETS

DESCRIPTION: These diets are composed of pureed food and formula or milk to meet the nutritional needs of infants from 4 to 9 months of age. In selecting an appropriate diet, the infant's age, physical development, and home eating patterns must be considered. For older infants who are capable of eating ground foods and finger foods, an advanced baby soft diet may be ordered.

ADEQUACY: Without some form of supplementation, these diets will be inadequate in iron.[1]

FOODS ALLOWED AND FOODS TO AVOID:

Food Group	Foods Allowed	Foods to Avoid
Beverages	Formula with iron or as ordered, human milk, whole milk (after age 6 months)	All others
Breads	Saltine or graham crackers, toasted bread, rusk, zwieback	All others
Cereals	Iron-fortified infant cereals	Other dry cereals, whole rice
Desserts	Pureed fruit, prepared strained desserts and puddings	All others
Dinners	Combination pureed vegetable-meat dinners, pureed high meat dinners	All others
Eggs	Cooked yolk, canned strained yolks	All others
Fats	Limited amounts	Excessive amounts

---

[1]The Committee on Nutrition of the American Academy of Pediatrics recommends that iron supplementation begin no later than 4 to 6 months of age in full-term infants and no later than 2 months of age in preterm infants. Supplementation should continue for the remainder of the first year of life. In breast-fed infants, the best source of iron supplementation is ferrous sulfate drops and iron-fortified infant cereal. In formula-fed infants, the most convenient sources of iron are iron-fortified commercial infant formula and iron-fortified infant cereal. An adequate dose of supplemental iron is about 1 mg/kg/day (of elemental iron) for term infants and 2 to 3 mg/kg/day for preterm infants, up to a maximum of 15 mg/day (American Academy of Pediatrics 1985, 216; Fomon 1986).

FOODS ALLOWED AND FOODS TO AVOID (continued):

Food Group	Foods Allowed	Foods to Avoid
Fruits, Fruit Juices	Strained fruit juice; smooth applesauce; pureed apricots, peaches, pears, plums, prunes; mashed banana	All others
Meat, Fish, Poultry, Cheese	Pureed beef, chicken, pork, veal, turkey, liver, lamb	Other meat and poultry, all fish and cheese
Potatoes and Substitutes	None	All
Soups	None	All
Sugar, Sweets	Limited amounts	Excessive amounts, honey[1]
Vegetables, Vegetable Juices	Pureed peas, green and wax beans, asparagus, beets[2], carrots, pumpkin, spinach[2], squash, sweet potato	All others

APPROXIMATE COMPOSITION OF SAMPLE MENU (milk or formula is not included in the calculations of the nutrients):

Baby Soft Diet #1:
Calories	147
Protein, g	3
Fat, g	1
Carbohydrate, g	35

Baby Soft Diet #2:
Calories	290
Protein, g	17
Fat, g	4
Carbohydrate, g	50

SAMPLE MENU FOR BABY SOFT DIETS:

Baby Soft Diet #1 (approximate age 4-6 months)

Breakfast	Luncheon	Dinner
3 tbsp baby cereal, enriched 3 tbsp pureed fruit	6 tbsp pureed vegetable	3 tbsp baby cereal, enriched 3 tbsp pureed fruit

---

[1] The intestinal tracts of some infants under 1 year of age are susceptible to infant botulism. Because the susceptibility of individual infants to the development of infant botulism remains unknown, it is reasonable to avoid use of nutritionally nonessential foods such as honey in infant feeding (Arnon et al. 1989).

[2] For use only after 5 months of age because of nitrate content.

Baby Soft Diet #2 (approximate age 7-9 months)

Breakfast	Luncheon	Dinner
1/4 cup strained orange juice 6 tbsp baby cereal, enriched	3 tbsp pureed meat 4 tbsp pureed vegetable 4 tbsp pureed fruit	3 tbsp pureed meat 4 tbsp pureed vegetable 4 tbsp pureed fruit

1-2 servings of toast, zwieback, or crackers may be given between meals.

D. INFANT FORMULAS AND FEEDINGS

DESCRIPTION: The age, size, and special requirements of a baby must be considered when ordering a formula. An ill baby may not tolerate the normal diet for age. A diet compatible with mental and physical development should be substituted.

The following table is a suggested guide for the feeding of infants.

Age	Calories/kg	Number of Feedings/24 hr	Oz/Feeding	Additional Food
Term	115	6-8	3-4	
Low birth weight	130	6-12	Individualized	
1-4 months	115	5-6	5-6	
4-6 months	95	4-5	6-7	Baby Soft #1 (optional)
6-12 months	92	3-4	6-8	Baby Soft #2 and Advanced Baby Soft

A formula must be ordered by name of product, calories per ounce of prepared feeding, number of ounces per feeding, and number of feedings per day. Normal dilution is 20 calories per ounce of formula.

A variety of formulas is available in premeasured, presterilized, hermetically sealed units known as "ready-to-feed disposable" formula. The remaining formulas are available only in concentrated liquid or powder form, with caloric values increased or decreased by variations in dilution.

The following table lists commercial formulas and other infant feedings commonly used at the University of Iowa Hospitals and Clinics. The information is current as of the press date.

Per 1000 cc	CHO gms/L	PRO gms/L	FAT gms/L	Cal/cc	Carbohydrate	Protein	Fat	mOsm/ Kg H$_2$O	Na mEq/L	K mEq/L	Ca mg/L
Milk-based											
Enfamil	69.0	15.0	38.0	0.68	Lactose	Reduced minerals whey, nonfat cow milk	Coconut and soy oils; coconut and corn oils (powder)	300	8	19	465
Milumil	82.0	18.0	31.0	0.68	Lactose, cornstarch, corn syrup solids	Nonfat cow milk	Coconut and soy oils	260	15	30	744
Similac	72.3	15.0	36.3	0.68	Lactose	Nonfat cow milk	Soy and coconut oils; corn and coconut oils (powder)	290	10	21	510
Similac PM 60/40 (liquid)	69.0	15.8	37.6	0.68	Lactose	Demineralized whey solids, sodium caseinate	Soy and coconut oils; corn and coconut oils (powder)	260	7	15	380
(prepared from powder)	69.0	15.0	37.8	0.68				260	7	15	380
SMA	72.0	15.0	36.0	0.68	Lactose	Reduced minerals whey, nonfat cow milk	Oleo, coconut, oleic, and soybean oils	300	6.5	14	420
Soy-based											
Advance	55.1	20.0	27.0	0.54	Corn syrup, lactose	Nonfat cow milk, soy protein isolate	Soy and corn oils	200	9	24	510
Isomil	68.3	18.0	36.9	0.68	Corn syrup, sucrose	Soy protein isolate + L-methionine	Soy and coconut oils	250	14	24	710
Isomil SF	68.3	20.0	36.0	0.68	Corn syrup, solids	Soy protein isolate + L-methionine	Soy and coconut oils	150	14	20	710
Nursoy	69.0	21.0	36.0	0.68	Sucrose; corn syrup solids and sucrose (powder)	Soy protein isolate + L-methionine	Oleo, coconut, oleic and soybean oils	296	9	18	600
Prosobee	67.7	20.3	35.9	0.68	Corn syrup solids	Soy protein isolate + L-methionine	Coconut and soy oils; coconut and corn oils (powder)	200	11	21	635
I-Soyalac	68.0	21.0	37.0	0.69	Sucrose, tapioca starch	Soy protein isolate + L-methionine	Soy oil	270	12	20	690
Soyalac	68.0	21.0	37.0	0.69	Sucrose, corn syrup solids	Soybean solids	Soy oil	240	13	20	635
Special											
Alimentum	68.9	18.6	37.5	0.68	Sucrose, tapioca starch	Casein hydrolysate	MCT oil, safflower oil, soy oil	370	13	20	710
Good Start H.A.	73.3	16.0	34.0	0.68	Lactose, maltodextrin	Hydrolyzed whey protein	Vegetable oils	--	7	17	426
Good Nature	88.0	20.0	26.0	0.68	Lactose, corn syrup solids	Nonfat cow milk	Palm oil, corn oil, safflower oil	--	11	23	900
Lofenalac	88.1	22.0	26.4	0.68	Corn syrup solids, modified tapioca starch	Specially processed casein hydrolysate	Corn oil	360	14	18	635
Nutramigen	91.0	19.0	26.4	0.68	Corn syrup solids, modified corn starch	Casein hydrolysate + L-cystine, L-tyrosine, and L-tryptophan	Corn oil	320	14	19	635

P ng/L	Vit. A I.U.	Vit. A mcg	Vit. D I.U.	Vit. D mcg	Vit. E I.U.	Vit. E mcg	Vit. K mcg/L	Thiamin mg/L	Riboflavin mg/L	Niacin mg/L	Vit. C mg/L	Fe mg/L	Zn mg/L	I mcg/L	Cu mg/L	Mg mg/L	Reference	Cost
320	2100	630	420	10.5	21	14.1	58	0.53	1.1	8.5	55	12.7[a]	5.3	69	0.63	53	2	Low
541	2522	757	406	10.1	8	5.4	54	0.27	0.6	6.8	54	10.8	4.2	50	0.42	74	3	Low
390	2030	609	410	10.2	20	13.4	54	0.68	1.0	7.0	60	12[b]	5.1	100	0.61	41	4	Low
190	2030	603	410	10.2	20	13.4	54	0.68	1.0	7.1	60	1.5	5.1	41	0.61	41	4	Low
190	2030	609	410	10.2	17	11.4	54	0.68	1.0	7.1	60	1.5	5.1	41	0.61	41	4	Low
280	2000	600	400	10.0	9.5	6.4	58	0.67	1.0	5.0	55	12.0[b]	5.0	60	0.47	45	5	Low
390	2160	648	410	10.2	20	13.4	54	0.76	0.92	10.0	50	10	4.9	59	0.59	65	4	Low
510	2030	609	410	10.2	20	13.4	100	0.41	0.61	9.1	60	12	5.1	100	0.51	51	4	Low
510	2030	609	410	10.2	20	13.4	100	0.41	0.61	9.1	60	12	5.1	100	0.51	51	4	Low
420	2000	600	400	10.0	9.5	6.4	100	0.67	1.0	5.0	55	11.5	5.0	60	0.47	67	5	Low
500	2100	630	420	10.5	21	14.1	106	0.53	0.63	8.5	55	12.7	5.3	69	0.63	74	2	Low
480	2110	633	420	10.5	16	10.7	53	0.63	0.63	8.4	80	13	5.3	53	0.79	74	1	Low
370	2110	633	420	10.5	16	10.7	53	0.53	0.64	8.4	80	13	5.3	53	0.53	80	1	Low
510	2030	609	410	10.2	20	13.5	100	0.41	0.61	9.1	60	12	5.1	100	0.51	51		Moderate
240	2000	600	400	10.0	8	5.4	55	0.40	0.90	5.0	53	10	5.0	53	0.53	45		Moderate
600	1667	500	433	10.8	5	3.4	54	0.53	0.64	8.5	53	12.7	4.2	38	0.51	56		Low
475	1691	507	420	10.5	10.5	7.1	106	0.53	0.63	8.5	55	12.7	4.2	48	0.63	74	2	Moderate
420	2100	630	420	10.5	21	14.1	106	0.53	0.63	8.5	55	12.7	5.3	48	0.63	74	2	Moderate

Per 1000 cc	CHO gms/L	PRO gms/L	FAT gms/L	Cal/cc	Carbohydrate	Protein	Fat	mOsm/ Kg H_2O	Na mEq/L	K mEq/L	Ca mg/L
Portagen	78.0	23.7	32.4	0.68	Corn syrup, solids, sucrose	Sodium caseinate	MCT oil (88%) and corn oil	220	15	22	635
Pregestimil	70.0	19.0	38.1	0.68	Corn syrup solids, modified tapioca starch, glucose	Casein hydrolysate + L-cystine, L-tyrosine, and L-tryptophan	Corn oil and MCT oil (60%)	300	14	19	635
Product 3232A	28.0	19.0	28.0	0.43[c]	Modified tapioca starch, added carbohydrate	Casein hydrolysate	MCT and corn oils	250[c]	13	19	635
Product 80056	84.4	0	26.4	0.58[d]	Corn syrup solids, modified tapioca starch	--	Corn oil	200[d]	4	10	365
RDF (Ross)	0+	20.0	36.0	0.405[c]	Varies according to carbohydrate added	Soy protein isolate + L-methionine	Soy and coconut oils	64[c]	14	20	710
Premature											
Enfamil Premature	89.0	24.3	41.4	0.81	Corn syrup solids, lactose	Reduced minerals whey, nonfat cow milk	MCT, soy, and coconut oils	300	14	23	950
Similac 24 LBW	85.3	22.0	44.9	0.81	Corn syrup solids, lactose	Nonfat cow milk	MCT, soy, and coconut oils	290	16	31	730
Similac Special Care	86.1	22.0	44.1	0.81	Corn syrup solids, lactose	Whey protein concentrate, nonfat cow milk	MCT, soy, and coconut oils	300	18	29	1460
SMA "Preemie"	86.0	20.0	44.0	0.81	Corn syrup solids, lactose	Whey protein concentrate, nonfat cow milk	Coconut, oleic, oleo, soy, and MCT oils	280	14	19	750
Human Milk Fortifier											
Similac Natural Care	86.1	22.0	44.1	0.81	Corn syrup solids, lactose	Whey protein concentrate, nonfat cow milk	MCT, soy, and coconut oils	300	18	29	1710
Enfamil Human Milk Fortifier (40 pkts = 38 g, to be added to 1 liter preterm human milk)	27.0	7.0	0.5	0.14	Corn syrup solids	Whey protein concentrate, casein	--	365[e]	3	4	600
Oral Electrolyte Solutions											
Lytren	25.0	0	0	0.10	Glucose, corn syrup solids	--	--	220	50	25	--
Pedialyte	25.0	0	0	0.10	Glucose	--	--	250	45	20	--
Pedialyte RS	25.0	0	0	0.10	Glucose	--	--	305	75	20	--
Resol	20.0	0	0	0.08	Glucose	--	--	269	50	20	80

Notes: I.U. Vitamin A ÷ 3.33 = mcg retinol; I.U. Vitamin D x 0.025 = mcg cholecalciferol; I.U. Vitamin E ÷ 1.49 = mg d-alpha-tocopherol.

Cost: Low = $0-3 per liter. Premature formulas are provided at no cost to hospitals only. Moderate = $3-6 per liter.

Reference: 1 = Loma Linda Foods, 11503 Pierce St., Riverside, CA 92515; 2 = Mead Johnson, Nutritional Division, Evansville, IN 47721; 3 = Milupa Corporation, 397 Boston Post Road, Darien, CT 06820; 4 = Ross Laboratories, 625 Cleveland Ave., Columbus, OH 43215; 5 = Wyeth Laboratories, P.O. Box 8299, Philadelphia, PA 19101.

[a]Low iron formula = 1.1.
[b]Low iron formula = 1.5.
[c]Without added carbohydrate.
[d]Without added protein, 111.2 g powder diluted to one quart.
[e]Fortifier added to human milk.

P mg/L	Vit. A I.U.	mcg	Vit. D I.U.	mcg	Vit. E I.U.	mcg	Vit. K mcg/L	Thiamin mg/L	Riboflavin mg/L	Niacin mg/L	Vit. C mg/L	Fe mg/L	Zn mg/L	I mcg/L	Cu mg/L	Mg mg/L	Reference	Cost
475	5280	1584	528	13.2	21	14.1	106	1.06	1.27	13.7	55	12.7	6.3	48	1.06	135	2	Moderate
420	2520	756	504	12.6	24.8	16.6	127	0.53	0.63	8.5	79	12.7	6.3	48	0.63	74	2	Moderate
420	2537	761	507	12.7	25	17.0	127	0.53	0.63	8.5	79	12.7	4.2	48	0.63	74	2	Moderate
353	1693	508	420	10.5	10.5	7.1	106	0.53	0.63	8.5	53	12.9	4.2	48	0.63	74	2	Low
510	2030	609	410	10.2	20	13.4	100	0.41	0.61	9.1	60	1.5	5.1	100	0.51	51	4	Low
476	9725	2918	2645	66.2	37	25.0	106	2.0	2.9	32.8	285	2.0	8.1	64	1.3	40	2	Low
570	2440	732	490	12.2	24	16.1	65	1.0	1.2	8.5	100	3.0	8.1	120	0.81	81	4	Low
730	5520	1656	1220	30.5	32	21.5	100	2.0	5.0	40.6	300	3.0	12.2	160	2.0	100	4	Low
400	2400	720	480	12.0	15	10.1	70	0.8	1.3	6.3	70	3.0	8.0	83	0.7	70	5	Low
850	5520	1656	1220	30.5	32	21.5	100	2.0	5.0	40.6	300	3.0	12.2	160	2.0	100	4	Low
330	7800	2340	2600	65.0	34	22.8	91	1.9	2.5	31.0	240	--	3.1	--	0.8	40	2	Moderate
-	--	--	--	--	--	--	--	--	--	--	--	--	--	--	--	--	2	Moderate
-	--	--	--	--	--	--	--	--	--	--	--	--	--	--	--	--	4	Moderate
-	--	--	--	--	--	--	--	--	--	--	--	--	--	--	--	--	4	Moderate
78	--	--	--	--	--	--	--	--	--	--	--	--	--	--	--	49	5	Moderate

E. WEIGHT CONTROL DIETS FOR CHILDREN

DESCRIPTION: A weight control diet provides for a decrease in caloric intake to promote weight loss or prevent weight gain. An approach that focuses on diet, exercise, and family counseling is recommended. The overall goal of the control program is to establish lifelong habits that will maintain desirable body weight.

PROCEDURE: Upon request for a weight control diet, the dietitian will interview the patient to calculate the present caloric intake and to assess the nutritional quality of the diet. Using information gathered from the interview, the dietitian will plan a weight reduction program based on specific changes in eating habits (usually reducing foods high in fat and/or sucrose). The patient is encouraged to choose a variety of appropriate servings from the basic four food groups. Establishing regular meal and snack times, increasing physical activity, and teaching the child to recognize satiety are emphasized. Behavior modification techniques are used (see page 157).

For most children, especially preadolescents, weight maintenance over several years is advisable; however, some children who are well above the 95th percentile in weight/height would need to reduce. Preadolescent children may be expected to lose up to 1 kg/month, whereas some adolescents can lose up to 0.5 to 1.0 kg/week.

WEIGHT REDUCTION IN PRADER-WILLI: A weight reduction regimen is nearly always indicated for children with the Prader-Willi Syndrome. This disorder is characterized by gross obesity, mental retardation, muscular hypotonia, hypogonadism, and short stature. Children with Prader-Willi display insatiable appetites and will go to extreme measures to obtain food. For this reason, environmental control of food supplies is essential.

F. CONSTANT CARBOHYDRATE DIET FOR CHILDREN WITH DIABETES MELLITUS

DESCRIPTION: A patient with insulin dependent diabetes admitted to a pediatric service at the University of Iowa Hospitals and Clinics is usually given a constant carbohydrate diet. On this program, the child eats a consistent amount of carbohydrate at regular times each day. The carbohydrate content of foods is determined by using the diabetic exchange lists (see pages 144-54) and supplemental lists of other usual American foods.[1] Substitutions from one exchange list to another may be made as long as the total grams of carbohydrate at a meal or snack is within the 5 g range of the carbohydrate pattern designed for the patient. Emphasis is placed on choosing a nutritionally adequate diet, with a limited amount of foods high in simple sugars. This diet is also low in cholesterol and fat. As a part of a complete diabetes education program, the patient and/or the family is thoroughly instructed in how diet can be managed to achieve good blood glucose control.

PROCEDURE: The initial carbohydrate pattern is based on the patient's diet history. If necessary, modifications are suggested to improve the nutritional quality of the diet. For example: if, prior to hospitalization, the patient was consuming a nutritionally well-balanced lunch containing 75 to 80 g carbohydrate, the proposed diet pattern will provide 75 to 80 g carbohydrate at lunch. Alterations in the carbohydrate pattern are made to meet growth needs; however, dietary alterations are not made on a daily basis to meet temporary appetite fluctuations. The patient is encouraged to reduce daily cholesterol intake to 200 to 300 mg and to reduce dietary fat to 30 to 35% of total calories. This can be achieved by eliminating or limiting egg yolks and organ meats and by consuming skim or lowfat milk and moderate amounts of meat, cheese, fried foods, salad dressings, and other concentrated fats.

The patient is taught the various symptoms that may indicate an insulin reaction and is instructed to carry a source of concentrated carbohydrate (such as sugar packets) so that insulin reactions can be promptly treated. The patient is also instructed to eat an additional 10 to 15 g carbohydrate in advance for each hour of anticipated increased activity. Through experience, the diabetic learns to adjust food intake to individual needs.

---

[1]Values are obtained from standard food composition tables and product labels.

SUPPLEMENTARY FOOD EXCHANGE LIST FOR CONSTANT CARBOHYDRATE DIET

Food	Portion	Carbohydrate (g)	Protein (g)	Fat (g)
Beans and frankfurters	1/2 cup	20	10	10
Brownie, unfrosted	3 x 1 1/2 in.	20	2	5
Burrito, frozen	6 oz	40	15	15
Cake, angel food, unfrosted	1/12 cake	30	5	--
Cake frosting	2 tbsp	20	--	5
Cake, plain	1/12 cake	30	5	10
Casseroles, homemade	1 cup	30	15	15
Catsup	1 tbsp	5	--	--
Chili con carne (with beans)	1/2 cup	15	10	10
Chocolate syrup	1 tbsp	10	--	--
Cocoa mix	1 oz pkg or 2 tbsp	20	5	--
Cookie, sandwich cream	2 cookies	20	2	5
Cottage cheese, creamed	1/2 cup	5	15	5
Egg roll	1 1/2 oz	15	5	5
Fudgsicle	2 1/2 oz bar	20	5	--
Gingersnaps	3 small	10	2	1
Granola	1/4 cup	15	3	5
Granola bar	1 small	15	2	5
Ice cream bar	2 1/2 oz bar	15	2	10
Ice cream cone (cone only)	1 (4 g)	5	1	--
Ice cream sugar cone (cone only)	1 (11 g)	10	2	--
Ice cream sandwich	2 oz	25	3	5
Jelly	1 tsp	5	--	--
Lasagna	1 cup	30	15	10
Macaroni and cheese	1 cup	30	10	10
Meat pot pie	8 oz	40	25	15
Milk, chocolate	1 cup	25	10	2-5
Pancake syrup	1 tbsp	15	--	--
Peanut butter	1 tbsp	5	5	10
Pizza (cheese), thin crust	1/4 of 15 oz or 1/4 of 10 in.	30	15	10
Pudding (butterscotch or chocolate)	1/2 cup (instant)	30	5	5
	1/2 cup (homemade)	35	5	5
Pudding (tapioca or vanilla)	1/2 cup (instant)	25	5	5
	1/2 cup (homemade)	20	5	5
Ravioli	1 cup	30	15	10
Sherbet	1/2 cup	30	1	2
Snack chips	1 oz	15	1	10
Soups:				
Bean or chunky	1 cup	20	10	5
Beef noodle or Chicken noodle	1 cup	10	5	--
Cream (made with water)	1 cup	15	--	5
Cream (made with milk)	1 cup	20	5	5
Vegetable	1 cup	15	--	--
Spaghetti in meat sauce	1 cup	30	15	10
Stew, beef with potato	1 cup	25	10	5
Sugar	1 tsp	4	--	--
Sweet pickle	3 1/3 oz - 1 large	35	--	--
Taco shell	1 average	10	2	--
Turnover	1 (3 1/3 oz)	30	2	20
Yogurt, fruit flavored	1/2 cup	20	5	--

Note: Nutrient values have been rounded. These values can be used when nutrient labels are not available. Although protein per se is not counted in the constant carbohydrate diet, the values are listed here for your information.

G. DISACCHARIDE RESTRICTED DIET

DESCRIPTION: This is a graduated diet for patients who cannot utilize disaccharides and polysaccharides. In the severe stages of this syndrome, only glucose and fructose are tolerated. As the patient improves, the diet may be liberalized, gradually adding starches, then foods containing sucrose, and finally foods containing milk solids (lactose). This progression is listed under Foods Allowed and Foods to Avoid.

If one of the carbohydrate "breakdown products" is not tolerated, the carbohydrates forming that product must be omitted. For example:

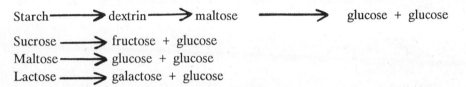

$$Starch \longrightarrow dextrin \longrightarrow maltose \longrightarrow glucose + glucose$$

$$Sucrose \longrightarrow fructose + glucose$$

$$Maltose \longrightarrow glucose + glucose$$

$$Lactose \longrightarrow galactose + glucose$$

A list of the more common carbohydrates in foods can be found in Appendix H.

ADEQUACY: The nutritional adequacy of this diet is variable, depending upon the number of foods tolerated.

FOODS ALLOWED AND FOODS TO AVOID:

Food Group	Low Disaccharide	Starches Tolerated	Sucrose Tolerated	Milk Solids Tolerated
Beverages	Kool-Aid or tea sweetened with dextrose or fructose, special formula containing mono-saccharides (RCF[1] or 3232A[2] with added dextrose or fructose)	Formulas containing corn syrup solids (Pregestimil, ProSobee, Isomil SF)	Beverages containing sucrose if it has been found to be tolerated	Milk
Breads	None	Breads made with dextrose but without sugar or milk, crackers that do not contain added sugar or milk	Breads and crackers that do not contain milk	Any

---

[1]Ross Carbohydrate-Free Protein Formula Base, Ross Laboratories, 625 Cleveland Ave., Columbus, OH 43215.

[2]3232A Mead Johnson, Evansville, IN 47721.

FOODS ALLOWED AND FOODS TO AVOID (continued):

Food Group	Low Disaccharide	Starches Tolerated	Sucrose Tolerated	Milk Solids Tolerated
Cereals	None	Farina, infant oat and rice cereals, oatmeal, puffed rice, shredded wheat, others that do not contain sugar or milk	Any that do not contain milk solids	Any
Desserts	Gelatin flavored with Kool-Aid and dextrose	Dextrose-sweetened lemon pudding	Any that do not contain milk or milk products	Any
Eggs	Any preparation to which milk is not added			
Fats	Butter, vegetable oils, margarine without milk solids, mayonnaise			Any
Fruits, Fruit Juices	Juice of allowed fruits. The following unsweetened fresh, frozen, or canned fruits containing <1.5% sucrose are allowed (dextrose may be used): boysenberries, blackberries, cranberries, currants, cherries, figs, concord or malaga grapes, gooseberries, lemons, loganberries, loquats, papayas, damson plums, pomegranates, raspberries, strawberries		Other fruits as tolerated	Any

FOODS ALLOWED AND FOODS TO AVOID (continued):

Food Group	Low Disaccharide	Starches Tolerated	Sucrose Tolerated	Milk Solids Tolerated
Meat, Fish, Poultry, Cheese	Fresh beef, chicken, lamb, liver, pork, turkey; fish and seafood that do not contain fillers, breading, lactose, or sucrose	Any that do not contain sucrose or milk solids	Any that do not contain milk solids	Any
Potatoes or Substitutes	None	Boiled or baked white potatoes, hominy, macaroni, noodles, spaghetti, rice	Sweet potato as tolerated	Others
Sugar, Sweets	Dextrose, fructose, honey (for child over 1 year)[1]	Corn syrup (for child over 1 year)	Sucrose	
Soups	Any made from allowed vegetables	Any made from allowed foods		Any
Vegetables, Vegetable Juices	Asparagus, green and wax beans, cabbage family vegetables, carrots, celery, cucumber, lettuce, rutabaga, summer squash, tomato; juices from allowed vegetables	Corn, lima beans, pumpkin, winter squash	Others	Any

---

[1]The intestinal tracts of some infants under 1 year of age are susceptible to infant botulism. Because the susceptibility of individual infants to the development of infant botulism remains unknown, it is reasonable to avoid use of nutritionally nonessential foods such as honey in infant feeding (Arnon et al. 1979).

215

FOODS ALLOWED AND FOODS TO AVOID (continued):

Food Group	Low Disaccharide	Starches Tolerated	Sucrose Tolerated	Milk Solids Tolerated
Miscellaneous	Herbs (read labels for other foods not listed above); vinegar	Carbohydrate supplements made from corn syrup solids (Moducal[1], Polycose[2], Sumacal[3])		

APPROXIMATE COMPOSITION OF SAMPLE MENU:

Calories	1520
Protein, g	72
Fat, g	75
Carbohydrate, g	142

SAMPLE MENU FOR DISACCHARIDE RESTRICTED DIET:

Breakfast	Luncheon	Dinner
1/2 cup unsweetened cranberry juice 1 egg, soft cooked 1 cup RCF with added dextrose	2 oz sliced chicken 1/2 cup green beans 1/2 sliced tomato on lettuce 1 tsp mayonnaise 1 tsp butter 1/2 cup fresh strawberries 1 cup RCF with added dextrose	3 oz roast beef 1/2 cup cooked carrots 3/4 cup tossed lettuce salad 1 tbsp vinegar and oil dressing 1 tsp butter 2 canned unsweetened figs 1 cup RCF with added dextrose

Midmorning Nourishment	Midafternoon Nourishment	Evening Nourishment
1/2 cup Kool-Aid sweetened with 2 tbsp dextrose	1/2 cup lemonade sweetened with 2 tbsp dextrose	1 cup RCF with added dextrose

[1]Mead Johnson, Evansville, IN 47721.

[2]Ross Laboratories, 625 Cleveland Ave., Columbus, OH 43215.

[3]Sherwood Medical, St. Louis, MO 63103.

H. GALACTOSE-FREE DIET

DESCRIPTION: This diet is used to treat individuals with galactosemia, an inborn error of galactose metabolism. Simply stated, an inborn error of metabolism is a genetically determined biochemical disorder in which a defect in an enzyme complex results in a metabolic block of pathological consequence. The goal of dietary restriction is to maintain erythrocyte galactose-1-phosphate concentration at or below 3 mg per 100 ml serum. Excluded are all sources of the monosaccharide galactose which is found primarily in the form of lactose, the disaccharide in milk and milk products. (Lactose is hydrolyzed within the intestinal mucosa to glucose and galactose.) Thus foods containing milk and milk products (whey and casein) are excluded. Lactate, lactic acid, and lactalbumin do not contain lactose and are therefore allowed. Because many processed foods contain milk, whey or casein, all ingredient labels should be read carefully. This precaution applies to medications as well, especially those in tablet form. Some of these medications do not list lactose on the label, even though the product contains lactose. The pharmacist, *Physician's Desk Reference,* or individual drug companies may be consulted to determine ingredients. The use of liquid medications and avoiding the purchase of over-the-counter medications that lack complete ingredient lists are other ways of avoiding lactose in medications.

Four enzymes are required for the normal metabolism of galactose to glucose-1-phosphate. Defects in 2 of the enzymes result in clinical symptoms that may be treated and/or prevented by dietary galactose restriction. Classical galactosemia, or transferase deficiency galactosemia, results from a deficiency of galactose-1-phosphate uridyltransferase, the enzyme which mediates the second step of the galactose metabolic pathway (see below). Galactokinase deficiency (the first enzymatic step in galactose metabolism) results in a less severe disorder associated with cataract formation only.

GALACTOSE METABOLIC PATHWAY

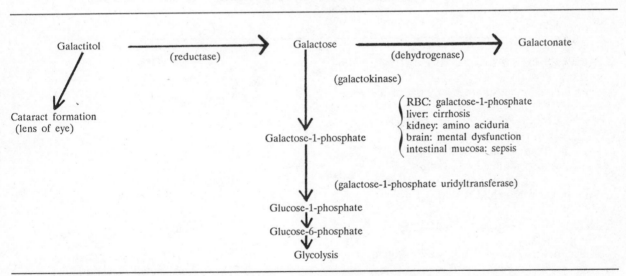

In classic galactosemia, galactose, galactose-1-phosphate, and galacticol accumulate in the body tissue. Untreated neonates present with vomiting and diarrhea within the first 3 days of life. Within the first week, jaundice, hepatomegaly, and cataracts occur. After several months developmental delay is observed. Shortly after the introduction of a galactose-free diet, signs and symptoms begin to regress. Because mental retardation is not reversible, the importance of early recognition and treatment is emphasized.

Because of the immediate onset of the galactosemia syndrome, it is imperative that an accurate diagnosis be made and dietary management begin immediately. Infants with galactosemia should consume a galactose-free formula (see table below) as their sole source of nutrition until approximately 4 to 6 months of age. The diet is then advanced in variety and texture according to the recommendations of the American Academy of Pediatrics. The galactose-free formula fed in infancy is also an appropriate source of protein, calories, and micronutrients for the older child. If adequate amounts of formula are not consumed beyond infancy, supplementation with calcium, zinc, phosphorus, riboflavin, and vitamin D must be considered.

The inclusion of certain legumes in the allowed foods lists remains controversial. Soybeans, navy beans, and lima beans contain galactose in the oligosaccharides raffinose and stachyose. It is thought that the enzymes in the intestinal mucosa are unable to break down these sugars. Intestinal microflora, however, do have this capability. Because the use of soy formula has not resulted in elevated erythrocyte galactose-1-phosphate concentrations, it remains an appropriate source of nutrition.

Mothers of patients with galactosemia are advised to restrict galactose intake during subsequent pregnancies in order to minimize fetal exposure to galactose and galactosemia sequelae. This is because some children, even though they are diagnosed and treated within the early neonatal period, already demonstrate cataract formation at birth and are intellectually compromised.

During the first year of life, dietary compliance is monitored by assay of erythrocyte galactose-1-phosphate every 2 to 3 months and by assessment of 3-day diet records, rate of linear growth, and weight gain. In subsequent years galactose-1-phosphate concentration, dietary intake information and growth parameters are obtained every 4 to 6 months.

INFANT FORMULAS USED IN THE TREATMENT OF GALACTOSEMIA

Product	Manufacturer/ Address	Description
ProSobee	Mead Johnson Nutritional Division Evansville, IN 47721	Galactose-free soy protein formula
Isomil	Ross Laboratories 625 Cleveland Ave. Columbus, OH 43215	Galactose-free soy protein formula
Nutramigen	Mead Johnson Nutritional Division Evansville, IN 47721	Casein hydrolysate formula, essentially galactose- and lactose-free

EXAMPLES OF GALACTOSE-FREE MENUS:

Sample menu for an infant 6 months of age:

    32 oz ProSobee formula (20 kcal/oz)
    2 tbsp rice cereal
    1-2 tbsp strained fruit
    1-2 tbsp strained vegetable

Sample menu for a child 4 years of age:

Breakfast	Luncheon	Dinner
8 oz ProSobee	8 oz ProSobee	8 oz ProSobee
1/2 cup cooked cereal	1 oz roast beef	1 oz baked chicken
1 tsp margarine	1 tsp mayonnaise	1 tsp milk-free margarine
4 oz juice	1 slice vienna bread	1/4 cup vegetable
	Carrot and celery sticks	1/4 cup rice
		1/2 cup gelatin with fruit

Sample menu for a child 4 years of age (continued):

Evening
Nourishment

4 oz ProSobee
Fresh fruit
Saltine crackers

APPROXIMATE COMPOSITION OF SAMPLE MENU (for adolescent or adult):

Calories	2209
Protein, g	86
Fat, g	65
Carbohydrate, g	319

Sample menu for an adolescent or adult:

Breakfast	Luncheon	Dinner
1/2 cup orange juice	1/2 cup tomato juice	3 oz roast beef
1/2 cup farina	2 oz sliced chicken	1/2 cup cubed white potato
1 egg, soft cooked	1/2 cup rice	1/2 cup cooked carrots
1 slice vienna bread, toasted	1/2 cup green beans	1 slice vienna bread
1 tsp milk-free margarine	1 slice vienna bread	2 tsp milk-free margarine
1 tbsp grape jelly	2 tsp milk-free margarine	1/2 cup canned pears
1 cup soy-based formula	1/2 cup canned peaches	1 cup soy-based formula
	1 slice angel food cake	
	1 cup soy-based formula	

Midafternoon
Nourishment

1/2 cup pineapple juice

Evening
Nourishment

3/4 cup Rice Krispies
2 tsp sugar
1/2 cup soy-based formula

FOODS ALLOWED AND FOODS TO AVOID:

Food Group	Foods Allowed	Foods to Avoid
Beverages	Soy-based formulas or casein hydrolysate formulas (Nutramigen or Pregestimil); carbonated beverages; fruit drinks; coffee and tea; nondairy milk substitute (Coffee Rich)	Milk or milk drinks, tableted or powdered soft drinks containing lactose, milk treated with Lact-Aid
Breads	Saltine and graham crackers, french and vienna breads, other breads made without milk or milk products	Bread, muffins, biscuits, or pancakes, containing milk, lactose, or other foods to avoid
Cereals	All cooked and prepared cereals free of milk or lactose	Any cereal, including instant, containing lactose or milk

FOODS ALLOWED AND FOODS TO AVOID (continued):

Food Group	Foods Allowed	Foods to Avoid
Desserts	Fruit pudding made without milk, flavored gelatin, cookies made without milk or butter, homemade baked products and puddings made of allowed ingredients, fruit ices, gelatin desserts, popsicles	All ice cream, ice milk, or sherbet; cakes, cookies, custard, puddings, pies, or pie crusts containing milk, butter, or lactose
Eggs	Any except preparations containing milk or butter	Scrambled, fondues, or omelets containing milk, milk products, or butter; creamed eggs
Fats	Margarine without milk solids; salad oils, shortening; mayonnaise; bacon fat; lard; peanut butter; cream substitutes free of milk, whey, or casein	Butter, cream, salad dressings made with milk, whey, or casein; margarines containing milk solids
Fruits, Fruit Juices	Any except those to avoid	Fruit drinks containing lactose, fruits processed with lactose
Meat, Fish, Poultry, Cheese	Baked, broiled, roasted, or stewed beef, fish, lamb, poultry, pork, veal	All creamed, breaded, or processed meats such as cold cuts; wieners containing lactose or milk; all organ meats; all cheese
Potatoes or Substitutes	White and sweet potatoes, hominy, macaroni, noodles, rice, spaghetti	Mashed potatoes containing milk or butter, dehydrated potatoes, french fries, and potato chips if lactose has been used in processing; creamed, scalloped, or buttered potatoes or substitutes
Soups	Clear soups, vegetable soups made from allowed foods, homemade cream soups made with allowed milk substitutes	Cream soups, chowders, commercial soups containing lactose

FOODS ALLOWED AND FOODS TO AVOID (continued):

Food Group	Foods Allowed	Foods to Avoid
Sugar, Sweets	Sugar, syrup, honey, hard candy, jelly, marshmallows, gum drops (read labels for foods to avoid), brown sugar, molasses	Candy containing lactose (milk sugar), milk or butter (butterscotch, caramels, milk chocolate)
Vegetables, Vegetable Juices	Juices made from allowed foods, all vegetables except those to avoid	Creamed vegetables or vegetables prepared with foods to avoid; possibly lima beans and navy beans
Miscellaneous	Catsup, mustard, carob powder, nuts and nut butters, olives, pickles, unbuttered popcorn, salt, vinegar, spices, flavorings without lactose, cocoa powder, cooking chocolate, semisweet chocolate, chewing gum	Cream sauce, milk gravy, corn curls, some spice blends (check labels), sugar substitutes containing lactose and other possible sources of lactose such as ascorbic acid and citric acid mixtures; dietetic and diabetic preparations; Easter egg dyes and dye carriers; penicillin and other antibiotics; pharmaceutical bulking agents, fillers, and excipients; tableted food and pharmaceuticals; tinctures, vitamin and mineral mixtures

I. PHENYLALANINE RESTRICTED DIET

DESCRIPTION: Simply stated, an inborn error of metabolism is a genetically determined biochemical disorder in which a defect in an enzyme or enzyme complex results in a metabolic block of pathological consequence. The goal of dietary treatment is to circumvent the biochemical defect and to maintain a normal physiological/biochemical environment. All newborns in the state of Iowa are tested for three inborn errors of metabolism, all of which require dietary management (phenylketonuria, galactosemia, and branched chain ketoacidemia). Positive blood tests are promptly reported to the attending physician and to the UIHC metabolic management team. The parents of the child are notified, and an appointment is made to confirm the diagnosis and initiate treatment. The infant may be hospitalized for observation while the parents are instructed in management of the disorder.

The phenylalanine (PHE) restricted diet is used in the treatment of infants, children, and young adults who have an abnormality in phenylalanine metabolism (phenylketonuria, hyperphenylalaninemia). The objective of the diet is to maintain serum PHE concentration between 2 and 10 mg/100 ml (mg/dl or mg%), while providing sufficient calories and nutrients to promote optimal growth and development. Because PHE is an essential amino acid, adequate amounts must be provided orally. Frequent blood PHE assessments must be performed to determine the adequacy of the diet. To prevent brain damage, dietary control should be instituted before 3 weeks of age and continued indefinitely.

DIETARY MANAGEMENT:

1. Estimate the child's daily requirement of PHE, protein, and calories according to age, weight, and metabolic history (previous blood PHE concentrations). A range is given for PHE and protein, allowing for individualization of the diet. The patient's history of PHE tolerance is the most important factor in determining the PHE content of the diet.

ESTIMATED DAILY REQUIREMENTS OF PHENYLALANINE, PROTEIN, AND CALORIES
FOR CHILDREN WITH PHENYLKETONURIA

Age	PHE (mg/kg)	Protein Total/day	Calories (kcal/kg)
0-2 months	40-70	2.5 g/kg	95-145
3-6 months	25-55	2.5 g/kg	95-145
7-12 months	15-50	2.2 g/kg	80-135
1-3 years	15-40	25 (1.8-2.0 g/kg)	90 (1300/day)
4-6 years	15-40	30 (1.6-1.8 g/kg)	85 (1700/day)
7-10 years	15-40	35 (1.2-1.6 g/kg)	85 (2400/day)
11-15 years	15-30	45-50 g	(2200-2700/day)
15-19 years	10-30	45-55 g	(1800-2100/day)

2. Select a low phenylalanine or phenylalanine-free formula powder to meet the majority of the individual's protein requirement (see table on page 224). When an infant is first diagnosed, a formula low in PHE (see table on page 224) is prescribed to promote endogenous utilization of the amino acid while meeting protein and calorie requirements for growth. When blood PHE concentration reaches 2 to 6 mg/dl, an additional source of PHE (infant formula, breast milk) is added to the specialty formula to meet the infant's requirement for continued growth. Each family is provided with a gram scale to facilitate accuracy of powder measurement. In general, solid foods are introduced according to the recommendations of the

American Academy of Pediatrics[1], except that meats and high protein cereals and dinners should be avoided due to their high PHE content. Solid foods will gradually replace formula or breast milk as the major source of phenylalanine. Once the child is able to consume a sufficient amount of low protein solid foods to meet the PHE requirement, usually around 3 years of age, a transition to a phenylalanine-free formula is initiated. The amount of solid food offered may be determined using phenylalanine exchange (equivalent) lists. These lists indicate the amount of various foods which provide 15 mg PHE. Protein and caloric content are also listed.

3. Monitor the dietary management of the disorder. As soon as the diagnosis of PKU is confirmed, the parents are instructed to keep accurate records of formula intake. Initially, diet records are kept daily to determine the infant's PHE, protein, and caloric requirements for growth and metabolic control. As consistent levels of blood PHE are achieved, diet records are required less frequently. Blood specimens for PHE analysis are initially performed twice a week and then weekly during the first year of life to assess the adequacy of the diet and the compliance to dietary restriction. Blood samples are required less frequently as good metabolic control is demonstrated. Plasma amino acid analysis is performed at the initial appointment and as indicated to assess PHE concentration in relation to other essential amino acids. Physical examinations, including height and weight measurements, are performed periodically[2] to assess the rate of growth, development, and the adequacy of the diet.

---

[1] To allow for the identification of food allergies, only 1 new food at a time is given, waiting 2 to 3 days before another is tried. Cereals are usually followed by fruits and then vegetables. In most cases formula is the only source of nutrition until 6 months of age.

[2] From 0 to 12 months of age, examine every month; from 12 to 24 months, every other month; from 24 to 36 months, every third month; over 36 months, every 4 months.

DIETARY PRODUCTS AVAILABLE FOR THE MANAGEMENT OF PKU

Product	Description/Comments
Analog XP[b]	Phenylalanine-free mixture of L-amino acids, designed for infants 0-1 year of age. Additional PHE must be provided by infant formula or breast milk.
Lofenalac[a]	Low PHE, nutritionally complete formula powder, designed for infants and young children with PKU. Additional PHE must be provided by standard infant formula, baby foods, or table foods.
Phenyl-Free[a]	Phenylalanine-free powder with a high protein to calorie ratio, designed for use by children and adults with PKU. PHE must be provided by other foods.
PKU 1[a]	Phenylalanine-free mixture of L-amino acids, sucrose, vitamins, and minerals, designed for use by infants and young children in combination with standard infant formula or foods. Sources of fat and carbohydrate must be provided to meet caloric requirements.
PKU 2[a]	Phenylalanine-free mixture of L-amino acids, sucrose, vitamins, and minerals, to be used in combination with solid foods for the management of PKU. Additional sources of PHE, fat, and calories must be provided.
PKU 3[a]	Phenylalanine-free mixture of L-amino acids, sucrose, vitamins, and minerals to be used in combination with table foods by pregnant women and older children. Additional sources of PHE, fat, and carbohydrate must be provided.
Maxamaid XP[b]	Phenylalanine-free mixture of amino acids, carbohydrate, vitamins, and minerals to be used in combination with sources of fat and vitamin K. This orange flavored drink is designed for children between 1 and 8 years of age.
Maxamum XP[b]	Phenylalanine-free mixture of amino acids, carbohydrate, vitamins, and minerals to be used in combination with sources of fat and vitamin K. This product is designed for individuals over 8 years of age and pregnant women.

[a]Mead Johnson, Nutritional Division, Evansville, IN 47721.
[b]Ross Laboratories, 625 Cleveland Ave., Columbus, OH 43215.

SUGGESTED SPECIALTY FORMULAS AND PHENYLALANINE SOURCES FOR INFANTS, CHILDREN, AND ADULTS WITH PKU

Age	Specialty Formula	Sources of Phenylalanine
0-6 months	Lofenalac, PKU 1, Analog XP	breast milk, commercial infant formula
6-12 months	Lofenalac, PKU 1, Analog XP	breast milk, commercial infant formula, baby foods
1-3 years	Lofenalac, PKU 1, Maxamaid XP	commercial infant formula, baby foods, table foods
3-4 years	transition to Phenyl-Free, PKU 2, or Maxamaid XP	table foods
> 4 years	Phenyl-Free, PKU 2, or Maxamaid XP	table foods
> 8 years	Phenyl-Free, PKU 3, or Maxamum XP	table foods

PROTEIN, PHENYLALANINE, AND CALORIE CONTENT
OF FORMULAS AND MILKS USED FOR PKU

Product	Protein (g)	Phenylalanine (mg)	Calories (kcal)
Lofenalac (g)	0.15	0.8	4.6
measure (9.5 g)	1.40	7.5	43.0
1 oz (20 kcal/oz)	0.65	3.5	20.0
Phenyl-Free (g)	0.20	–	4.0
measure (9.8 g)	2.00	–	40.0
1 oz (20 kcal/oz)	1.00	–	20.0
PKU 1 (g)	0.50	–	2.7
PKU 2 (g)	0.67	–	3.0
PKU 3 (g)	0.68	–	2.8
Analog XP (g)	0.13	–	4.75
Maxamaid XP (g)	0.25	–	3.6
Maxamum XP (g)	0.40	–	3.1
Enfamil			
powder (g)	0.12	5.1	5.3
scoop (8.3 g)	1.00	42.3	43.0
1 oz (20 kcal/oz)	0.45	19.0	20.0
1 oz (40 kcal/oz)	0.90	38.0	40.0
Similac			
powder (g)	0.10	5.2	4.8
scoop (8.74 g)	0.90	46.0	40.0
1 oz (20 kcal/oz)	0.49	21.6	20.0
1 oz (40 kcal/oz)	0.90	43.2	40.0
Isomil			
powder (g)	0.12	6.4	4.6
scoop (8.74 g)	1.06	56.2	40.0
1 oz (20 kcal/oz)	0.45	31.7	20.5
1 oz (40 kcal/oz)	0.90	63.3	41.0
SMA			
powder (g)	0.11	6.3	4.8
1 oz (20 kcal/oz)	0.45	24.0	20.0
1 oz (40 kcal/oz)	0.91	48.0	40.0
Milk (oz)			
whole	1.00	50.0	18.0
2%	1.00	50.0	16.0
skim	1.00	50.0	10.0
Breast Milk (oz)	0.31	13.9	21.2

AVERAGE PHE, PROTEIN, AND CALORIE CONTENT
OF PHE FOOD EXCHANGES

Food Group	PHE (mg)	Protein (g)	Calories (kcal)
Vegetables			
Strained and Junior	15	0.6	20
Table Foods	15	0.5	10
Fruits			
Strained and Junior	15	0.5	60
Table Foods	15	0.6	60
Breads/Cereals	15	0.3	10
Fats	15	0.3	180

SAMPLE CALCULATION OF DIET USING LOFENALAC:

1. Note infant's age and weight.

   Age 4 months; wt = 6.2 kg

2. Calculate estimated PHE, protein, and calorie requirements per kg body weight. See table on page 222. In this example, 40 mg PHE/kg and 3.3 g protein/kg are used. Round to the nearest tenth of a gram for protein, and whole number for PHE.

   PHE @ 40 mg/kg = 248 mg
   Protein @ 3.3 g/kg = 20.46 g (Round to 20.5 g)

   Calories @ 110 kcal/kg = 682 kcal

3. 80 to 85% of the protein requirement should be provided by Lofenalac. 85% is used in this example.

   0.85 x 20.5 g = 17.4 g protein from Lofenalac

4. Determine the grams of Lofenalac needed to provide the protein (from step 3). See table on page 225. Round to the nearest 5 g for ease of measurement.

   $$\frac{17.4 \text{ g protein}}{0.15 \text{ g protein/g Lofenalac}} = 116 \text{ g Lofenalac}$$

   (Round to 115 g Lofenalac)

5. Determine the number of calories and mg of PHE provided by the amount of Lofenalac calculated in step 4. See table on page 225.

   115 g Lofenalac x 4.6 kcal/g Lofenalac = 529 kcal

   115 g Lofenalac x 0.8 mg PHE/g Lofenalac = 92 mg PHE

6. Determine the amount of other infant formula needed to meet the estimated PHE requirement: Subtract the PHE in Lofenalac from the estimated requirement, and divide the answer by the mg PHE/g formula. See table on page 225. Enfamil powder is the other infant formula in this example. Round to the nearest 5 g for ease of measurement.

Estimated PHE requirement	248 mg
PHE in Lofenalac	- 92 mg
PHE to be supplied by other infant formula	156 mg

   $$\frac{156 \text{ mg PHE}}{5.1 \text{ mg PHE/g Enfamil}} = 30.6 \text{ g Enfamil (Round to 30 g)}$$

7. Determine the calories and protein provided by the other infant formula. See table on page 225.

   30 g Enfamil x 5.25 kcal/g Enfamil = 157.5 kcal
   30 g Enfamil x 0.12 g protein/g Enfamil = 3.6 g protein

	PHE (mg)	Protein (g)	Calories (kcal)
8. Total the amount of PHE, protein, and calories provided by the formulas. Compare these to the estimated requirements.			
115 g Lofenalac	92	17.4	529
30 g Enfamil	+156	3.6	157.5
Total	248	21.0	686.5
Requirement	248	20.5	682

9. Water should be added to the formula powders to make a dilution of 20 to 24 calories per oz. The infant's volume tolerance and rate of growth determine the concentration of the formula. In this example, water is added to make a total of 34 oz, yielding a 20 kcal/oz formula.

SAMPLE CALCULATION OF DIET USING PHENYLALANINE-FREE FORMULA AND TABLE FOODS:

1. Note the child's weight and age.

   Age 5 years; wt = 20 kg

2. Calculate estimated PHE, protein, and calorie requirements per kg body weight. See table on page 222. In this example, 20 mg PHE/kg and 1.7 g protein/kg are used. Round to the nearest tenth of a gram for protein, and whole number for PHE.

   PHE @ 20 mg/kg = 400 mg
   Protein @ 1.7 g/kg = 34 g

   Calories @ 85 kcal/kg = 1700 kcal

3. Determine the number of PHE food exchanges needed to provide the estimated requirement. (One food exchange equals approximately 15 mg PHE.) Round to the nearest whole number.

   400 mg PHE ÷ 15 mg PHE/exchange = 26.7 exchanges

   (Round to 27 exchanges)

4. Designate the number of PHE exchanges for each food group by noting the child's preferences and the relative PHE content of the food groups. (Bread contains much more PHE than fruit or vegetables, and therefore a greater percentage of the exchanges should be allotted to bread.)

   9 fruit, 8 vegetable, 10 bread, 2 fat

5. Determine the PHE, protein and calorie content of the food exchanges using average values from the table on page 222.

Food Exchanges	PHE (mg)	Protein (g)	Calories (kcal)
9 Fruit	135	5.4	540
8 Vegetable	120	4.0	80
10 Bread	150	3.0	100
2 Fat	0	0.6	360
Total	405	13.0	1080

6. Calculate the protein to be provided by formula. Subtract the protein provided by food (step 5) from the estimated protein requirement.

Protein requirement	34 g
Protein in food	- 13 g
Protein to be provided as formula	21 g

7. Calculate the amount of formula needed to meet the estimated protein requirement. Divide protein supplied from formula (step 6) by protein supplied per gram of product. See table on page 222. Round answer to the nearest 5 g for ease of measurement. Phenyl-Free, containing 0.2 g protein/g powder, is the product used in this example.

   $$\frac{21 \text{ g protein to be supplied by Phenyl-Free}}{0.2 \text{ g protein/g Phenyl-Free}} =$$

   105 g Phenyl-Free

8. Calculate the calories provided by the amount of formula needed in step 7. Phenyl-Free, used in this example, contains 4 kcal/g. Round to the nearest 5 calories.

105 g Phenyl-Free x 4 kcal/g = 420 kcal

9. Determine the calories to be provided from free foods by subtracting the sum of calories from formula (step 8) and exchanges (step 5) from the estimated need (step 2).

Calories from formula	420
Calories from exchanges	+1080
Calories from formula and exchanges	1500
Estimated calorie need	1700
Calories from formula and exchanges	-1500
Calories to be provided from free foods	200

10. Calculate the calories, protein, and PHE/kg child's weight. Compare these to the requirements.

Final Diet:	PHE (mg)	Protein (g)	Calories (kcal)
105 g Phenyl-Free	--	21.0	420
9 Fruit	135	5.4	540
8 Vegetable	120	4.0	80
10 Bread	150	3.0	100
2 Fat	--	0.6	360
Free Foods	--	--	200
Total	405	34.0	1700
Total/kg	20.3	1.7	85
Requirements/kg	20	1.7	85

Food	Grams/Tbsp	Amount	Phenylalanine (mg)	Protein (g)	Calories
List A. Strained and Junior Foods					
(approximately 15 mg phenylalanine per serving)					
Fruits	14.3				
Applesauce		11 tbsp	15	0.3	69
Applesauce/apricots		10 tbsp	15	0.4	124
Applesauce/pineapple		10 tbsp	15	0.3	62
Apricots/tapioca		12 tbsp	14	0.7	124
Bananas/tapioca		7 tbsp	14	0.5	69
Peaches		6 tbsp	15	0.4	69
Pears		10 tbsp	15	0.6	73
Pears/pineapple		11 tbsp	15	0.6	74
Plums/tapioca		11 tbsp	15	0.5	143
Prunes/tapioca		8 tbsp	14	0.7	90
Bananas/pineapple/tapioca		10 tbsp	14	0.4	109
Free Fruit in amounts listed					
Applesauce/raspberry[a]		5 tbsp	4	0.1	49
Apple/blueberry[b]		4 tbsp	4	0.1	39
Fruit Juices	15				
Apple		16 oz	14	0.5	226
Apple/apricot		16 oz	14	0.5	336
Apple/cherry		10 oz	15	0.6	147
Apple/grape		16 oz	14	0.5	250
Mixed fruit		6 oz	14	0.5	108
Orange		4 oz	16	0.6	59
Orange/apple		6 oz	14	0.7	97
Orange/apple/banana		4 oz	16	0.5	67
Orange/apricot		3 oz	14	0.6	43
Orange/pineapple		4 oz	16	0.7	67
Vegetables (strained and junior)	14.3				
Mixed vegetables		2 tbsp	17	0.3	12
Garden vegetables		1 tbsp	16	0.4	5
Beets		4 tbsp	14	0.7	21
Carrots		5 tbsp	15	0.5	21
Creamed corn		1 tbsp + 2 tsp	17	0.3	18
Creamed green beans		2 tbsp	15	0.3	13
Creamed spinach		2 tbsp	13	0.3	5
Green beans		2 tbsp	18	0.4	7
Peas		2 tsp	15	0.4	5
Squash		3 tbsp	15	0.4	12
Sweet potato		2 tbsp	15	0.3	28
(approximately 30 mg of phenylalanine per serving)					
Cereal (dry)	2.4				
Barley		2 tbsp	28	0.5	19
Mixed cereal		2 tbsp	28	0.6	19
Oatmeal[c]		2 tbsp	37	0.7	16
Rice cereal		4 tbsp	31	0.6	37
Mixed cereal/banana		2 tbsp	24	0.6	19
Oatmeal/banana		2 tbsp	30	0.6	19
Rice cereal/banana		4 tbsp	34	0.7	34
Cereal (jar) (strained and junior)	14.3				
Mixed/applesauce/banana		3 tbsp	27	0.6	40
Oatmeal/applesauce/banana		2 tbsp	27	0.6	30
Rice/applesauce/banana		14 tbsp	28	0.8	140
Rice/mixed fruit		4 tbsp	34	0.6	36

Food	Grams/Tbsp	Amount	Phenylalanine (mg)	Protein (g)	Calories
List B. Table Food					
		(approximately 15 mg phenylalanine per serving)			
Fruits					
Apple, raw		2 1/2 small	15	0.5	145
Apple juice		16 oz	16	0.4	236
Applesauce	19	3/4 cup	14	0.5	207
Apricots, raw		1 1/2 medium	14	0.6	31
Apricots, canned		3 halves	14	0.6	86
Apricots, dried		2 halves	14	0.6	31
Apricot nectar		18 oz	12	1.8	321
Avocado	9.5	3 tbsp	14	0.6	48
Banana, raw		1/2 small or 1/3 cup sliced	17	0.6	43
Blackberries, canned/syrup	15.6	5 tbsp	16	0.6	71
Blackberries, raw	9	6 tbsp	17	0.6	31
Blueberries, raw	8.8	10 tbsp	16	0.6	55
Blueberries, frozen, unsweetened	10	9 tbsp	16	0.6	50
Blueberries, canned/syrup	15	10 tbsp	15	0.6	151
Cantaloupe, raw	15	5 tbsp	16	0.5	23
Cherries, sour	13	4 tbsp	16	0.6	30
Cherries, sweet, canned/syrup	13	5 tbsp	15	0.6	53
Cranberries, raw	6	1 1/2 cups	14	0.6	44
Cranberry juice cocktail		12 oz	12	0.3	243
Cranberry sauce	20	1 2/3 cups	16	0.5	780
Cranberries, sweetened, cooked	13	1 1/2 cups	16	0.6	555
Dates	11	2 tbsp + 1 tsp	15	0.6	69
Fig, raw		1 large	15	0.6	40
Figs, canned/syrup		4 small	16	0.6	105
Fig, dried		1 small	16	0.6	41
Fruit cocktail	13	3/4 cup	16	0.6	119
Grapefruit, raw	12	3/4 cup or 1/2 large	14	0.7	59
Grapes, Thompson seedless	10	1/2 cup or 12 grapes	14	0.5	54
Grape juice		8 oz	15	0.5	165
Grapefruit juice		4 oz	15	0.7	53
Guava, raw		1 small	16	0.6	47
Honeydew, raw	13	5 tbsp	16	0.5	21
Mango, raw		1/2 medium	18	0.7	66
Mulberries, black, red, white		3 tbsp	15	0.3	15
Nectarines, raw		2 large	15	0.8	80
Orange, raw		1 medium (3 in. diam)	18	1.5	74
Orange juice		5 oz	15	1.2	77
Papaya, raw	16	1/3 medium or 6 tbsp + 1 tsp	16	0.6	39
Peaches, raw	11	1 large or 3/4 cup	16	0.8	50
Peaches, canned/syrup	16	4 medium halves	16	0.8	156
Peaches, dried	10	2 1/2 tbsp	16	0.8	66
Peach nectar		12 oz	15	0.9	180
Pear, raw		1/2 medium	17	0.7	61
Pears, canned/syrup	16	5 small halves	15	0.5	190
Pear, dried		1/2 pear	12	0.4	35
Pear nectar		5 oz	15	0.5	88
Pineapple, raw	8	1 cup	14	0.5	67
Pineapple, canned/syrup	16	2 large slices	16	0.6	148
Pineapple juice		5 oz	15	0.5	75
Pineapple-grapefruit drink		15 oz	12	0.3	216

231

Food	Grams/Tbsp	Amount	Phenylalanine (mg)	Protein (g)	Calories
List B. Table Food (cont'd)					
Fruits (cont'd)					
Plums, damson, raw	13	2 whole	13	0.5	66
Plums, prune-type, raw	13	1 1/2 whole	17	0.4	38
Plums, canned/syrup	14	4 whole	13	0.5	110
Prunes, dried		3 medium	18	0.4	54
Prune juice		3 oz	15	0.4	68
Raisins, seedless	10	2 tbsp	15	0.5	58
Raspberries, black, raw	11	1/4 cup	17	0.7	32
Raspberries, red, raw	8	6 tbsp	15	0.6	27
Raspberries, black, canned/syrup	13	4 tbsp	15	0.6	27
Raspberries, red, canned/syrup	13	7 tbsp	16	0.6	32
Rhubarb, cooked, added sugar	15	6 tbsp	15	0.5	141
Strawberries, raw	9	10 large	17	0.7	37
Strawberries, frozen, whole	15	15 large	15	0.6	138
Tangerine		1 small or 1/2 large	12	0.4	23
Watermelon	12.5	2/3 cup	17	0.7	36
Soups (Campbell's condensed, prepared with equal volume of water)					
Asparagus		3 tbsp	15	0.5	12
Beef Broth		2 tbsp	17	0.6	4
Beef Noodle		2 tbsp	19	0.5	8
Celery		3 tbsp	15	0.3	16
Chicken Gumbo		2 tbsp	14	0.4	7
Clam Chowder/Tomato		3 tbsp	14	0.4	15
Cream of Chicken		2 tbsp	15	0.4	12
Minestrone		3 tbsp	18	0.8	17
Mushroom		2 tbsp	15	0.3	17
Onion		3 tbsp	19	0.9	11
Tomato		3 tbsp	17	0.4	16
Vegetable/Beef Broth		4 tbsp	16	0.5	15
Vegetarian Vegetable		3 tbsp	14	0.3	12
Vegetables					
Asparagus, cooked	9	3 tbsp or 1 1/2 stalk	17	0.6	5
Beans, green, cooked	8	3 tbsp	14	0.4	6
Beans, yellow, cooked	8	1/4 cup	16	0.4	7
Bean sprouts, mung, cooked	8	1 tbsp + 1 cup	16	0.3	3
Beets, cooked	10	2/3 cup	16	1.2	34
Beet greens, cooked	13	3 tbsp	15	0.6	6
Broccoli, cooked	10	1 tbsp + 1 tsp	14	0.4	3
Brussels sprouts, cooked		1 medium	13	0.4	4
Cabbage, raw	6	1/2 cup	15	0.6	12
Cabbage, cooked	10	1/3 cup	14	0.6	11
Carrots, raw		1/2 large or 1 small	18	0.6	21
Carrots, cooked		1/3 cup	15	0.5	16
Cauliflower, cooked		3 tbsp	17	0.5	5
Celery, raw	6	6 tbsp or 2 stalks	15	0.3	6
Celery, cooked	8	6 tbsp	18	0.4	7
Chard leaves, cooked	10	3 tbsp	14	0.5	5
Collards, cooked	11	1 tbsp	13	0.4	4
Cucumber, pared, raw		1 whole	14	0.6	14
Eggplant, raw	13	2 tbsp	13	0.3	7
Eggplant, cooked	13	3 tbsp	17	0.4	7
Green pepper, raw	10	3 tbsp	17	0.4	7

Food	Grams/Tbsp	Amount	Phenylalanine (mg)	Protein (g)	Calories
List B. Table Food (cont'd)					
Vegetables (cont'd)					
Kale, cooked	7	2 tbsp	18	0.4	4
Lettuce		2 leaves	14	0.4	5
Mushrooms, raw		3 small	17	0.8	8
Mushrooms, canned	13	3 tbsp	16	0.4	7
Mushrooms, sauteed	17	1/2 large	13	0.2	10
Mustard greens, cooked	13	1 tbsp + 2 tsp	16	0.5	5
Okra, cooked		3 tbsp	17	0.7	10
Onion, raw	10	1/4 cup	15	0.6	15
Onion, cooked	13	1/4 cup	16	0.6	15
Parsley, raw	3	4 tbsp	17	0.4	5
Parsnips, cooked	13	3 tbsp	18	0.6	26
Pickle, dill		1 large	16	0.7	11
Pickle, sweet	13	1 large	16	0.7	146
Pickle, sweet relish	13	8 tbsp	14	0.5	144
Pumpkin, cooked	14	4 tbsp	16	0.6	18
Radishes, raw		3 small	13	0.3	5
Sauerkraut	15	1/4 cup	15	0.6	11
Scallions, raw		2 whole	15	0.6	14
Spinach, cooked	11	1 tbsp	15	0.3	3
Squash, summer, cooked	13	5 tbsp	16	0.6	9
Squash, winter, cooked	13	1/4 cup	16	0.6	20
Tomato, raw	17	1/2 small	14	0.6	11
Tomatoes, canned	17	1/4 cup	17	0.7	14
Tomato catsup	17	2 tbsp	17	0.7	36
Tomato juice	14	1/4 cup	16	0.6	13
Tomato puree	6	6 tbsp	15	0.6	14
Tomato sauce	18	3 tbsp	18	0.7	52
Turnip greens, cooked	9	2 tbsp	18	0.4	4
Turnips, cooked	10	9 tbsp	15	0.7	21

(approximately 30 mg phenylalanine per serving)

Food	Grams/Tbsp	Amount	Phenylalanine (mg)	Protein (g)	Calories
Cereals (prepared)					
All-Bran		1 tbsp	28	0.5	11
Alpha Bits		3 tbsp	27	0.6	23
Apple Jacks		6 tbsp	32	0.7	47
Boo Berry		5 tbsp	27	0.5	39
Cap'n Crunch		5 tbsp	29	0.7	65
Cap'n Crunchberries		1/4 cup	31	0.5	47
Cap'n Crunch Peanut Butter		3 tbsp	32	0.6	38
Cheerios		2 tbsp	27	0.5	15
Cocoa Krispies		1/2 cup	29	0.5	48
Cookie Crisp		1/2 cup	25	0.5	55
Corn Chex		1/2 cup	29	0.6	30
Cornflakes		1/4 cup	28	0.6	31
Count Chocula		6 tbsp	28	0.6	42
Crispy Critters		1/4 cup	32	0.8	28
Franken Berry		7 tbsp	30	0.6	50
Froot Loops		5 tbsp	36	0.6	40
Fruity Pebbles		10 tbsp	30	1.0	80
Golden Grahams		1/4 cup	25	0.5	28
Granola		1 tbsp	32	0.6	19
Grape-Nuts Flakes		3 tbsp	29	0.7	30
Grapenuts		1 tbsp	27	0.6	26
Honeycomb Corn		7 tbsp	28	0.6	35
Kaboom		6 tbsp	30	0.6	42
King Vitamin		1/2 cup	32	0.6	63
Kix		1/2 cup	28	0.6	32
Lucky Charms		3 tbsp	29	0.5	23
Puffed Rice		10 tbsp	31	0.6	40
Puffed Wheat		1/4 cup	32	0.9	12

Food	Grams/Tbsp	Amount	Phenylalanine (mg)	Protein (g)	Calories
List B. Table Food (cont'd)					
Cereals (prepared) (cont'd)					
Quaker Life		1 tbsp	30	0.6	12
Quisp		1/2 cup	31	0.8	68
Raisin Bran		3 tbsp	33	0.6	27
Rice Chex		6 tbsp	31	0.6	44
Rice Krinkles		1/2 cup	28	0.5	63
Rice Krispies		1/4 cup	28	0.5	30
Shredded Wheat		1/4 biscuit	29	0.6	21
Special K		2 tbsp	29	0.6	11
Sir Grapefellow		5 tbsp	27	0.5	39
Sugar Frosted Flakes		1/2 cup	30	0.6	62
Sugar Pops		1/2 cup	30	0.6	43
Sugar Smacks		7 tbsp	31	0.7	55
Super Sugar Crisp		1/4 cup	28	0.4	36
Team Flakes		10 tbsp	30	0.6	39
Trix		6 tbsp	30	0.7	45
Wheat Chex		7 biscuits	31	0.7	25
Wheaties		1/4 cup	31	0.7	25
Cereals (cooked)					
Cornmeal		4 tbsp	29	0.7	30
Cream of Rice		5 tbsp	31	0.6	38
Cream of Wheat		2 tbsp	28	0.6	17
Farina		3 tbsp	31	0.6	19
Malt-O-Meal		2 tbsp	30	0.6	20
Oatmeal		2 tbsp	33	0.6	17
Pettyjohns		2 tbsp	32	0.7	23
Ralston		2 tbsp	31	0.6	16
Rice, white		3 tbsp	28	0.5	29
Rice, brown		2 tbsp	28	0.5	25
Wheatena		2 tbsp	31	0.6	22
Wheat Hearts		2 tbsp	31	0.7	17
Crackers					
Animal crackers		5	33	0.7	43
Arrowroot cookies		2	30	0.6	45
Bacon Flavored Thins		3	27	0.6	20
Bugles		9	27	trace	45
Cheese Flavored Flings		4	32	0.8	40
Cheese Nips		6	30	0.6	30
Cheese Tid-Bits		8	32	0.8	32
Chicken-in-a-Biskit		4	28	0.4	40
Corn chips		8	32	trace	40
Graham crackers		1	28	0.6	21
Meal Mates		1	25	0.5	24
Mr. Salty 3-Ring Pretzels		2	30	0.6	24
Oyster crackers		9	27	0.9	27
Ritz cheese crackers		2	30	0.6	36
Ritz crackers		3	35	0.7	45
Saltines		2	27	0.5	26
Tortilla, corn		1/4 (6 in. diam)	33	0.7	27
Tortilla, flour		1/4 (6 in. diam)	35	0.7	27
Triscuit wafers		1 1/2	30	0.6	31
Vanilla wafers		4	32	0.6	60
Waverly wafers		2	24	0.4	36
Wheat Thins		4	34	0.7	32
Miscellaneous					
Chocolate sauce, Hershey's		1 tbsp	25	0.5	49
Corn, cooked		2 tbsp	29	0.5	17
Corn-on-cob		1/6 med. ear	33	0.6	16

Food	Grams/Tbsp	Amount	Phenylalanine (mg)	Protein (g)	Calories
List B. Table Food (cont'd)					
Miscellaneous (cont'd)					
Hominy grits, cooked		6 tbsp	32	0.7	31
Jello		1/3 cup	30	0.6	65
Macaroni, cooked		2 tbsp	32	0.6	20
Marshmallows		6 (62/lb)	38	0.8	60
Noodles, cooked		2 tbsp	32	0.7	20
Popcorn, popped, plain		5 tbsp	29	0.6	19
Spaghetti, cooked		2 tbsp	32	0.6	20
Potatoes					
Baked, no skin		1/3 (2 1/2 in. diam)	38	0.9	32
Boiled in skin		1/3 (2 1/2 in. diam)	31	0.7	25
Boiled, no skin		1/3 (2 1/2 in. diam)	28	0.6	22
Chips		6 (2 in. diam)	29	0.6	68
French fried		3 (1/2 in. x 1/2 in. x 2 in.)	30	0.6	41
Instant (no milk), dry		1 1/2 tsp	27	0.6	28
Sweet Potatoes					
Baked in skin		1/4 small	29	0.5	35
Boiled, no skin		1/2 small	27	0.6	54
Canned, syrup pack		1/2 small	27	0.5	57
Instant (no milk), dry		2 tbsp (10 g)	23	0.4	38

(approximately 5 mg phenylalanine per serving)

Food	Grams/Tbsp	Amount	Phenylalanine (mg)	Protein (g)	Calories
Desserts (Comstock)					
Apple Pie Filling		1/4 cup	1	<0.05	89
Apricot Pie Filling		1/4 cup	8	0.4	79
Blackberry Pie Filling		1/4 cup	1	<0.05	109
Blueberry Pie Filling		1/4 cup	6	0.2	83
Boysenberry Pie Filling		1/4 cup	11	0.4	93
Cherry Pie Filling		1/4 cup	11	0.4	83
Peach Pie Filling		1/4 cup	4	0.2	78
Pineapple Pie Filling		1/4 cup	4	0.1	70
Raspberry Pie Filling		1/4 cup	8	0.3	106
Strawberry Pie Filling		1/4 cup	5	0.2	79
Fats					
Butter		1 tbsp	4	0.1	100
French dressing, commercial		5 tbsp	5	0.2	442
Margarine		1 tbsp	5	0.1	108
Miracle Whip		1 tbsp	5	0.1	68
Olives, green		2 tbsp	5	0.2	16
Olives, ripe		2 tbsp	5	0.2	18
Mayonnaise		2 tbsp	5	0.1	72
Nondairy Creams					
Coffee Rich		1 tbsp	3	trace	23
Cool Whip		1 tbsp	2	trace	14
D-Zerta Whip, liquid		1 tbsp	9	0.2	44
Rich's Topping		1 tbsp	trace	trace	43
Mocha Mix		1 tbsp	2	trace	13

Food	Grams/Tbsp	Amount	Phenylalanine (mg)	Protein (g)	Calories
List B. Table Food (cont'd)					
Aproten[d] Low Protein Products					
Low Protein Bread		1/2 slice	4	0.2	110
Pastas					
Anellini, cooked		1/2 cup	4	0.2	98
Ditalini, cooked		1 cup cooked	4	0.2	114
Rigatini, cooked		1 cup cooked	4	0.2	114
Spaghettini		1/2 cup cooked	4	0.2	107
Tagliatelle		1/2 cup cooked	4	0.2	107
Rusks		1 slice	2	0.1	43
dp Low Protein					
Chocolate Chip Cookies[d]		1 cookie	2	0.1	70
Miscellaneous					
Cake flour		1 tbsp	29	0.6	29
Cornstarch		1 tbsp	1	trace	29
Tapioca, granulated		1 tbsp	2	0.1	35
Wheat starch		1 tbsp	1	trace	25

Note: Less than 0.04 g protein = trace.
[a]Phenylalanine estimated as 3% of protein.
[b]Phenylalanine estimated as 3.7% of protein.
[c]Phenylalanine content is higher than in other cereals, so alternate it with other cereals.
[d]From Dietary Specialties, Inc., P.O. Box 227, Rochester, NY 14601.

FOOD EXCHANGE LIST FOR PHENYLKETONURIA: FREE FOODS

Food	Amount	Calories
(contain little or no phenylalanine)		
Apple juice	6 oz	85
Candies		
Butterscotch	1 piece	20
Cream mints	1 piece	7
Fondant, patties or mint	1 piece	40
Gum drops	1 large	35
Hard candy	2 pieces	39
Jelly beans	10	110
Lollipops	1 medium (2 1/2 in. diam)	108
Carbonated beverages, regular	6 oz	78
Corn syrup	1 tbsp	58
Danish Dessert	1/2 cup	123
Diet margarine	1 tbsp	50
Fruit butter	1 tbsp	37
Fruit ices	1/2 cup	69
Jellies	1 tbsp	55
Kool-Aid, regular	4 oz	48
Lemonade, regular	4 oz	53
Maple syrup	1 tbsp	50
Molasses	1 tbsp	46
Popsicle, regular	1 twin bar	95
Prono[a]	1/3 cup	55
Shortening	1 tbsp	123
Start, liquid	4 oz	60
Sugar, brown	1 tbsp	46
Sugar, granulated	1 tbsp	43
Sugar, white, powdered	1 tbsp	59
Tang, liquid, regular	4 oz	59

Note: These foods may be used as desired to meet caloric needs.
[a]From Dietary Specialties, Inc., P.O. Box 227, Rochester, NY 14601.

SECTION 8

Test Diets and Test Meals

A. GLUCOSE TOLERANCE TEST DIET (300-GRAM CARBOHYDRATE DIET)

DESCRIPTION: The glucose tolerance test (GTT) is used occasionally as one indication of the ability to utilize carbohydrate appropriately. The test consists of administering an oral glucose solution of 75 g carbohydrate. Plasma glucose levels are then checked at 30 minutes, 60 minutes, 90 minutes, 2 hours, 3 hours, and in some instances, blood may be drawn at 4 and 5 hours as well. The test diet is based on the premise that eating a diet containing an inadequate amount of carbohydrate results in low insulin stores in the pancreas. Thus, a diet containing approximately 300 g carbohydrate per day is necessary for 3 days prior to a glucose tolerance test to prevent false positive results.

PROCEDURE: The 300-gram Carbohydrate Diet is given for a period of 72 hours (3 days) prior to a GTT. The dietary intake of carbohydrate is estimated after each meal and snack; replacements are offered as necessary to attain the goal of 300 g carbohydrate per day. An estimate of the amount of carbohydrate consumed for each of the 3 days is recorded in the patient's medical record.

B. 100-GRAM FAT TEST DIET

DESCRIPTION: The 100-gram Fat Test Diet is used in diagnosing fat malabsorption. The test may be indicated in a variety of conditions such as Crohn's disease, idiopathic ulcerative colitis, irritable bowel syndrome, short bowel syndrome, gluten-induced enteropathy, pancreatic disease, and cystic fibrosis. The test is usually ordered for a 6-day period. The first 3 days are preparatory for fecal collections which occur on the final 3 days of the test. Stools are analyzed for fat content, and the presence and severity of steatorrhea is determined. The results can be used to assess the nutritional consequences of the intestinal disorder. When the diet includes 100 g fat per day, a normal value is less than 6 g fat per 24 hours as an average of a 3-day collection.

PROCEDURE: The patient's food selections are monitored by the dietitian to insure that 100 ± 10 g fat per day are included. The diabetic food exchange system (see pages 144-54) and the department's nutrition analysis booklet of menu items are used to calculate the total amount of fat offered. After each meal, the patient's fat intake is estimated. Replacements are offered as needed to insure that the patient consumes the minimum level of 90 g fat required for the test.

C. HIGH FAT TEST FORMULA

DESCRIPTION: The High Fat Test Formula is a screening test for fat malabsorption. Following a fatty meal, there is normally an increased serum turbidity due to the presence of chylomicrons, which is measurable as a change in serum optical density. A normal response is regarded as a maximum increase in optical density of greater than 0.100. When malabsorption is a prominent clinical factor, the maximum rise in serum optical density is lower. The test is affected not only by the postabsorptive capacity of the intestinal cell, but also by other factors such as gastric emptying time, rate of utility or storage, and activity of beta lipoprotein lipase.

PROCEDURE: The fasted patient is given an oral formula consisting of 50 cc (50 g fat) corn oil blenderized with 240 cc skim milk. The changes in a patient's serum (or plasma) optical density are measured prior to and at 4- and 6-hour intervals after ingestion of the formula.

D. FAT-FREE TEST MEAL

DESCRIPTION: Historically, a fat-free test meal was given to patients prior to a gallbladder series. This is no longer routinely done. The present protocol for a cholecystography indicates that after the dinner meal the evening before the test, only water is allowed until the test is completed. For a cholangiography, a regular dinner may be consumed the evening before a test and a clear liquid diet the day of examination.

PROCEDURE: A fat-free meal is ordered for 1 meal only unless specified otherwise. If breakfast is ordered, it will consist only of fruit or fruit juice; toast; jelly; coffee, tea, or decaffeinated coffee; and sugar. If the meal is ordered for lunch or dinner, it consists only of fruit or fruit juice; steamed or baked potato or fat-free substitute; fat-free vegetable (from the Soft Diet); sherbet or fruit-flavored gelatin; bread and jelly; coffee, tea, or decaffeinated coffee; and sugar and salt.

E. 5-HYDROXYINDOLE-ACETIC ACID TEST DIET (5-HIAA)

DESCRIPTION: The patient is given a diet eliminating foods that contain large amounts of serotonin. Serotonin, an amino acid derived from tryptophan, is metabolized mainly to 5-HIAA, which is excreted in the urine. Some patients with carcinoid tumors excrete high amounts of 5-HIAA as a result of increased serotonin synthesis by the tumor.

PROCEDURE: Unless specified otherwise, the diet is prescribed for a period of 72 hours (3 days). A 24-hour urine sample is collected on the final day.

FOODS TO AVOID: Avocado, banana, kiwi fruit, pineapple, plums, tomato, walnuts, butternuts, hickory nuts, and pecans.

F. VANILLYLMANDELIC ACID (VMA) TEST DIET

DESCRIPTION: 4-hydroxy-3-methoxymandelic acid (VMA) is a major urinary metabolite of the catechol-amines, epinephrine, and norepinephrine. Measurement of urinary VMA is widely used in establishing the diagnosis of neurogenic tumors (pheochromocytomas associated with hypertension, and neuroblastomas). If urine chromatography studies are used as the diagnostic test, a diet eliminating food items that may give a falsely elevated VMA level in the urine is necessary. Use of the prevailing fluorescence assays, which are more specific, eliminates the need for dietary modification.

PROCEDURE: If needed, the diet is prescribed for a period of 72 hours (3 days). A 24-hour urine sample is collected on the final day.

FOODS TO AVOID: Caffeine-containing beverages such as coffee, tea, and cola; banana, citrus fruit, chocolate, nuts, raisins, and vanilla.

G. PRIMARY ALDOSTERONISM TEST DIET

DESCRIPTION: This diet consists of two 5-day phases and is used to diagnose primary aldosteronism. For the first phase (days 1 to 5) designed to stimulate renin secretion, the patient is given a diet of 230 mg (10 mEq) sodium and 3120 to 3900 mg (80 to 100 mEq) potassium. Volume depletion, resulting from salt restriction, provides a powerful stimulus to renin secretion in normal persons and in patients with essential hypertension. In primary aldosteronism, volume depletion does not occur and renin concentrations remain low.

For the second phase (days 6 to 10) designed to suppress aldosterone secretion, the patient is given a diet of 8050 mg (350 mEq) sodium and 3120 to 3900 mg (80 to 100 mEq) potassium. Normally, the increased blood volume associated with a high salt diet and adequate potassium intake causes aldosterone secretion to be very low as a result of the suppression of renin secretion. Only in primary aldosteronism will the plasma aldosterone concentration remain elevated.

PROCEDURE: The most reliable method of meeting the diet prescription for either phase is by using a special formula with supplementary foods. For the first phase a low sodium formula from the Clinical Research Center is used, supplemented with low sodium foods (see sample diet). For the second phase, a formula, broth of known sodium content, and supplemental foods are provided.

For both phases of this diet, the patient's diet can be calculated using the renal exchange system (see pages 84-98). This method can be used provided some variability can be tolerated, since natural foods contain widely different amounts of sodium and potassium. The first phase of the diet (very low sodium) is the most difficult to provide using food versus formula. Low sodium foods have unexpectedly variable sodium content (especially canned and frozen items), therefore only fresh fruits and vegetables and carefully controlled baked products are provided. The second phase of the diet (very high sodium) could be provided using salted foods, however these products are also highly variable in sodium content. Using broth as a concentrated source of sodium is more reliable than calculating food sodium.

The patient's intake of sodium and potassium is estimated after each meal, and replacements are offered if necessary. An estimate of the amount of sodium and potassium consumed is recorded daily in the patient's chart.

SAMPLE PROCEDURE FOR CALCULATING A PRIMARY ALDOSTERONE TEST DIET:

1. Determine patient's caloric need by nomogram or BEE (basal energy expenditure) formula. The BEE is calculated from patient's height, weight, and age. See Appendix E for the nomogram and page 246 for the BEE.

2. Interview patient to obtain choices for supplemental foods and flavor of formula.

3. Total amounts of potassium (phase one) and sodium and potassium (phase two) provided by formula and supplemental foods. Subtract these amounts from the total amounts prescribed.

4. Calculate the amount of 100 mg/ml mineral (KCl or NaCl) solution to be added to formula. (Pharmacy provides these solutions.) Do *not* add NaCl solution to formula for phase one.

Example:

Step 1: 23-year-old male, 191 cm, 95 kg, physical activity level 30% above basal.

$$BEE = 66 + 13.7 \, (95) + 5(191) - 6.8(23) =$$
$$66 + 1302 + 955 - 156 = 2167$$
$$2167 \times 1.3 = 2817$$
Round to 2800 calories

Step 2: See sample diets for phases one and two.

Step 3: (Phase One) Total amount of K in formula and supplemental foods:

	K
6 1/2 c LS chocolate formula	180 mg
4 slices LS Bread	105 mg
4 pats LS margarine	5 mg
4 pkgs jelly	40 mg
1 apple	160 mg
1 orange	235 mg
1 banana	450 mg
4 tsp coffee powder	130 mg
Total potassium	1305 mg

Subtract amount of K in food and formula from K prescribed.

3900 mg K prescribed
1305 mg in food and formula
2595 mg K from KCl solution

Step 4: (Phase One) Divide mg K needed by mg K in KCl solution.

$$\frac{2595 \text{ mg K needed}}{100 \text{ mg K/ml}} = 25.95 \text{ ml KCl solution}$$

Round to nearest whole number, 26 ml.

Example (continued):

Step 3: (Phase Two) Total amount of Na and K in formula and supplemental foods.

	Na	K
6 1/2 cups LS chocolate formula	100 mg	180 mg
Chicken broth powder	5575 mg	90 mg
4 slices wheat bread	525 mg	275 mg
4 pats margarine	160 mg	5 mg
2 pkgs jelly	5 mg	20 mg
1 apple	0 mg	160 mg
1 orange	0 mg	235 mg
1 banana	0 mg	450 mg
4 tsp coffee powder	0 mg	130 mg
	Total Na 6365 mg	Total K 1545 mg

Subtract amount of Na and K in food and formula from amounts prescribed.

8050 mg Na prescribed	3900 mg K prescribed
- 6365 mg Na in food and formula	- 1545 mg K in food and formula
1685 mg Na from NaCl solution	2355 mg K from KCl solution

Step 4: (Phase Two) Divide mg Na and mg K needed by mg Na and mg K in NaCl and KCl solutions respectively.

$$\frac{1685 \text{ mg Na needed}}{100 \text{ mg Na/ml}} = 16.85 \text{ ml NaCl solution}$$

$$\frac{2355 \text{ mg K needed}}{100 \text{ mg K/ml}} = 23.55 \text{ ml KCl solution}$$

Round to nearest whole number, 17 ml.   Round to nearest whole number, 24 ml.

FORMULAS FOR PRIMARY ALDOSTERONISM TEST DIET:

Low Sodium Vanilla Formula

43 g calcium caseinate (Casec)
68 g sugar
66 g corn syrup
37 g salt-free butter
15 g corn oil
 6 g frozen sugared egg yolk mix[1]
10 g vanilla
594 g distilled water

Low Sodium Chocolate Formula

42 g calcium caseinate (Casec)
68 g sugar
45 g corn syrup
26 g salt-free butter
14 g corn oil
 6 g frozen sugared egg yolk mix[1]
10 g vanilla
602 g distilled water
26 g semisweet chocolate

---

[1]Or substitute 5 g frozen egg yolk plus 1 g sugar for 6 g sugared egg yolk mix.

Directions:

1. Weigh all ingredients directly into a 1-gallon blender.
2. Cover and blend for 10 minutes.
3. Transfer to a labeled storage container. (Formula will keep 3 to 5 days in refrigerator and 3 months in freezer.)
4. Shake well before serving.

One recipe yields approximately 800 g (about 3 1/4 cups).

Approximate Nutrient Composition:

Formulas (g)	Amount	Weight (g)	Kcal	Na (mg)	K (mg)
LS Vanilla Formula	3 1/4 c	800	1000	65	15
LS Chocolate Formula	3 1/4 c	800	1000	50	90

SAMPLE DIET FOR PHASE ONE OF PRIMARY ALDOSTERONE TEST DIET:

Prescription: 2800 Calories
            <10 mEq (230 mg) Sodium
            100 mEq (3900 mg) Potassium

Food	Amount	Weight (g)	Calories	Na (mg)	K (mg)
LS chocolate formula	6 1/2 c	1600	2000	100	180
KCl solution[1]	26 ml	28	0	0	2600
LS bread	4 slices	100	270	60	105
LS margarine	4 pats	20	145	0	5
Jelly	4 pkgs	56	160	10	40
Apple (weighed with core)	1 medium	150	80	0	160
Orange (weighed without peel)	1 medium	130	60	0	235
Banana (weighed with peel)	1 medium	175	105	0	450
Coffee powder	4 tsp	4	5	0	130
Distilled water	ad lib		0	0	0
			2815	170	3905

SAMPLE DIET FOR PHASE TWO OF PRIMARY ALDOSTERONE TEST DIET:

Prescription: 2800 Calories
            350 mEq (8050 mg) Sodium
            100 mEq (3900 mg) Potassium

[1] 100 mg/ml K.

Food	Amount	Weight (g)	Calories	Na (mg)	K (mg)
LS chocolate formula	6 1/2	1600	2000	100	180
NaCl solution[1]	17 ml	19	0	1700	0
KCl solution[2]	24 ml	26	0	0	2400
Chicken broth powder	5 tbsp	30	80	5575	90
Water	ad lib				
Wheat bread	4 slices	100	245	525	275
Margarine	4 pats	20	145	160	5
Jelly	2 pkgs	28	75	5	20
Apple (weighed with core)	1 medium	150	80	0	160
Orange (weighed without peel)	1 medium	130	60	0	235
Banana (weighed with peel)	1 medium	175	105	0	450
Coffee powder	4 tsp	4	5	0	130
Water	ad lib				
			2795	8065	3945

[1] 100 mg/ml Na.

[2] 100 mg/ml K.

243

H. MINIMUM RESIDUE TEST DIET

DESCRIPTION: The Minimum Residue Test Diet is used in preparation for the barium enema examination. Ideally, 3 days are needed to prepare the bowel for the examination: 2 days of the minimum residue test diet are followed by 1 day of a clear liquid diet. The patient is NPO the day of the examination until it is completed.

FOODS ALLOWED AND FOODS TO AVOID: Foods allowed and foods to avoid are the same as listed for the Minimum Residue Diet (pages 23-24) with the following *additional* restrictions:

Food Group	Foods Allowed	Foods to Avoid
Beverages	Coffee, tea, decaffeinated coffee, carbonated beverages	Cereal beverages, milk, nondairy creamer
Breads	None	All
Cereals	Cooked refined farina, Cream of Rice; prepared cereals made from refined rice	All others
Desserts	Arrowroot cookies, angel food cake, plain gelatin desserts, puddings made with strained fruit juice or water, popsicles, fruit ices and frappés made without milk, sugar and vanilla wafers	Sponge cake, sugar cookies, and all others
Eggs	Any prepared without milk or cheese	Any prepared with milk or cheese
Fats	1-2 tbsp butter, margarine or oil, 1 oz nondairy creamer/day	Butter, margarine, or oil in excess of 1-2 tbsp; all others
Fruits, Fruit Juices	Strained juices only	All others
Meat, Fish, Poultry, Cheese	Canned, pureed baby meats; baked skinless fish; finely chopped canned tuna; dry cottage cheese	All others
Sugar, Sweets	Plain candy, honey, jelly, marshmallows, sugar, syrup (all used in moderation)	All others

244

FOODS ALLOWED AND FOODS TO AVOID (continued):

Food Group	Foods Allowed	Foods to Avoid
Vegetables, Vegetable Juices	Tomato juice	All others
Miscellaneous	Salt, mild spices in moderation, dilute vinegar	All others

Nutritional Assessment and Recommendations for Special Needs

A. NUTRITIONAL ASSESSMENT

The aim of nutritional assessment is to detect patients who have malnutrition or are at risk of developing it. Malnutrition occurs in 33 to 65% of all hospitalized patients, with only the advanced cases obvious on inspection.

Nutritional assessment is indicated for hospitalized and ambulatory care patients with one or more of the conditions identified in 3c. on page 247. These conditions result in increased or decreased nutrient requirements and affect the patient's ingestion, absorption, utilization, synthesis, or storage of essential nutrients.

DESCRIPTION: A nutritional assessment includes the following parameters:

1. Diet History

   This includes obtaining a typical day's intake of food plus information about weight change, patterns of eating, changes in appetite, taste, food intolerance, and digestive disorders. Educational needs and potential drug-nutrient interactions are also evaluated.

2. Nutrient Intakes

   When a nutritional assessment is ordered, a 3-day nutrient intake is automatically performed. This includes calculation of calories, protein, fat, and carbohydrate from all food, formula, and IV solutions. Nutrient intakes may also be ordered separately for 3-day periods for patients suspected of having a poor dietary intake.

3. Nutritional Needs

   In order to determine a patient's caloric and protein needs, 4 factors are calculated:

   a. BEE (basal energy expenditure): a factor calculated from the patient's weight, height, and age.

   The following Harris-Benedict equations are used:

   Male = 66 + [13.7 x Wt (kg)] + [5 x Ht (cm)] - [6.8 x Age (yrs)]

   Female = 655 + [9.6 x Wt (kg)] + [1.7 x Ht (cm)] - [4.7 x Age (yrs)]

b. Activity Needs: a factor added to the BEE based on the patient's physical activity level.

Percentage above Basal	Classification	Groups of Individuals
20	Limited Activity	Bed-rest, anorexia nervosa
30	Minimum Activity	Up and about, but inactive, women > 50 years old
40	Average Activity	Most women, men > 50 years old
50	Average Activity	Most men
60	Exercisers	Those who engage in physical exercise daily (20-30 minutes or more)
70	Heavy Work	Physical laborers

c. Metabolic Needs: a factor added to the BEE based on the patient's clinical status.

Percent above Basal	Condition
13	Fever (increase 13% for each 1°C above normal)
20	Minor operation
35	Skeletal trauma (long bones)
40-60	Major sepsis
20-40	Moderate infection
20	Mild infection
5-25	Peritonitis
30	Soft tissue trauma
25	Cancer
10	Need for weight gain

d. Protein Needs: a factor calculated from the patient's weight (gm pro/kg) and based on the patient's metabolic state.

Metabolic State	Protein Needs (g/kg/day)
Nonstress	0.8 - 1.0
Elective surgery	1.5
Polytrauma	1.5-1.75
Sepsis	2.0
Burn	1.5-2.0

4. Laboratory Data

The following laboratory tests should be ordered to obtain biochemical data on nutritional status:

a. Serum Albumin
b. Serum Trasferrin
c. Hemoglobin
d. Hematocrit
e. Total Lymphocyte Count
f. Serum Glucose

5. Anthropometric Measurements

To determine the extent of depletion, specific physical parameters may also be evaluated. The following 3 parameters are measured:

a. Height/weight - compared with ideal weight.
b. Mid-arm muscle circumference - a measure of the patient's lean body mass or the degree of protein depletion.[1]
c. Triceps skinfold - an indirect measure of body fat.[1]

6. Delayed Hypersensitivity Skin Testing[1]

Four skin tests for cell-mediated immunity are sometimes utilized for evaluating nutritional status. Lack of response to the antigen indicates anergy, or failure of the body's defense system to recognize foreign protein and to fight infection. The 4 antigens are:

a. PPD
b. Mumps
c. Candida albicans
d. Streptokinase/Streptodornase (not performed at UIHC)
   (Note: Skin tests must be ordered separately from the nutritional assessment and are read by nursing personnel.)

7. Prognostic Nutrition Index (PNI)[2]

PNI is a formula developed to preoperatively predict the risk of postoperative complications. If time permits, this may allow a patient's nutritional status to be improved prior to surgery. The formula is a percentage based on the following indicators:

a. Albumin (Alb) - g/dl
b. Triceps skinfold (TSF) - mm
c. Serum transferrin (TFN) - mg/dl
d. Delayed hypersensitivity skin testing (DH)

$$PNI(\%) = 158 - [16.6 \times Alb] - [.78 \times TSF] - [.20 \times TFN] - [5.8 \times DH]$$

Risk of postoperative morbidity and mortality:
<30% PNI = low risk
30-59% PNI = intermediate risk
>59% PNI = high risk

8. Summary Recommendations

Upon completion of the assessment[3], the dietitian will summarize the parameters measured and make recommendations to improve the patient's nutritional status.

---

[1] Optimal parameters.

[2] Optional for preoperative patients.

[3] Detailed instructions and feeding protocols can be found in the Enteral Nutrition Handbook (1989), available for purchase from the Dietary Department, University of Iowa Hospitals and Clinics.

B. CRITICAL CARE NUTRITION

The critically ill patient presents a unique set of nutritional challenges. Because this patient is often hypermetabolic and sometimes septic, differing CVN formula types are utilized to meet the specific needs of individual cases.

Objectives of nutrition support are to meet the level of stress, prevent protein loss, and avoid overfeeding. A nutritional assessment is performed to estimate the patient's basal energy expenditure (BEE) by the Harris-Benedict equation. See page 246. The CVN should be formulated to meet the estimated calorie, protein, and electrolyte needs. Protein goals can be achieved by providing between 0.8 g and 2.0 g protein kg/day (0.1 g to 0.3 g N_2/kg/day). Basic electrolytes are added from the beginning. Vitamins and trace elements are added after 1 week. See Appendix I, page 329 for standard solutions.

In a previously well-nourished patient with no surgical complications, oral intake can be resumed when bowel function returns. In a patient suffering from multiple fractures, major injury, infection, or malnutrition, nutritional support is instituted 48 to 72 hours after the surgery/injury.

The endocrine response to trauma/injury involves an initial decrease in metabolic rate in conjunction with glucose intolerance. Therefore, excessive glucose can cause hyperglycemia and glucosuria resulting in dehydration. Amino acids administered during the acute phase of stress will be utilized as energy, with the end product NH_3 excreted in the urine. For this reason it is important to supply the patient with sufficient glucose (100 to 200 gm/d) to obtain a maximal protein sparing effect and to cover the needs of glucose-dependent tissues. Ten percent dextrose infused at a rate of 50cc/hr will supply 120 gm glucose, thus meeting these requirements.

Alterations in glucose metabolism continue to occur in the critically ill patient after the initial stress phase. The administration of large amounts of glucose can cause increases in resting CO_2 production and O_2 consumption. The use of fat emulsions as an energy source as well as a source of essential fatty acids appears to alleviate glucose intolerance in certain patients. In addition, when ventilated patients are changed from a dextrose-based CVN to a lipid/dextrose system, dramatic improvements in PCO_2 have been noted.

Fatty acids in the form of lipid emulsions are excellent sources of calories and are nitrogen sparing. However, the breakdown of fatty acids cannot provide the carbohydrates necessary for the glucose-dependent tissues. Consequently, at least 100 g dextrose should be infused per day. Generally, 50% of the nonprotein calories are provided as fat and 50% are derived from dextrose. The 20% fat emulsions are popular since they provide a richer calorie load per ml than 10% fat emulsions and are cleared at essentially the same rate. This principle becomes important in fluid overloaded patients when a volume restriction is warranted.

Studies of several septic, mechanically ventilated, critically ill patients have revealed that overfeeding can cause additional stress on the body systems.

MONITORING:

Protein - A 24-hour urine collection for urine urea nitrogen can be obtained in order to approximate protein utilization. An increase in the BUN concentration may signal protein overload.

Fat   - Lipid clearance should be monitored by measuring the serum triglyceride level. Prior to the initiation of lipid infusions a baseline value is obtained. Four hours after the termination of lipids, serum triglycerides are remeasured and compared to the baseline to determine clearance. For serum triglycerides > 300 to 500 mg/L, fat may be limited to essential fatty acid needs.

Glucose- If hyperglycemia or glucosuria occur, lower glucose concentrations are used and/or insulin is added to the TPN.

C. NUTRITIONAL MANAGEMENT OF BURN PATIENTS

Nutritional assessment and support is essential to promote wound healing and prevent weight loss in patients with burn injury. The increase in energy expenditure that accompanies burns exceeds that of any other injury. These patients appear to become and remain hypermetabolic in response to a characteristic set of hormonal signals. This postburn elevated metabolic rate is proportional to the size of the thermal injury and lasts until the majority of the wound is closed. If the increased protein and caloric requirements are not supplied externally through nutritional support, the patient's skeletal muscle is broken down for fuel. Inadequate nutritional support can result in weight loss, loss of lean body mass, negative nitrogen balance, delayed wound healing, skin graft failure, decreased immunologic response, burn wound sepsis, and increased mortality.

Many methods exist for estimating the nutritional requirements of burn patients. All have some limitations. The Curreri formula is widely used to determine caloric requirements and is probably best at estimating peak energy expenditure:

Adult: (25 calories x kg preburn weight) + (40 calories x percentage of body burned)

Child (≤ 12 years of age): (60 calories x kg preburn weight) + (35 calories x percentage of body burned)

Protein should be supplied in amounts to provide a nonprotein calorie to nitrogen ratio of 150 to 1. Additional protein may be required for patients with severe burns (> 40 to 50% of body surface area). A goal of 1.5 to 2.0 g protein per kilogram of body weight can be used as a guideline.

Patients should receive a high calorie, high protein diet. Most also receive therapeutic vitamin and mineral supplementation. Adequacy of nutrient intake should be monitored by daily weights and calorie counts. Oral dietary supplements, tube feedings, and/or parenteral nutrition are included as needed.

No benefits to overfeeding have been demonstrated. Maintaining the patient's weight within 10% of preburn weight is suggested as a guideline to prevent the problems associated with over- or underfeeding.

D. NUTRITION AND CANCER

Nutrition is an important concern for patients with cancer. They often have anorexia (a lack or loss of appetite) and many develop cachexia, a profound disorder marked by general ill health, weight loss, and malnutrition. If untreated, the severe malnutrition from these conditions may contribute as much as the illness itself to the death of the patient.

NUTRITIONAL EFFECTS OF CANCER:

1. Altered Metabolism

An alteration in metabolism may result from the systemic effects of many types of tumors. Abnormalities in the metabolism of carbohydrates, proteins, and lipids, as well as increases in basal metabolic rate and energy expenditure have been shown to occur.

2. Fluid and Electrolyte Imbalances

Imbalances frequently occur in patients with hepatic or central nervous system metastases; obstruction of the urinary, lymphatic, or venous tracts; or with hormone-secreting neoplasms. Vomiting, induced by obstruction of the gastrointestinal tract; diarrhea; or intracranial pressure from a cancerous tumor may also cause imbalances.

3. Malabsorption

Malabsorption may be precipitated by cancers of the pancreas, small bowel, or stomach.

4. Anorexia

The etiology of anorexia has many postulated causes. Abnormal taste perceptions, sensations of satiety, and derangement in central nervous system serotonin metabolism have been suggested. Dysgeusia (perversion of the sense of taste) and learned food aversions are also implicated.

5. Psychological Stress

The diagnosis itself, uncertainties of the disease process, and treatments may cause mood swings, difficulty in concentrating, and anorexia.

NUTRITIONAL EFFECTS OF TREATMENT:

1. Surgery

Certain surgical procedures can have a profound impact on the nutritional status of the patient. Examples include resection in the head and neck region, esophagectomy, gastrectomy, pancreatectomy, and bowel resections. Without careful nutritional management patients can suffer from malabsorption, diarrhea, and dumping syndrome.

2. Radiation

A consequence of radiation therapy is obligatory damage to healthy tissue within the irradiated field. Radiation damage to the salivary glands, oral cavity, and esophagopharyngeal area may lead to nutritional problems such as loss of taste, mouth dryness, oral infections, dysphagia, nausea, and vomiting. Radiation to the small bowel epithelium leads to altered function in the form of diarrhea, abdominal pain, nausea, vomiting, fistulas, and malabsorption.

3. Chemotherapy

Numerous nutritional consequences are associated with chemotherapy. Most of these effects are the result of interference with metabolic reactions. Among the most common side effects are diarrhea, nausea, vomiting, anorexia, and mucositis. Various antiemetic drugs can be useful in managing the nausea and vomiting associated with chemotherapy and radiotherapy.

NUTRITIONAL MANAGEMENT OF THE PATIENT WITH CANCER:

The single most common nutritional problem in patients with cancer is protein-calorie malnutrition, a direct consequence of anorexia and altered host metabolism. The goals of nutritional management of patients with cancer are twofold: (1) achievement and maintenance of reasonable weight and (2) prevention or correction of nutritional imbalances and deficiencies.

1. Nutritional Assessment

Adequate calories, protein, fats, minerals, vitamins, and fluids must be supplied in appropriate amounts. A simple, rapid screening of nutritional status should be performed on every patient within 48 hours of admission to a health care facility. If the patient appears to be at risk for malnutrition, a more extensive assessment may be in order.

2. Types of Feeding

Although nausea, vomiting, and diarrhea commonly limit nutrient intake, the gastrointestinal tract should be used whenever possible. Liquid formula feedings are often better tolerated than solid food, and may be used to replace or supplement the usual diet.

Oral feeding of either food or formula may be impossible because of pain while swallowing, weakness, obstruction, or anorexia. In many instances, adequate nutrition can be supplied by enteral tube feedings (see chart on pages 288-94).

Total parenteral nutrition permits the nutritional repletion of patients who cannot be adequately nourished enterally. Although it is a very useful method, it must be monitored quite closely and is extremely expensive. It should be used only if the gut is not available.

E. ANOREXIA NERVOSA AND BULIMIA

The two eating disorders, anorexia and bulimia, have unknown causes, although biological, environmental, and psychological mechanisms are involved. Individuals with these disorders utilize food in an attempt to gain control of their lives and relieve emotional distress. Even though the symptomatology of these eating disorders is similar, the underlying causes and personalities vary greatly, necessitating individualized therapy. The most effective treatment appears to be a multidisciplinary team approach to correct electrolyte imbalances, replete nutrient stores, normalize eating patterns, teach proper eating habits, prescribe appropriate psychotropic medication, and resolve underlying psychological issues. Because severe weight loss interferes with cognitive ability, weight gain may be necessary before therapy can be effective.

<u>Anorexia Nervosa</u>

This disorder often begins as a moderate effort to lose weight, but results in self-imposed starvation, an obsession with diet and exercise, and a profound change in eating habits.

Patients with anorexia nervosa lose weight by drastic food deprivation, self-induced vomiting, excessive exercise, laxative and/or diuretic abuse, or a combination of these. The mortality rate from this psychiatric disorder is estimated to be between 5 to 10%.

Psychological/behavioral characteristics of anorexia nervosa include altered body image, a relentless pursuit of thinness, rigorous exercise despite emaciation and fatigue, denial of appetite, peculiar eating habits and rituals, rigid exclusion of certain foods, extreme guilt after eating, and attempts to control self and others by disciplined dieting.

Physical Signs and Symptoms of Anorexia Nervosa

Sleep disturbances
Increased weakness
Gastrointestinal disturbances
Decreased sexual interest
Hyperacuity to noise and light
Edema
Hypothermia
Decreased basal metabolic rate
Hypotension
Amenorrhea
Lanugo
Electrolyte imbalances

Bulimia

This disorder often begins as an effort to control weight by purging after binge eating. Patients with bulimia attempt to control their weight by dieting, self-induced vomiting, and use of cathartics or diuretics. Most of these individuals are within their normal weight range, but some are underweight and others are overweight.

Typically a large quantity of food is consumed in a short period of time, followed by self-induced vomiting. Emotions experienced after the episode are guilt, shame, and feeling "out of control." Isolation from others, sometimes by sleeping, usually completes the cycle.

Physical Signs and Symptoms of Bulimia
Abdominal pain
Enlarged parotid glands
Esophageal inflammation
Dental lesions
Hypokalemia
Metabolic acidosis
Dehydration
Electrolyte imbalances
Sleep disturbances
Depression

DIETARY TREATMENT:

Anorexia Nervosa

An ideal weight is set and caloric needs are estimated using a nomogram for each patient. A contract is signed specifying expectations and consequences of failure to comply.

The patient is interviewed to obtain information about food preferences, allergies, and why certain foods are avoided. Due to misinformation and food phobias, many patients have excluded whole categories of foods such as red meat, breads, cereals, milk, or desserts. If dental problems are present such as enamel erosion from self-induced vomiting, foods with firm textures may be avoided to prevent painful chewing. The patient is allowed to choose only 2 foods that will not be served. Changes in these foods are not allowed, since manipulation can become a major problem.

Taking these food preferences into consideration, the dietitian selects the patient's menus, emphasizing balance. All food groups are represented, including at least 3 cups of 2% milk/day, and no "diet" foods are used. Three meals and 3 snacks are planned to meet estimated caloric needs. Daily calorie counts document the intake.

At the beginning of treatment the patient often chooses to eat less than 1000 calories/day. Rapid increases are common as the patient learns to gain weight to earn privileges and eventual discharge. The patient is expected to gain an average of 0.2 kgs/day. If this is not achieved within 5 days of treatment, the patient is tube fed to assure adequate intake of calories and nutrients.

When the target weight is reached, the maintenance phase of treatment begins. The patient then selects food from family style service and may eat meals away from the hospital as long as the weight stays within 1 kg of target. In this phase the patient learns what an appropriate intake is in order to maintain weight. The dietitian offers suitable suggestions to meet and maintain this goal.

Bulimia

A desirable weight is determined for each patient based on height, body structure, sex, and age. If the weight is normal, the patient must maintain it within 1 kg. If the patient is underweight or overweight, the target weight must be achieved within 1 kg. Caloric needs are estimated using a nomogram. A contract is signed specifying expectations and consequences of failure to comply.

The dietitian interviews the patient to obtain information about food preferences and allergies. The patient is allowed to choose only 2 foods that will not be served. If dental problems are present such as enamel erosion from self-induced vomiting, foods with firm textures may be avoided to prevent painful chewing.

Taking these food preferences into consideration, the dietitian selects the patient's menus emphasizing balance. All food groups are represented, including at least 3 cups of milk. Three meals or 3 meals and 3 snacks are planned to meet estimated caloric needs. Daily calorie counts document intake.

When the patient reaches target weight, the maintenance phase of treatment begins. The patient then selects food from family style service and may eat meals away from the hospital. The patient must maintain the target weight within 1 kg for 7 days or the program is reinstated. The purpose of the maintenance phase is to teach appropriate caloric intake to maintain the desirable weight. The dietitian offers appropriate suggestions to meet and maintain this goal.

F. NUTRITION IN SPORTS AND EXERCISE

In recent years Americans have become more aware of fitness and health. As a result, dietitians have been challenged to provide appropriate nutrition information to both the casual exerciser and the serious athlete. Although the dietitian's approach to the individual or group will vary, basic nutrition information to benefit the exerciser/athlete involves nutrient requirements based on age, sex, body size and composition, rate of metabolism, and state of health. More specifically, the dietitian can (1) determine nutritional adequacy of the diet; (2) evaluate body composition; (3) make recommendations for energy needs and distribution of calories; (4) provide information on fluid replacement; and (5) suggest appropriate preexercise feedings.

NUTRITIONAL ADEQUACY OF THE DIET:

The greatest difference in food requirements of the athlete versus the nonathlete is the total number of calories consumed. The need for nutrients which function as cofactors in energy metabolism--thiamin, riboflavin, niacin, and chromium--is proportional to energy intake and utilization. Therefore, the extra calories and cofactors needed can be met by consuming a varied diet with liberal intake from the bread, cereal, and grain group. For the athlete who has an extremely high energy need and difficulty consuming large volumes of food, an increased intake of fats and sugars may be warranted. It is rarely necessary or advantageous to provide the athlete with supplemental vitamins, minerals, protein, or amino acids provided he/she is consuming a well-balanced diet.

Iron may be the exception. The female athlete of childbearing age requires extra iron due to losses through menstruation and perspiration. Long distance runners may have increased hemolysis and decreased iron absorption. Serum ferritin and hemoglobin levels determined every 3 to 4 months can detect those who need supplemental iron. Training tends to increase red blood cell mass and plasma volume disproportionately, and can result in a decreased hematocrit. This drop in hematocrit may be of minor consequence; however, low serum ferritin reflects a prelatent stage in iron deficiency. Nutrition counseling and/or iron supplementation may be warranted.

Protein requirements for athletes are controversial. Strenuous exercise, especially for the growing individual in the early stages of training, may increase the need for dietary protein. The recommended protein allowance of 0.8 g/kg may be inadequate for some athletes. For those engaged in strength/power and endurance activities, the suggested protein intake is 1.5 to 2.0 g/kg and 1.2 g/kg respectively. The typical athlete's diet provides this level of protein. However, the athlete who has an eating disorder or inadequate caloric intake may not be obtaining sufficient protein.

BODY COMPOSITION:

Body composition assessment is important for determining a desirable weight. The most common methods for determining percentage of body fat are hydrostatic (underwater) weighing, skinfold measurements, and bioelectrical impedance. Hydrostatic weighing is regarded as an accurate estimate of body fat; however, many athletes do not have access to the special facilities required.

Bioelectric impedance is a rapid, noninvasive, and convenient method for determining body fat. However, clinicians using this method should verify that the equations used are appropriate for the population tested.

Skinfold measurements are a simple, less expensive, and convenient method for determining body fat. Practice is required before reliable results can be obtained. Skinfold measurements can be used in 2 ways. One application is to monitor changes in body composition by taking the sum of 5 measurements at various intervals during a training program. The most common skinfold measurements used are biceps and subscapula, and at the suprailiac, abdominal, and upper thigh sites. Another method uses mathematical equations designed to predict body density or percentage of body fat. These equations are population specific and predict body fat only in subjects who are similar to the population from which the equations were derived. Sample equations for predicting body fat for men and women are shown on the next page.

<u>Women</u>

Body Density = $1.1125025 - 0.0013124\ (x_1) + 0.0000055\ (x_1)^2 - 0.0002440\ (x_2)$

> x_1 = sum of chest, triceps, and subscapular skinfolds
> x_2 = age in years

<u>Men</u>

Body Density = $1.089733 - 0.0009245\ (x_1) + 0.0000025\ (x_1) - 0.0000973\ (x_2)$

> x_1 = sum of triceps, suprailium, and abdominal skinfolds
> x_2 = age in years

The following table provides guidelines for assessing an individual's body composition:

PERCENTAGE OF BODY FAT FOR MEN AND WOMEN

Body Fat Description	Male	Female
Essential	2-5	6-12
Average	12-17	19-25
Borderline Obese	18-24	26-30
Obese	25+	30+
Athletes	4-18	6-30

DETERMINING BODY WEIGHT: Accurate assessment of the body weight of exercisers and athletes requires more than the traditional height and weight tables. A more accurate method of identifying ideal body weight is to use percentage body fat in the following formula:

$$\text{Desired Weight} = \frac{\text{Lean Body Mass}^*}{(1 - \%\ \text{fat desired})}$$

For example, suppose a 150-pound woman with 30% body fat wishes to lose weight in order to attain a body fat of 20%. She wants to know how many pounds of fat she needs to lose. The computation would be:

Fat = 150 pounds x 0.30 = 45 pounds
Lean body mass = 150 pounds - 45 pounds = 105 pounds

$$\text{Desirable body weight} = \frac{105\ \text{pounds}}{(1 - 0.20)} = \frac{105\ \text{pounds}}{0.8} = 131.25\ \text{pounds}$$

150 pounds - 131.25 pounds = 18.75 pounds

Accordingly, this woman needs to lose approximately 19 pounds in order to attain a body fat of 20%.

It is important to realize that the optimum level of body fat varies from individual to individual and is influenced by a variety of factors such as genetics. It does appear that it is desirable to maintain body fat at 15% or less for male athletes and 25% or less for women athletes. In general, the leanest women in the population do not have body fat levels less than 10 to 20% of body weight, probably representing the lower limits of fatness for most women in good health. The lower limit of percentage body fat for men is probably 3%.

---

*Lean body mass refers to that part of the total body weight which remains after all of the body fat is removed. It is composed of muscle, skin, bone, organs, and all other nonfat tissue.

ENERGY NEEDS AND DISTRIBUTION OF CALORIES: Energy requirements for an exerciser/athlete vary not only with the individual's metabolic needs, but also with the duration, intensity, and frequency of the activity.

A recommended calorie level for the exerciser/athlete must be determined individually, based on the amount of food required to maintain desired body weight/body composition. The recommended distribution of calories is 55 to 60% as carbohydrate, 10 to 15% as protein, and 30% or less as fat, which is generally the same distribution recommended for the rest of the population, with slightly more carbohydrate and less fat. To prevent a progressive reduction in muscle glycogen, levels up to 70% carbohydrate have been suggested for athletes engaged in strenuous training. However, many athletes cannot consume the large volume of food associated with this diet. Foods high in both carbohydrate and protein and low in fat such as legumes and skim milk are needed to provide adequate protein in a diet with 70% of the calories as carbohydrate.

The fuel sources for muscle activity are primarily carbohydrate and fat. Events requiring short bursts of intensive activity (anaerobic events) rely solely on carbohydrate as the fuel choice. Endurance events requiring prolonged muscular work (aerobic events) use fat and carbohydrate for energy. In addition, recent research has identified amino acids as a fuel source during intense endurance activities, but more study is needed regarding this.

The amount of carbohydrate stored in muscle as glycogen is one limiting factor in an athlete's ability to perform endurance exercise. As glycogen stores near depletion, the working muscle fibers fail to contract, resulting in the onset of exhaustion. Glycogen supercompensation, more commonly known as "carbohydrate loading," is a practice which increases the glycogen stores in both muscle and liver. Many investigators have shown that carbohydrate loading can increase endurance only when an event exceeds 90 minutes. Carbohydrate loading is of no advantage to the athlete in intensive, short-term competition and is especially contraindicated for athletes engaged in weight control sports, since 2.7 g water are stored with each gram of extra glycogen. The increase in weight may be as much as 2.5 kg.

Research now indicates that it is not necessary to perform the depletion phase of carbohydrate loading, which consists of a low carbohydrate diet prior to the high carbohydrate regimen. To increase body glycogen for endurance events, the athlete should consume a high carbohydrate diet and avoid exhaustive workouts 3 to 4 days prior to competition. In addition, carbohydrate loading should be restricted to important competitions.

FLUID REPLACEMENT: Of primary concern to the athlete is maintenance of an adequate state of hydration, especially during exercise in hot weather. During athletic competition or practice, thirst is not a sufficient indicator of fluid needs. The dehydrated athlete is at risk for heat stroke. The following are general guidelines to use regarding fluid replacement:

1. Two hours prior to an event, the athlete in endurance competition should attempt to drink 600 ml of fluid.

2. Ten to 15 minutes before the event, 400 to 500 ml of water should be consumed.

3. During the event, the athlete should be offered small amounts of water (100-200 ml) every 10 to 15 minutes.

4. After the event, the athlete should continue to drink fluids at frequent intervals.

Plain water at 45°F is the best choice for rehydration, in spite of the common use of salt tablets and/or electrolyte drinks. The potassium, sodium, and chloride consumed in a mixed diet usually replaces that lost in sweat. If dilute solutions of ade-type drinks are given during an exercise workout or an endurance event, sugar should not exceed 5 to 10%; sodium, 10 mEq/liter; and potassium, 5 mEq/liter.

PREEXERCISE FEEDINGS: Replenishing liver glycogen stores is the primary purpose of preexercise meals. However, the stomach should be empty at the time of competition in order to prevent gastrointestinal distress. In addition, if food is present in the small intestine, blood flow to the working muscles is reduced. Most investigators support the recommendation of a high carbohydrate, moderate protein, lowfat meal 1 1/2 to 4 hours prior to an event. Although carbohydrate should be the major constituent of the preexercise meal, the ingestion of sugar less than an hour before competition is contraindicated. The blood glucose will actually be lower and less available to the athlete due to an insulin response.

SECTION 10

Enteral Formulas
and Supplements

Enteral formulas and supplements are used to nourish the patient who is physically or psychologically unable to consume adequate food. Formulas may be fed orally or by tube. A great variety of commercial preparations is available, but not all are stocked at the University of Iowa Hospitals and Clinics. At least one formula from each of the enteral hyperalimentation categories is provided. Occasionally it is necessary to formulate a special tube feeding for a particular patient. In most instances, the commercial feedings supply all of the Recommended Dietary Allowances in 1000 to 2000 ml.

Nutritional supplements are used to supply additional calories and/or other nutrients to patients who are able to consume some food by mouth. Some of the tube feedings are palatable and may serve as a nutritional supplement to those patients who are eating. A comparison of the nutritive values and features of the formulas and supplements is found on pages 288-99.

Several complications are associated with the administration of tube feedings. Diarrhea, dehydration, and aspiration can be lethal if adequate safeguards are not met. Lactase deficiency in the hospitalized patient is a routine concern. Many of the commercial formulas are lactose-free, eliminating this frequent complication. In addition, electrolyte imbalance, glucosuria, azotemia, and constipation are problems that can arise. Refer to tube feeding complications and suggested treatments on pages 264-65 to determine possible solutions.

It is important to note that the osmolality of the solution is often associated with tube feeding complications. Osmolality refers to the number of osmoles (mOsm: the measure of osmotically active particles) per kilogram of solvent (usually water). It is frequently confused with osmolarity, but the two are not synonymous. Osmolarity refers to the number of osmoles per liter of solution (solvent plus solute). Osmolarity is thus influenced by the volumes of all the solutes contained in the solution, and by the temperature, while osmolality is not. While there are only small clinical differences between the terms osmolality and osmolarity, osmolality is generally considered the correct and preferable term. Isotonic formulas have an osmolality of 300 mOsm/kg water which closely approximates the osmolality of blood, thereby theoretically avoiding hyperosmolar diarrhea.

FACTORS TO CONSIDER IN SELECTING A FORMULA: The first step in selecting a tube feeding is defining the patient's major nutritional problem(s) and assessing any digestive or metabolic disorders. Nutritional assessments or consultations are recommended to assist in the process. The enteral hyperalimentation category can then be determined and a formula with features to meet the needs of the patient can be selected. If the primary problem is a physical or psychological inability to consume food orally, a lactose-free standard formula is usually indicated. Many formulas specifically designed for digestive and absorptive disorders, stress, trauma, renal, or hepatic disease are available. Once the formula is selected, the mode of administration, the rate, the concentration, and the feeding advancement schedule must be developed. It is helpful to determine the final rate and concentration needed to meet the patient's calculated calorie, nutrient, and water requirements. Monitoring is an integral and ongoing part of the selection and administration process so that changes can be made when appropriate.

The following checklists are useful in selecting the appropriate formula.

Assessment of Patient:

        Past medical history and present problems
        Caloric and protein needs
        Gastrointestinal function
        Renal function
        Hepatic function
        Hydration status

Assessment of Formula:

        Osmolality
        Caloric density
        Calorie to nitrogen ratio
        Protein quality and bioavailability
        Balanced composition of carbohydrate, protein, and fat
        Adequate vitamin, mineral, and trace element content
        Suitable viscosity and homogenization
        Convenience and ease of administration
        Bacteriologic safety
        Cost

TYPE OF FORMULAS AND SUPPLEMENTS:

Standard Feedings

    Standard feedings are indicated for patients who have essentially normal gastrointestinal function, but who are unable to consume a regular diet. Formulas in this group are milk-based, lactose-free, and meat-based (blenderized). They all contain approximately 1 calorie/cc. Milk-based formulas contain intact sources of protein, come in a variety of flavors, and are designed to be given orally or by tube. Lactose-free formulas contain caseinates, soy protein isolates, or egg albumin as their protein sources. Generally, milk-based and lactose-free formulas are lower in cost than meat-based formulas. Meat-based formulas are blended food made from meat, vegetables, fruits, cereals, and sometimes egg. The lactose-containing meat-based formulas include nonfat milk; the lactose-free, caseinates. Meat-based formulas are designed specifically for tube feedings and are not recommended for oral use. The standard adult tube feeding at the University of Iowa Hospitals and Clinics is a meat-based, lactose-free liquid diet (Compleat Modified) because it closely approximates a normal mixed diet.

Nutritional Supplements

    A variety of commercial supplements is available to provide one or more specific nutrients. To decide which product is suitable for a particular patient, the nutrients ingested in less than adequate amounts must be determined. A supplement which furnishes these nutrients in accordance with the patient's needs can then be selected. For example, frequently a patient's need for more calories must be met within protein or electrolyte restrictions.

    If the problem is mainly one of insufficient quantity of food, the diet is typically inadequate in calories and low in protein, vitamins, and minerals. Many of the standard feedings previously described are quite palatable and therefore useful in providing well-balanced nutrition in a concentrated and easily ingested form. Two products designed specifically for general supplementation are Carnation Instant Breakfast and Citrotein. See the chart on pages 288-89 and 292-93 for a complete analysis.

FORMULAS AND SUPPLEMENTS FOR DIGESTIVE AND ABSORPTIVE PROBLEMS: Lactose-free, low residue, and high fiber products are available for patients with diarrhea, constipation, cramps, and distention due to carbohydrate intolerance. Secondary lactose intolerance is not uncommon in hospitalized patients.

    The type or amount of fat may be altered if fat malabsorption is present. Medium-chain triglycerides replace some or all of the fat in various products. Partially predigested and chemically defined formulas (elemental and/or peptide formulations) are suggested only when further refinements are necessary due to malabsorption.

Elemental and/or Peptide Formulations

These types of formulas were developed for digestive and malabsorptive complications. Nutrients are presented in simple form so that they can be readily absorbed in the proximal small bowel. Carbohydrate is provided in the form of glucose or maltodextrins; and protein, in the form of amino acids or peptides. Fat is present in very small quantities and/or in the form of medium-chain triglycerides (MCT). Essential fatty acid deficiency may develop without supplementation. The osmolality of these formulas tends to be high, ranging from 300 to 810 mOsm/kg water. These formulas are often used as a transition diet between parenteral nutrition and a lactose-free formula or standard feeding. They may also be used for the patient suffering from severe allergy symptoms or for whom the elimination diets fail to isolate the allergen(s). (See page 169.) Defined formula diets come in powder form and must be mixed with water prior to use. They may be given orally in a variety of flavors; however, patient acceptance is often low. These formulas are costly (approximately three times that of standard feedings) and should therefore be prescribed only when indicated by disease conditions.

High Caloric Density Formulas

High caloric density formulas are lactose-free and contain 1.5 to 2.0 calories per cc. They are indicated for patients with high metabolic needs or fluid restrictions. These formulas are generally less palatable than the 1 calorie per cc standard formulas. The osmolality ranges from 500 to 600 mOsm/kg water. Particular attention to the patient's state of hydration is necessary when these formulas are used, since adequate calories can be supplied in volumes much lower than levels normally recommended to maintain fluid balance. Fluid from other sources (intravenous, flushing NG tubing, and by mouth) should be totaled and additional fluids supplemented as necessary. (See table on page 262.)

Specialty Formulas for Stress and Trauma

Patients with multiple physical stresses or trauma as indicated in the chart below may benefit by receiving formulas high in branched chain amino acids. These amino acids, isoleucine, leucine, and valine are primarily metabolized in peripheral muscle tissue. They may be preferentially utilized for energy under stress conditions. The rationale for using stress formulas is based on these findings and studies of parenteral administration of branched chain amino acids. These studies indicate that administration of these amino acids can inhibit the release of endogenous amino acids from the muscle, thus decreasing muscle protein catabolism and stimulating muscle protein synthesis. A study of postoperative patients showed more efficient nitrogen utilization when compared to a standard amino acid injection.

These formulas meet the RDA for all nutrients when 3000 calories are given.

CONDITIONS WARRANTING USE OF HIGH STRESS FORMULAS

	Polytrauma	Sepsis
Urinary Excretion of N_2 (g/dl)	10-15	>15
Blood Sugar Level (mg%)	150 ± 25	250 ± 50
Blood Lactate Level (uM/l)	1,200 ± 200	3,000 ± 500
Glucagon/Insulin Ratio	3 ± 0.7	8 ± 1.5
O_2 Consumption Index (ml/m^2)	140 ± 6	170 ± 10

Note: If two or more indicators are present, a high stress formula may be advisable.

Specialty Formulas for Renal and Liver Disease

Amin-Aid and Travasorb Renal can be used to meet caloric requirements while limiting protein intake. Essential amino acids supply the protein in Amin-Aid. This formulation promotes lowering and stabilizing of blood urea nitrogen levels as, theoretically, the nonessential amino acids are synthesized from the urea in the blood. Travasorb Renal includes essential and nonessential amino acids to enhance nitrogen balance and weight gain. Another characteristic of these formulas is that they contain negligible amounts of electrolytes, since renal patients often have elevated serum potassium, magnesium, and phosphorus levels. Careful monitoring of electrolytes is especially important when using Amin-Aid or Travasorb Renal. Supplements of vitamins, and possibly minerals and essential fatty acids, may be needed, depending upon the length of time the patient receives the formula. Amin-Aid contains *no* vitamins or minerals, whereas Travasorb Renal contains water-soluble vitamins, but not fat-soluble ones. A variety of flavors is available.

Hepatic-Aid II and Travasorb Hepatic are used to provide sufficient calories and protein in patients with chronic liver disease. These formulas do not exacerbate or promote hepatic encephalopathy in protein-intolerant patients. The product contains increased amounts of branched chain amino acids and arginine (an ammonia-processing amino acid) and decreased amounts of aromatic amino acids and methionine to reflect the balance needed. The precise mechanisms of hepatic encephalopathy are not known, but dietary studies indicate that the amino acid composition of ingested protein is important. Some proteins seem to precipitate encephalopathy more than others: the amino acid pattern of increased plasma concentrations of the aromatic amino acids phenylalanine, tyrosine, and tryptophan; increased concentrations of methionine and decreased concentrations of the branched chain amino acids valine, leucine, and isoleucine are characteristic. Hepatic-Aid II contains negligible amounts of vitamins, minerals, and electrolytes which may need to be supplemented depending upon the length of time the patient receives the product. Travasorb Hepatic contains vitamins, minerals, and electrolytes. Careful monitoring of electrolytes is especially important when Hepatic-Aid or Travasorb Hepatic is used.

Portagen, a formula containing medium-chain triglycerides, is useful in the treatment of patients with bile acid deficiency who do not efficiently digest and absorb conventional long-chain food fats. The product may be used as a supplementary beverage with the MCT Diet (see pages 124-26) or as a complete formula for infants.

Modular Components

Modular components are energy sources limited primarily to carbohydrate, protein, or fat. They may be used singly or in combination with one another to provide calories in a certain distribution or concentration. For example, they may be added to formulas or foods to change the percentage concentration of a nutrient or the caloric concentration of the diet.

Modular components may also be combined to create a formula specifically designed for a particular patient's need. The composition and features of these modules are described in the chart on pages 296-99.

Other low protein formulas and food substitutes have been developed for patients who need high calorie, low protein, low electrolyte supplements.

Nutrisource is a modular system of individual nutrient components. This system provides the freedom and flexibility to alter nutrient content and source, control caloric density, and regulate fluid and electrolyte balance to tailor nutritional support to the patient's specific disease state or metabolic need.

DETERMINING VOLUME AND CALORIC DENSITY OF FORMULA NEEDED: The amount of carbohydrate, protein, and fat will determine the caloric content of the formula. The standard dilution is 1 calorie per cc. The caloric density and calorie-to-nitrogen ratio are important considerations. Adequate amounts of water must be given to excrete the metabolic end products of protein digestion. Extra fluid is usually not necessary with the 1 calorie/cc dilution unless the patient has an elevated body temperature, an unusual fluid loss, or is dehydrated. High caloric density formulas containing 1.5 to 2.0 calories per cc are useful for patients in hypermetabolic states or those with volume restrictions. Special attention to the patient's state of hydration is necessary when high caloric density formulas are used. (See "Guidelines for Free Fluids in Tube Feedings" and "Maintenance Fluid Allowances" below.) Formulas which provide the patient with the principal source of calories have a calorie-to-nitrogen ratio of about 130 to 150:1. Adequate nonprotein calories must be provided so that amino acids are used for anabolic processes rather than as a source of energy. Products designed primarily for supplementation have a calorie-to-nitrogen ratio of about 80:1.

To calculate caloric and protein needs, a nutritional assessment is done (See Section 9, pages 246-48).

GUIDELINES FOR FREE FLUIDS IN TUBE FEEDINGS

Caloric Density (Kcal/cc)	Percent Free Fluid
1.0	80
1.5	70
2.0	60

MAINTENANCE FLUID ALLOWANCES

Patients	Fluid (cc/Kg)
Infant	100-120
Child, 1-10 years	60-80
Adolescent, 11-18 years	41-55
Adult, 19+ years	20-30

Source: Adapted from Segar (1972).
Note: For fever add 360 cc/degree Centigrade/day.

ADMINISTRATION OF ENTERAL FEEDINGS: To determine the appropriate concentration of formula to initiate, a general rule is to start the product at a concentration of 300 mOsm/kg water to avoid hyperosmolar diarrhea.

General rules for the administration of an enteral feeding, unless otherwise indicated are:

1. Challenge the gastrointestinal tract with a normal saline solution at a rate of 50 cc/hour. Check residuals and gastric emptying hourly for 6 hours.

2. Initiate the formula at 1/2 strength at a rate of 50 cc per hour. The concentration of the formula should not exceed 300 mOsm to avoid hyperosmolar diarrhea.

3. Increase the rate by 25 cc an hour or every 12 hours until the desired rate is achieved.

4. Increase the strength every 12 hours *only after* the desired rate is achieved in gradations of 1/2 to 3/4 to full strength *as tolerated*.

5. Flush the feeding tube with 100 cc water every 4 hours if on continuous drip or after each feeding and delivery of oral medications.

TUBE FEEDING COMPLICATIONS AND SUGGESTED TREATMENTS

Complication	Possible Reason	Suggested Treatment
Diarrhea	Medications	Medications which can cause diarrhea are antibiotics and quinine. Change to another drug if possible. If not, treat diarrhea with antidiarrheal agent.
	Osmotic overload (especially with transpyloric feeding)	Dilute formula with water or reduce rate of administration or change to isotonic formula.
	Volume overload	Reduce flow rate.
	Lactose intolerance	Use lactose-free formula.
	Tube placement too low in stomach causing gastric distention with increased gastric emptying	Check tube placement.
	Liquid stools around impaction	Check for impaction. An enema may be indicated. Adequate water intake or a bulking agent should be used to prevent impaction.
	Decreased bulk	Change to formula which provides more bulk. One to 3 times daily use a bulking agent (1 tsp Metamucil in 50 cc water) and give immediately via bolus feeding. Flush tube with 20 cc water.
	Inadequate intestinal flora due to antibiotic therapy	Give thinned yogurt or acidophilus milk twice a day. For acute cases, discontinue formula for 24 hours and give 50/50 mixture of plain yogurt and acidophilus milk at 50 cc/hr.
	Fat malabsorption	Decrease fat content of feeding and/or use MCT oil.
	Insufficient osmotic pressure for absorption as indicated by low serum albumin (≤ 2.2 mg/dl)	Reduce enteral feeding and supplement with peripheral albumin, or administer TPN until albumin reaches 2.5 mg/dl.
	Bacterial contamination	Change feeding container and administration tubing every 24 hours. Use clean technique when transferring formula. Hang only 4 hours of formula.
Constipation	Impaction	Physician performs rectal examination. Give patient a laxative or an enema.
	Decreased bulk	Change to formula which provides more bulk. Use a bulking agent as described above.

Complication	Possible Reason	Suggested Treatment
Constipation (cont'd)	Insufficient free fluid	Increase free fluid administered with formula. (See tables on page 274 "Guidelines for Free Fluids in Tube Feedings" and "Maintenance Fluid Allowances.")
	Medications which decrease intestinal motility	Change medications if possible or give stool softener, additional fluid, or laxative.
	Decreased intestinal motility due to inactivity	Increase patient's activity or treat symptomatically.
	Complete absorption of elemental formula resulting in minimal waste products	Provide patient education and reassurance.
Aspiration	Incorrect tube selection and placement	Use small tubing to avoid compromise of lower esophageal sphincter and use transpyloric feedings.
	Too high a flow rate	Decrease rate.
	Incorrect position of patient	Position head at 30–45 degree angle and lay patient on right side.
	Decreased gastric motility	Use metaclopramide to increase gastric motility.
Electrolyte Imbalance	Composition of formula Excessive losses Insufficient excretion Water depletion or excess	Increase or decrease affected electrolytes. Adjust free water.
Dehydration	Renal impairment Administration of concentrated formulas Diarrhea or other abnormal losses Glucosuria leading to diuresis Fever Inadequate administration of water along with the formula	Correct any abnormal losses, provide increased free water, or adjust the formula to decrease renal solute load.
Glucosuria	Increased carbohydrate load (especially in defined formula diets) Diabetic patients with inadequate insulin intake Steroid therapy Stress-induced glucose intolerance	Decrease carbohydrate content of formula or give insulin.
Azotemia	High protein formula	Reduce amount of protein in formula.
	Insufficient water to excrete products	Increase free water for excretion.
	Renal impairment	Change to special renal formula.
	Gastrointestinal bleeding	Determine and treat cause.

Bibliography

GENERAL

Adams, C. F.: Nutritive Value of American Foods in Common Units. USDA Handbook 456. Washington, DC, 1975.

Agricultural Research Service: Composition of Foods: Raw, Processed, Prepared. USDA Handbook 8, Sections 1-16. Washington, DC, 1976-1988.

The American Dietetic Association: Handbook of Clinical Dietetics. New Haven: Yale University Press, 1981.

The American Dietetic Association: Manual of Clinical Dietetics. Chicago: The American Dietetic Association, 1988.

Anderson, L., Mitchell, H. S., Rynbergen, H., Dibble, M., and Turkki, P.: Nutrition in Health and Disease. Philadelphia: Lippincott, 1982.

Food and Nutrition Board: Recommended Dietary Allowances (9th ed.). Washington, DC: National Academy of Sciences, 1980.

Glanz K.: Compliance with dietary regimens: Its magnitude, measurement, and determinants. Prev Med 9:787, 1980.

Goodhart, R. S., and Shills, M. E.: Modern Nutrition in Health and Disease (6th ed.). Philadelphia: Lea & Febiger, 1980.

Guyton, A. C.: Textbook of Medical Physiology (7th ed.). Philadelphia: Saunders, 1986.

Krause, M. V., Mahan, L. K.: Food, Nutrition and Diet Therapy (7th ed.). Philadelphia: Saunders, 1984.

Leveille, G. A., Zabik, M. E., and Morgan, K. J.: Nutrients in Foods. Cambridge: The Nutrition Guild, 1984.

Luigi, B., Porro, G. B., Rodolfo, C., and Lipkin, M.: Nutrition in Gastrointestinal Disease. New York: Raven Press, 1987.

Pennington, J. A., and Church, H. N. (eds): Food Values of Portions Commonly Used (14th ed.). Philadelphia: Lippincott, 1985.

Present Knowledge in Nutrition (5th ed.). New York: Nutrition Foundation, 1984.

Robinson, C. H., and Lawler, M.: Normal and Therapeutic Nutrition (16th ed.). New York: Macmillan, 1982.

Schneider, H. A., Anderson, C. E., and Coursin, D. B.: Nutritional Support of Medical Practice (2nd ed.). New York: Harper and Row, 1983.

Shils, M. E., and Young, V. R. (eds): Modern Nutrition in Health and Disease. Philadelphia: Lea & Febiger, 1988.

Zeman, F. J.: Clinical Nutrition and Dietetics. Lexington, MA: Collamore Press, 1983.

SECTION 1

GENERAL

American Heart Association: Dietary guidelines for healthy American adults. A statement for physicians and health professionals by the Nutrition Committee, American Heart Association, Dallas, TX, 1986.

HIGH PROTEIN--HIGH CALORIE

Bistrian, B. R.: Nutritional assessment and therapy of protein-calorie malnutrition in the hospital. J Am Diet Assoc 71:393, 1977.

Blackburn, G. L., and Bistrian, B. R.: Nutritional care of the injured and/or septic patient. Surg Clin North Am 56:1195, 1976.

Curreri, P. W., Richmond, D., Marvin, J., and Baxter, C. R.: Dietary requirements of patients with major burns. J Am Diet Assoc 65:415, 1975.

Imes, S., Pinchbeck, B. R., and Thomson, A. B. R.: Diet counseling modifies nutrient intake of patients with Crohn's disease. J Am Diet Assoc 87:457, 1987.

MATERNAL

American College of Obstetricians and Gynecologists. Standards for Ambulatory Obstetric Care. Washington, DC: American College of Obstetricians and Gynecologists, 1977

American College of Obstetricians and Gynecologists. Standards for Obstetric-Gynecologic Services (6th ed.). Washington, DC: American College of Obstetricians and Gynecologists, 1985.

Black, A. E., Wiles, S. J., and Paul, A. A.: The nutrient intakes of pregnant and lactating mothers of good socio-economic status in Cambridge, UK: Some implications for recommended daily allowances of minor nutrients. Br J Nutr 56:59, 1986.

Carruth, B. R.: Adolescent pregnancy and nutrition. NY State J Med 1288, 1981.

Ceresa, C., Theiss, T., and Sinibaldi, T.: Nutritional aspects of diabetes care and pregnancy. Diabetes Educ 9:21, 1983.

Committee on Adolescence--American Academy of Pediatrics: Statement on teenage pregnancy. Pediatrics 63:795, 1979.

Dwyer, J.: Nutritional support during pregnancy and lactation. Prim Care 9:475, 1982.

Elster, A. B.: The effect of maternal age, parity, and prenatal care on perinatal outcome in adolescent mothers. Am J Obstet Gynecol 149:845, 1984.

Ferris, A. M., Dalidowitz, C. K., Ingardia, C. M., Reece, E. A., Fumia, F. D., Jensen, R. G., and Allen, L. H.: Lactation outcome in insulin-dependent diabetic women. J Am Diet Assoc 88:317, 1988.

Gardner, D. F.: More vigilance is needed during pregnancy. Diabetes Care 8:349, 1982.

Levin, M. E., Rigg, L. A., and Marshall, R. E.: Pregnancy and diabetes, team approach. Arch Intern Med 146:758, 1986.

Lindheimer, M.: Current concepts of sodium metabolism and use of diuretics in pregnancy. Contemp Ob Gyn 15:207, 1980.

Maternal and newborn nutrition. In Brann, A. W., Jr., and Cefalo, R. C., eds.: Guidelines for Perinatal Care. Evanston, IL, and Washington, DC: American Academy of Pediatrics and American College of Obstetricians and Gynecologists, 1983.

Oakes, G. K., Jones, P., Williams, J., and Schoensiegel, B. B.: Management of diabetes mellitus in pregnancy. Mt Sinai J Med 54:261, 1987.

Orstead, C., Arrington, D., Kamath, S. K., Olson, R., and Kohrs, M. B.: Efficacy of prenatal nutrition counseling: Weight gain, infant birth weight, and cost effectiveness. J Am Diet Assoc 85:40, 1985.

Pitkin, R. M.: Assessment of nutritional status of mother, fetus, and newborn. Am J Clin Nutr 34:658, 1981.

Rosso, P.: A new chart to monitor weight gain during pregnancy. Am J Clin Nutr 41:644, 1985.

Rudolf, M. C. J., and Sherwin, R. S.: Maternal ketosis and its effect on the fetus. Clin Endocrinol Metab 12:413, 1983.

Suter, C., and Ott, D.: Maternal and infant nutrition recommendations: A review. J Am Diet Assoc 84:572, 1984.

Williams, E. J.: Pregnancy and insulin-dependent diabetes. Diabetes Educ 12:264, 1986.

Williams, J.: Gestational diabetes. Nurs Times 82:48, 1986.

Worthington-Roberts, B.: Nutritional support of successful reproduction: An update. J Nutr Educ 19:1, 1987.

Zuckerman, B., Albert, J. J., Dooling, E., Hingson, R., Kayne, H., Morelock, S., and Oppenheimer, E.: Neonatal outcome: Is adolescent pregnancy a risk factor? Pediatrics 71:489, 1983.

OSTOMY

Abrams, J. S., and Willard, C. J.: Aftercare of the patient with an ileostomy. Prim Care 1:691, 1974.

Anderson, H., Bosaeus, I., Brummer, R. J., Fasth, S., Hulten, L., Magnusson, O., and Strauss, B.: Nutritional and metabolic consequences of extensive bowel resection. Dig Dis 4:193, 1986.

Barer, A.: Stoma care in conventional ileostomy. Clin Gastroenterol 11:275, 1982.

Emerson, A. P.: Foods high in fiber and phytobezoar formation. J Am Diet Assoc 87:1675, 1987.

Hessov, I., Hasselblad, C., Fasth, S., and Hulten, L.: Magnesium deficiency after ileal resections for Crohn's disease. Scand J Gastroenterol 18:643, 1983.

Hill, G. L.: Ileostomy: Surgery, Physiology, and Management. New York: Grune and Stratton, 1976.

Hill, G. L.: Metabolic complications of ileostomy. Clin Gastroenterol 11:260, 1982.

Kennedy, H. J., Callender, S. T., Truelove, S. C., and Warner, G. T.: Haematological aspects of life with an ileostomy. Br J Haematol 52:445, 1982.

Kirsner, J. B., and Shorter, R. G.: Recent developments in nonspecific inflammatory bowel disease. N Engl J Med 306:775, 1982.

Metcalf, A. M., and Phillips, S. F.: Ileostomy diarrhea. Clin Gastroenterol 15:705, 1986.

Nilsson, L. O., Myrvold, H. E., Swolin, B., and Ojerskog, B.: Vitamin B_{12} in plasma in patients with continent ileostomy and long observation time. Scand J Gastroenterol 19:369, 1984.

Schwarz, K. B., Ternberg, J. L., Bell, M. J., and Keating, J. P.: Sodium needs of infants and children with ileostomy. J Pediatr 102:509, 1983.

Todd, I. P.: Mechanical complications of ileostomy. Clin Gastroenterol 11:268, 1982.

Tornquist, H., Rissanen, A., and Andersson, H.: Balance studies in patients with intestinal resection: How long is enough? Br J Nutr 56:11, 1986.

ORAL, MAXILLOFACIAL, AND PHARYNGEAL

Sobol, S. M., Conoyer, J. M., Zill, R., Thawley, S. S., and Ogura, J. H.: Nutritional concepts in the management of the head and neck cancer patient. I. Basic concepts. Laryngoscope 89:794, 1979.

Sobol, S. M., Conoyer, J. M., Zill, R., Thawley, S. S., and Ogura, J. H.: Nutritional concepts in the management of the head and neck cancer patient. II. Management concepts. Laryngoscope 89:962, 1979.

FIBER

Anderson, J. W.: Plant Fiber in Foods. Lexington, KY: HCF Diabetes Research Foundation, Inc., 1986.

Cummings, J.H.: Nutritional implications of dietary fiber. Am J Clin Nutr 31:(S)21, 1978.

ESHA Research: Sources of Vitamins and Minerals, Section D. Salem, OR, 1985.

Klurfeld, D. M.: The role of dietary fiber in gastrointestinal disease. J Am Diet Assoc 87:1172, 1987.

Lanza, E., and Butrum, R.: A critical review of food fiber analysis and data. J Am Diet Assoc 86:732, 1986.

Position of the American Dietetic Association: Health implications of dietary fiber. J Am Diet Assoc 88:216, 1988.

Position of the American Dietetic Association: Health implications of dietary fiber--technical support paper. J Am Diet Assoc 88:217, 1988.

Rydning, A., Aadland, E., Berstad, A., and Odegaard, H.: Prophylactic effect of dietary fibre in duodenal ulcer disease. Lancet 2:736, 1982.

Schneeman, B. O.: Dietary fiber: Comments on interpreting recent research. J Am Diet Assoc 87:1163, 1987.

Slavin, J. L.: Dietary fiber: Classification, chemical analyses, and food sources. J Am Diet Assoc 87:1164, 1987.

Watts, J. H., Graham, D. C. W., Jones, Jr., F., Adams, F. J., and Thompson, D. J.: Fecal solids excreted by young men following the ingestion of dairy foods. Am J Dig Dis 8:364, 1963.

BLAND DIET--ESOPHAGEAL REFLUX/HIATAL HERNIA

Jewett, T. C., and Siegel, M.: Hiatal hernia and gastroesophageal reflux. J Pediatr Gastroenterol Nutr 3:340, 1984.

Ulshen, M. H.: Treatment of gastroesophageal reflux: Is nothing sacred? J Pediatr 110:254, 1987.

BLAND DIET--PEPTIC ULCER

Borland, J. L.: Rational management of peptic ulcer disease. Hosp Pract 11:33, 1976.

Council on Foods and Nutrition, American Medical Association: Diet as Related to Gastrointestinal Function. Chicago: American Medical Association, 1984.

Eating and ulcers. Br Med J 280:205, 1980.

Isenberg, J. I.: Therapy of peptic ulcer. JAMA 233:540, 1975.

Richardson, C. T.: Pharmacotherapy: A perspective. South Med J 72:260, 1979.

Rydning, A., Aadland, E., Berstad, A., and Odegaard, B.: Prophylactic effect of dietary fibre in duodenal ulcer disease. Lancet 2:736, 1982.

Taylor, K. B.: Gastrointestinal disease and nutritional status. Compr Ther 12:45, 1979.

CLEAR LIQUID

Andersson, H., Bosaeus, I., Brummer, R., Fasth, S., Hulten, L., Magnusson, O., and Strauss, B.: Nutritional and metabolic consequences of extensive bowel resection. Dig Dis 4:193, 1986.

Fletcher, J. P., and Little, J. M.: High calorie and protein clear fluid regime for pre-operative bowel preparation. Aust N Z J Surg 56:693, 1986.

Hellberg, R., Hulten, L., and Bjorn-Rasmussen, E.: The nutritional and haematological status before and after subsequent resectional procedures for classical Crohn's disease and Crohn's colitis. Acta Chir Scand 148:453, 1982.

MacDonald, R. F., and Byrd, C. W.: Early postoperative oral feeding. Surg Gynecol & Obstet 25:510, 1960.

Stickler, G. B., and Simmons, P. S.: Rx: "Clear liquid diet"--clear to whom? [letter], Clin-Pediatr (Phila.) 25:114, 1986.

SECTION 2

LOW CALCIUM

Stewart, A. F.: Therapy of malignancy-associated hypercalcemia: 1983. Am J Med 74:475, 1983.

IRON

Arthur, C. K., and Isbister, J. P.: Iron deficiency, misunderstood and mistreated. Drugs 33:171, 1987.

Brittin, H. C., and Nossaman, C. E.: Iron content of food cooked in iron utensils. J Am Diet Assoc 86:897, 1986.

Burroughs, A. L., and Chan, J. J.: Iron content of some Mexican-American foods. J Am Diet Assoc 60:123, 1972.

Carmel, R., Weiner, J. M., and Johnson, C. S.: Iron deficiency occurs frequently in patients with pernicious anemia. JAMA 257:1081, 1987.

Clydesdale, F. M.: Physicochemical determinants of iron bioavailability. Food Technol 37:133, 1983.

Cook, J. D., and Monsen, E. R.: Food iron absorption in human subjects. III. Comparison of the effect of animal proteins on nonheme iron absorption. Am J Clin Nutr 29:859, 1976.

Cook, J. D., and Reusser, M. E.: Iron fortification: An update. Am J Clin Nutr 38:648, 1983.

Dallman, P. R., Yip, R., and Johnson, C.: Prevalence and causes of anemia in the United States, 1976 to 1980. Am J Clin Nutr 39:437, 1984.

Disler, P. B., Lynch, S. R., Charlton, R. W., Torrance, J. D., Bothwell, T. H., Walker, R. B., and Mayet, F.: The effect of tea on iron absorption. Gut 16:193, 1975.

Farley, M. A., Smith, P. D., Mahoney, A. W., West, D. W., and Post, J. R.: Adult dietary characteristics affecting iron intake: A comparison based on iron density. J Am Diet Assoc 87:174, 1987.

Hallberg, L., Brune, M., and Rossander, L.: Effects of ascorbic acid from different types of meals, studies with ascorbic acid rich food and synthetic ascorbic acid given in different amounts with different meals. Hum Nutr Appl Nutr 40A:97, 1986.

Layrisse, M., Martinez-Torres, C., and Gonzales, M.: Measurement of the total daily dietary iron absorption by the extrinsic tag model. Am J Clin Nutr 27:152, 1974.

Mertz, W.: Mineral elements: new perspectives. J Am Diet Assoc 77:258, 1980.

Monsen, E. R., and Balintfy, J. L.: Calculating iron bioavailability: Refinement and computerization. J Am Diet Assoc 80:307, 1982.

Monsen, E. R., Hallberg, L., Layrisse, M., Hegsted, D. M., Cook, J. D., Mertz, W., and Finch, C. A.: Estimation of available dietary iron. Am J Clin Nutr 31:134, 1978.

POTASSIUM CONTROLLED

Corrigan, S. A., and Langford, H. G.: Dietary management of hypertension. Compr Ther 13:62, 1987.

Langford, H. G.: Potassium in hypertension--the case for its role in pathogenesis and treatment. Postgrad Med 74:227, 1983.

SODIUM RESTRICTED

American College of Obstetricians and Gynecologists: Standards for ambulatory care. Washington, DC: American College of Obstetricians and Gynecologists, 1977.

BDA Renal Dialysis Group: Update paper: dietary treatment of chronic renal failure in adults. Hum Nutr Appl Nutr 38A:390, 1984.

Burton, B. T.: Nutritional implications of renal disease. J Am Diet Assoc 70:479, 1977.

Clinical nutrition cases: Cystinuria is reduced by low-sodium diets. Nutr Rev 45:79, 1987.

Connolly, G. N., Winn, D. M., Hecht, S. S., Henningfield, J. E., Walker, B., and Hoffman, D.: The re-emergence of smokeless tobacco. N Engl J Med 314:1020, 1986.

Corrigan, S. A., and Langford, H. G.: Dietary management of hypertension. Compr Ther 13:62, 1987.

Crocco, S. C.: The role of sodium in food processing. J Am Diet Assoc 80:36, 1982.

Department of Health and Human Services, Food and Drug Administration: Food labeling, declaration of sodium content of foods and label claims for foods on the basis of sodium content. Federal Register 49:15510, 1984.

Engstrom, A. M., and Tobelman, R. C.: Nutritional consequences of reducing sodium intake. Ann Intern Med 98:870, 1983.

Fagerberg, B., Anderson, O. K., Isaksson, B., and Bjorntorp, P.: Blood pressure control during weight reduction in obese hypertensive men: Separate effects of sodium and energy restriction. Br Med J 288:11, 1984.

Feldman, R. D., Lawton, W. J., and McArdle, W. L.: Low sodium diet corrects the defect in lymphocyte B-adrenergic responsiveness in hypertensive subjects. J Clin Invest 79:290, 1987.

Fleming, J. L., and Reed, J. S.: Ascites, a diagnostic and therapeutic approach. J Kans Med Soc 83:579, 1982.

Grobbee, D. E., and Hofman, A.: Does sodium restriction lower blood pressure? Br Med J 293:27, 1986.

Hunt, J. C.: Sodium intake and hypertension: A cause for concern. Am Intern Med 98:724, 1983.

Jackson, C. G., Glasscock, M. E., III, Davis, W. E., Hughes, G. B., and Sismanis, A.: Medical management of Meniere's disease. Ann Otol Rhinol Laryngol 90:142, 1981.

Jaeger, P., Portmann, L., Saunders, A., Rosenberg, L. E., and Thier, S. O.: Anticystinuric effects of glutamine and of dietary sodium restriction. N Engl J Med 315:1120, 1986.

Jefferson, J. W., and Greist, J. H.: Some hazards of lithium use. Am J Psychiatry 138:93, 1981.

Kaplan, N. M.: Nonpharmacologic therapy of hypertension. Med Clin North Am 71:921, 1987.

Karppanen, H., Tanskanen, A., Tuomilehto, J., Puska, P., Vuori, J., Jantti, V., and Seppanen, M.: Safety and effects of potassium- and magnesium-containing low sodium salt mixtures. J Cardiovasc Pharmacol 6:S236, 1984.

Klein, L. W., and Visocan, B. J.: The role of restriction of sodium intake in the treatment of heart failure in the elderly. J Am Geriatr Soc 32:353, 1984.

Kristinsson, A., Hardarson, T., Palsson, K., Petursson, M. G., Snorrason, S. P., and Thorgeirsson, G.: Additive effects of moderate dietary reduction and captopril in hypertension. Acta Med Scand 223:133, 1988.

Langford, H. G., Schlundt, D., Levine, K.: Sodium restriction in hypertension. Compr Ther 10:6, 1984.

MacGregor, G. A., Markandu, N. D., Best, F. E., Elder, D. M., Cam, J. M., Sagnella, G. A., and Squires, M.: Double-blind randomised crossover trial of moderate sodium restriction in essential hypertension. Lancet 1:351, 1982.

McLaughlin, B., and Kevany, J.: A pilot investigation into the effect of a short-term restriction in sodium intake on blood pressure, sodium chloride taste threshold and the problems associated with such a dietary restriction. I J Med Sc 152:399, 1983.

Marsh, A. C., Klippstein, R. N., and Kaplan, S. D.: The sodium content of your food. USDA Home and Garden Bulletin No. 233. Washington, DC, 1980.

Moss, S., Gordon, D., Forsling, M. L., Peart, W. S., James, V. H., and Roddis, S. A.: Water and electrolyte composition of urine and ileal fluid and its relationship to renin and aldosterone during dietary sodium deprivation in patients with ileostomies. Clin Sc 61:407, 1981.

Muldowney, F. P., Freaney, R., and Moloney, M. F.: Importance of dietary sodium in the hypercalciuria syndrome. Kidney Int 22:292, 1982.

Nugent, C. A., Carnahan, J. E., Sheehan, E. T., and Myers, C.: Salt restriction in hypertensive patients: comparison of advice, education, and group management. Arch Intern Med 144:1415, 1984.

Poindexter, S. M., Dear, W. E., and Dudrick, S. J.: Nutrition in congestive heart failure. Nutr Clin Prac 1:83, 1986.

Riccardella, D., and Dwyer, J.: Salt substitutes and medicinal potassium sources: Risks and benefits. J Am Diet Assoc 85:471, 1985.

Schroeder, K. L., and Chen, M. S.: Smokeless tobacco and blood pressure (correspondence). N Engl J Med 312:919, 1985.

Subcommittee on Nonpharmacological Therapy of the 1984 Joint National Committee on Detection, Evaluation, and Treatment of High Blood Pressure: Nonpharmacological approaches to the control of high blood pressure. Hypertension 8:444, 1986.

Tobin, J. R.: The treatment of congestive heart failure: Digitalis glycosides are still the primary mode of therapy. Arch Intern Med 138:453, 1978.

Varda, V. A., Bartak, B. R., and Slowie, L. A.: Nutritional therapy of patients receiving lithium carbonate. J Am Diet Assoc 74:149, 1979.

Wassertheil-Smoller, S., Langford, H. G., Blaufox, M. D., Oberman, A., Hawkins, M., Levine, B., Cameron, M., Babcock, C., Pressel, S., Caggiula, A., Cutter, G., Curb, D., and Wing, R.: Effective dietary intervention in hypertensives: Sodium restriction and weight reduction. J Am Diet Assoc 85:423, 1985.

Weinberger, M. H.: Dietary sodium and blood pressure. Hosp Pract 21:55, 1986.

SECTION 3

PROTEIN RESTRICTED AND RENAL

Acchiardo, S. R., Moore, L. W., and Cockrell, S.: Does low protein diet halt the progression of renal insufficiency? Clin Neph 25:289, 1986.

Alverstand, A., Ahlberg, M., Bergstrom, J.: Retardation of the progression of renal insufficiency in patients treated with low-protein diets. Kidney Int 24, Suppl. 16:S-268, 1983.

Attman, P. O., Bucht, H., Larsson, O., and Uddebom, G.: Protein-reduced diet in diabetic renal failure. Clin Nephrol 19:217, 1983.

Bannister, D. K., Acchiardo, S. R., Moore, L. W., and Kraus, Jr., A. P.: Nutritional effects of peritonitis in continuous ambulatory peritoneal dialysis (CAPD) patients. J Am Diet Assoc 87:53, 1987.

Barsotti, G., Guiducci, A., Ciardella, F., and Giovannetti, S.: Effects on renal function of a low-nitrogen diet supplemented with essential amino acids and ketoanalogues and of hemodialysis and free protein supply in patients with chronic renal failure. Nephron 27:112, 1981.

Barsotti, G., Morelli, E., Giannoni, A., Guiducci, A., Lupetti, S., and Giovannetti, S.: Restricted phosphorus and nitrogen intake to slow the progression of chronic renal failure: A controlled trial. Kidney Int Suppl 16, 16:S278, 1983.

BDA Renal Dialysis Group: Update paper: Dietary treatment of chronic renal failure in adults. Hum Nutr Appl Nutr 38A:390, 1984.

Beaudette, F., et al.: Nutritional aspects of chronic renal disease. Nutrition in Practice 1:5, 1982.

Berger, M.: Dietary management of children with uremia. J Am Diet Assoc 70:498, 1977.

Bergstrom, J.: Discovery and rediscovery of low protein diet. Clin Nephrol 21:29, 1984.

Berlyne, G. M.: Calcium carbonate treatment of uremic acidosis. Isr J Med Sci 7:1235, 1971.

Blackburn, S. L.: Dietary compliance of chronic hemodialysis patients. J Am Diet Assoc 70:31, 1977.

Blumenkrantz, M., et al.: Nutritional management of the adult patient undergoing peritoneal dialysis. J Am Diet Assoc 73:251, 1978.

Blumenkrantz, M., et al.: Protein losses during peritoneal dialysis. Kidney Int 19:593, 1981.

Bouma, S. F., and Dwyer, J. T.: Glucose absorption and weight change in 18 months of continuous ambulatory peritoneal dialysis. J Am Diet Assoc 84:194, 1984.

Brenner, B., Meyer, J. W., and Hostetter, T. H.: Dietary protein intake and the progressive nature of kidney disease: The role of hemodynamically mediated glomerular injury in the pathogenesis of progressive glomerular sclerosis in aging, renal ablation and intrinsic renal disease. N Engl J Med 307:652, 1982.

Bricker, N. S.: Sodium homeostasis in chronic renal disease. Kidney Int 21:886 1982.

Burton, B. T., and Hirschman, G. H.: Current concepts of nutritional therapy in chronic renal failure: An update. J Am Diet Assoc 82:359, 1983.

Butler, B.: Dietary phosphorus. J Neph Nurs 69, 1985.

Campbell, J., et al.: Chronic illness and its effect on dietary compliance. Nephrotic News 3:5, 1979.

Comty, C. M., and Collins, A. J.: Dialytic therapy in management of chronic renal failure. Med Clin North Am 68:399, 1984.

Davis, M., Comty, C., and Shapiro, F.: Dietary management of patients with diabetes treated by hemodialysis. J Am Diet Assoc 75:265, 1979.

Gardner, J.: "Hyperdietism"--its prevention, control, and relation to compliance in dialysis and transplant patients. Dialysis and Transplantation 10:57, 1981.

Giordana, C.: The place of dietetic treatment in chronic renal failure (concluding remarks). Contrib Nephrol 34:29, 1982.

Golper, T. A.: Therapy for uremic hyperlipidemia. Nephron 38:217, 1984.

Greenburger, N. J., Carley, J., Schenker, S., Bettinger, I., Stamnes, C., Beyer, P.: Effect of vegetable and animal protein diets in chronic hepatic encephalopathy. Dig Dis 22:845, 1977.

Grodstein, G. P., Blumenkrantz, M. J., Kopple, J. D., Moran, J. K., and Coburn, J. W.: Glucose absorption during continuous ambulatory peritoneal dialysis. Kidney Int 19:564, 1981.

Harvery, K. B., Blumenkrantz, M. J., Levine, S. E., and Blackburn, G. L.: Nutritional assessment and treatment of chronic renal failure. Am J Clin Nutr 33:1586, 1980.

Hegsted, D. M.: Minimum protein requirements of adults. Am J Clin Nutr 21:352, 1968.

Henry, R.: Nutrition assessment in renal disease: An overview. RD 1:5, 1981.

Hirsch, D. J.: The effect of protein intake on renal disease. The Renal Family 9:35, 1983.

Hirsch, D. J.: Limited-protein diet: a means of delaying the progression of chronic renal disease? Can Med Assoc J 132:913, 1985.

Ibels, L. S., Alfrey, A. C., Haut, L., and Huffer, W. E.: Preservation of function in experimental renal disease by dietary restriction of phosphate. N Engl J Med 298:122, 1978.

Kaysewn, G. A., Gambertoglio, J., Jimenez, I., Jones, H., and Hutchison, F. N.: Effect of dietary protein intake on albumin homeostasis in nepthrotic patients. Kidney Int 29:572, 1986.

Klahr, S., Buerkert, J., and Purkerson, M. L.: Role of dietary factors in the progression of chronic renal disease. Kidney Int 24:579, 1983.

Kluthe, R., Luttgen, F. M., Capetianu, T., Heinze, V., Katz, N., and Sudhoff, A.: Protein requirements in maintenance hemodialysis. Am J Clin Nutr 31:1812, 1978.

Kopple, J. D.: Nutritional management of chronic renal failure. Postgrad Med 64:135, 1978.

Kopple, J. D.: Nutritional therapy in kidney failure. Nutr Rev 39:193, 1981.

Levine, S. E.: Nutritional care of patients with renal failure and diabetes. J Am Diet Assoc 81:261, 1982.

Liddle, V., et al.: Diet in transplantation. Dialysis and Transplantation 6(5):9, 1977.

Lopes, G. S.: A dietary approach to chronic renal failure. Iss Compr Ped Nurs 6:23, 1983.

Makoff, D. L., Gordon, A., Franklin, S. S., Gerstein, A. R., Maxwell, M. H.: Chronic calcium carbonate therapy in uremia. Arch Intern Med 123:15, 1969.

Maschio, G., Oldrizzi, L., Tessitore, N., D'Angelo, A., Valvo, E., Lupo, A., Loschiavo, C., Fabris, A., Gammaro, L., Rugiu, C., and Panzella, G.: Effects of dietary protein and phosphorus restriction on the progression of early renal failure. Kidney Int 22:371, 1982.

Migone, L., Bono, F., and Zanelli, P.: The place of dietetic treatment in chronic renal failure (cons). Contrib Nephrol 34:8, 1982.

Miller, R., and Milton, S.: Compliance with renal diets: A review and analysis. Dialysis and Transplantation 9:968, 1980.

Mitch, W. E., and Sapir, D. G.: Evaluation of reduced dialysis frequency using nutritional therapy. Kidney Int 20:122, 1981.

Mitch, W. E., and Wilcox, C. S.: Disorders of body fluids, sodium and potassium in chronic renal failure. Am J Med 72:536, 1982.

Mitch, W. E., Walser, M., Steinman, T. I., Hill, S., Zeger, S., and Tungsange, K.: The effect of a keto acid-amino supplement to a restricted diet on the progression of chronic renal failure. N Engl J Med 311:623, 1984.

Morgan, M. Y.: Amino acids in hepatic failure. In Williams, R., ed.: Liver Failure. New York: Churchill Livingstone, 1986.

Norwood, K.: An expanded role for the dietitian in the treatment of renal osteodystrophy and secondary hyperparathyroidism. Contemporary Dialysis and Nephrology: August, 1987.

Oldrizzi, L., Rugiu, C., Valvo, E., Lup, A., Loschiavo, C., Gammaro, L., Tessitore, N., Fabris, A., Giovanni, P., and Maschio, G.: Progression of renal failure in patients with renal disease of diverse etiology on protein-restricted diet. Kidney Int 27:553, 1985.

Piper, C. M.: Very low protein diets in chronic renal failure: nutrient content and guidelines for supplementation. J Am Diet Assoc 85:1344, 1985.

Rampton, D. S., Cohen, S. L., Crammond, V. B., Gibbons, J., Lilburn, M. F., Rabet, J. Y., Vince, A. J., Wagner, J. D., and Wrong, O. M.: Treatment of chronic renal failure with dietary fiber. Clin Nephrol 21:159, 1984.

Rosman, J. B., Meijer, S., Sluiter, W. J., Wee, P. M., Peirs-Becht, T., and Donker, J. M.: Prospective randomised trial of early dietary protein restriction in chronic renal failure. Lancet 2:1291, 1984.

Shaw, S., Warner, T. M., and Liever, C. S.: Comparison of animal and vegetable protein sources in the dietary management of hepatic encephalopathy. Am J Clin Nutr, 38:59, 1983.

Slatopolsky, E., Weerts, C., Lopez-Hiker, S., Norwood, K., Zink, M., Windus, D., and Delmex, J.: Calcium carbonate as a phosphate binder in patients with chronic renal failure undergoing dialysis. N Engl J Med 315:157, 1986.

Spinozzi N. S., and Grupe, W. E.: Nutritional implications of renal disease. J Am Diet Assoc 70:493, 1977.

Tsaltas, T. T.: Dietetic management of uremic patients. I. Extraction of potassium from foods for uremic patients. Am J Clin Nutr 22:490, 1969.

Tsukamoto, Y., Okubo, M., Yoneda, T., Marumo, F., and Nakamure, H.: Effects of a polyunsaturated fatty acid-rich diet on serum lipids in patients with chronic renal failure. Nephron 31:236, 1982.

Walser, M.: Does diet therapy have a role in the predialysis patient? Am J Clin Nutr 33:1629, 1980.

Walser, M.: Nutrition in renal failure. Ann Rev Nutr 3:125, 1983.

Wineman, R. J., Sargent, J. A., and Piercy, L.: Nutritional implications of renal disease. J Am Diet Assoc 70:483, 1977.

SECTION 4

MODIFICATION OF FAT

Andersson, H.: Fat-reduced diet in the symptomatic treatment of patients with ileopathy. Nutr Metabol 17:102, 1974.

Andersson, H.: Low fat diet in the short-gut syndrome. Lancet 2:347, 1983.

Andersson, H., Bosaeus, I., Hellberg, R., and Hulten, L.: Effect of a low fat diet and antidiarrhoeal agents on bowel habits after excisional surgery for classical Crohn's disease. Acta Chir Scand 148:285, 1982.

Bach, A. C., and Babayan, V. K.: Medium chain triglycerides: An update. Am J Clin Nutr 36:950, 1982.

Bosaeus, I., Andersson, H., and Nystom, C.: Effect of a low fat diet on bile salt excretion and diarrhoea in the gastrointestinal radiation syndrome. Acta Radiol Oncol 18:460, 1979.

Hurley, R. S., and Mekhjian, H. S.: Dietary habits of patients with cholelithiasis: Do we need to instruct? J Am Diet Assoc 87:209, 1987.

Keith, R. G.: Effect of a low fat elemental diet on pancreatic secretion during pancreatitis. Surg Gynecol Obstet 151:337, 1980.

Robbins, C., and Walker, C.: Practical low-fat diets. Lancet I:505, 1982.

Simko, V., and Michael, S.: Rise in fecal fat not always steatorrhea. Gastroenterology 92:557, 1987.

LOW CHOLESTEROL

American Heart Association: Counseling Adolescents for Dietary Change. Dallas: American Heart Association Office of Communications, 1982.

American Heart Association: Counseling the Patient with Hyperlipidemia. Dallas: American Heart Association Office of Communications, 1984.

American Heart Association: Dietary Treatment of Hypercholesterolaemia: A Handbook for Counsellors. Dallas: American Heart Association, 1988.

American Heart Association: Eating for a Healthy Heart. Dallas: American Heart Association Office of Communications, 1984.

Castelli, W. P.: Epidemiology of coronary heart disease: The Framingham study. Am J Med 4:12, 1984.

Connor, S. L., Artaud-Wild, S. M., Classick-Kohn, C. J., Gustafson, J. R., Flavell, D. P., Hatcher, L. F., and Connor, W. E.: The cholesterol/saturated-fat index: an indication of the hypercholesterolaemic and atherogenic potential of food. Lancet 1:1229, 1986.

Connor, S. L., and Connor, W. E.: The New American Diet. New York: Simon & Schuster, 1986.

Connor, W. E., and Bristow, J. D. (eds): Coronary Heart Disease, Prevention, Complications, and Treatment. Philadelphia: Lippincott, 1985.

Connor, W. E.: Hypolipidemic effects of dietary omega-3 fatty acids in normal and hyperlipidemic humans: Effectiveness and mechanisms. In Simopoulos, A. P., ed.: Health Effects of Polyunsaturated Fatty Acids in Seafoods. NY: Academic Press, 1986.

Consensus Conference: Lowering blood cholesterol to prevent heart disease. JAMA 253:2080, 1985.

Ernst, N.D., Cleeman, J., Mullis, R., Sooter-Bochenek, J., Van Horn, L.: The National Cholesterol Education Program: Implications for Dietetic Practitioners from the Adult Treatment Panel Recommendations. J Am Diet Assoc 88:1401-11, 1988.

The Expert Panel, Goodman, D. C., chairman: Report of the National Cholesterol Program Expert Panel on Detection, Evaluation, and Treatment of High Blood Cholesterol in Adults. Arch Intern Med 148:36-69, 1988.

Goodnight, Jr., S. H., Harris, W. S., Connor, W. E., and Illingworth, D. R.: Polyunsaturated fatty acids, hyperlipidemia and thrombosis. Arteriosclerosis 2:87, 1982.

Grundy, S. M., Bilheimer, D., Blackburn, H., Brown, W. V., Kwiterovich, P. O., Mattson, F., Schonfeld, G., and Weidman, W. H.: Rationale of the diet-heart statement of the American Heart Association. Report of the Nutrition Committee. Circulation 65:839A, 1982.

Grundy, S. M.: Cholesterol and coronary heart disease: A new era. JAMA 256:2849, 1986.

Grundy, S. M.: Comparison of monounsaturated fatty acids and carbohydrates for lowering plasma cholesterol. N Engl J Med 314:745, 1986.

Hoeg, J. M., Gregg, R. E., and Brewer, H. B.: An approach to the management of hyperlipoproteinemia. JAMA 255:512, 1985.

Inter-society Commission for Heart Disease Resources: Optimal resources for primary prevention of atherosclerotic diseases. Circulation 70:153A, 1984.

Kuske, T. T., and Feldman, E. B.: Hyperlipoproteinemia, atherosclerosis risk, and dietary management. Arch Intern Med 147:357, 1987.

Lipid Research Clinics Program: The lipid research clinics coronary primary prevention trial results: I. The relationship of reduction in incidence of coronary heart disease to cholesterol lowering. JAMA 251(3):365-74 1984.

National Institutes of Health Consensus Conference: Lowering blood cholesterol to prevent heart disease. JAMA 253:2080, 1985.

National Institutes of Health: Treatment of hypertriglyceridemia. JAMA 251:1196, 1984.

Nutrition Coding Center: Elemental items: Food table information listing primary nutrients and food units. Minneapolis, MN, 1987.

Perry, R. S.: Therapy reviews: Contemporary recommendations for evaluating and treating hyperlipidemia. Clin Pharm 5:113, 1986.

Phillipson, B. E., Rothrock, D. W., Connor, W. E., Harris, W. S., and Illingworth, D. R.: Reduction of plasma lipids, lipoproteins, and apoproteins by dietary fish oils in patients with hypertriglyceridemia. N Engl J Med 312:1210, 1985.

Posner, B. M., DeRusso, P. A., Norquist, S. L., and Erick, M. A.: Preventive nutrition intervention in coronary heart disease: Risk assessment and formulating dietary goals. J Am Diet Assoc 86:1395, 1986.

Schaefer, E. J., and Levy, R. I.: Pathogenesis and management of lipoprotein disorders. N Engl J Med 312:1300, 1985.

U.S. Department of Health and Human Services: Heart to Heart. NIH Publication No. 83-1528, Washington, D.C.: Public Health Service National Institutes of Health, 1983.

MCT

Bach, A. C., and Babayan, V. K.: Medium-chain triglycerides: An update. Am J Clin Nutr 36:950, 1982.

Hermann-Zaidins, M. G.: Malabsorption in adults: Etiology, evaluation, and management. Continuing Education 86:1171, 1986.

SECTION 5

DIABETIC DIETS

American Diabetes Association: Glycemic effects of carbohydrates policy statement. Diabetes Care 7:607, 1984.

American Diabetes Association, Inc., and American Dietetic Association: The exchange lists for meal planning. Alexandria, VA, and Chicago, IL: American Diabetes Association and American Dietetic Association, 1986.

Anderson, J. W., Gustafson, N. J., Bryant, C. A., and Tietyen-Clark, J.: Dietary fiber and diabetes: A comprehensive review and practical application. J Am Diet Assoc 87:1189, 1987.

Arky, R., et al.: Examination of current dietary recommendations for individuals with diabetes mellitus. Diabetes Care 5:59, 1982.

Beebe, C. A.: Self blood glucose monitoring: An adjunct to dietary and insulin management of the patient with diabetes. J Am Diet Assoc 87:61, 1987.

Coulston, A. M., Hollenbeck, C. B., Swislocki, A. L. M., Chen, Y-D. I., and Reaven, G. M.: Deleterious metabolic effects of high-carbohydrate sucrose-containing diets in patients with non-insulin-dependent diabetes mellitus. Am J Med 82:213, 1987.

Crapo, P.: The nutritional therapy of non-insulin dependent (type II) diabetes. Diabetes Educator 9:13, 1983.

Crapo, P., and Vinik, A. I.: Nutrition controversies in diabetes management. J Am Diet Assoc 87:25, 1987.

Franz, M.: Glycemic effects of carbohydrates. Diabetes Educator 11:69, 1985.

Franz, M. J., Barr, P., Holler, H., Powers, M. A., Wheeler, M. L., and Wylie-Rosett, J.: Exchange lists: Revised 1986. J Am Diet Assoc 87:28, 1987.

Harold, M. R., Reeves, R. D., Bolze, M. S., Guthrie, R. A., and Guthrie, D. W.: Effect of dietary fiber in insulin-dependent diabetics: insulin requirements and serum lipids. J Am Diet Assoc 85:1455, 1985.

Hauenstein, D. J., Schiller, M. R., and Hurley, R. S.: Motivational techniques of dietitians counseling individuals with Type II diabetes. J Am Diet Assoc 87:37, 1987.

Horwitz, D. L.: Management of diabetes mellitus. Surv Ophthalmol 31:111, 1986.

Kabadi, U. M.: Nutritional therapy in diabetes: Rationale and recommendations. Postgrad Med 79:145, 1986.

McFarland, K. F., and Baker, C.: Diabetes management: An update. Am Fam Physician 34:143, 1986.

Nuttall, F. Q.: Diet and the diabetic patient. Diabetes Care 6:197, 1983.

Subcommittee on Nonpharmacological Therapy of the 1984 Joint National Committee on Detection, Evaluation, and Treatment of High Blood Pressure: Nonpharmacological approaches to the control of high blood pressure. Hypertension 8:444, 1986.

WEIGHT LOSS

Beaudette, T.: Obesity: Pathogenesis, Consequences and Treatment. Littleton, CO: Seminars in Nutrition, 1985.

Bennett, W., and Gurin, J.: Do diets really work? Science 82:42, 1982.

Brownell, K. D.: Obesity: Understanding and treating a serious, prevalent, and refractory disorder. J Consult Clin Psychol 50:820, 1982.

Callaway, C. W.: Weight standards: Their clinical significance. Ann Intern Med 100:296, 1984.

Edelman, B.: Developmental differences in the conceptualization of obesity. JAMA 80:122, 1982.

Hertzler, A. A.: Obesity--impact of the family. JAMA 79:525, 1981.

Mahalko, J. R., and Johnson, L. K.: Accuracy of predictions of long-term energy needs. J Am Diet Assoc 77:557, 1980.

Rock, C. L., and Coulston, A. M.: Weight control approaches: A review by the California Dietetic Association. J Am Diet Assoc 88:44, 1988.

Schulz, L. O.: Obese, overweight, desirable, ideal: Where to draw the line in 1986? JAMA 86:1702, 1986.

Steffee, W. P.: The medical syndrome of obesity. Prim Care 9:581, 1982.

Thompson, J. K., Jarvie, G. J., Lahey, B. B., and Cureton, K. J.: Exercise and obesity: Etiology, physiology, and intervention. Psychol Bull 91:55, 1982.

Weinsier, R. L., Wadden, T. A., Ritenbaugh, C., Harrison, G. G., Johnson, F. S., and Wilmore, J. H.: Recommended therapeutic guidelines for professional weight control programs. Am J Clin Nutr 40:865, 1984.

VBG

Bukoff, M., and Carlson, S.: Diet modifications and behavioral changes for bariatric gastric surgery. J Am Diet Assoc 78:158, 1981.

Bukoff Priddy, M. L.: Gastric reduction surgery: A dietitian's experience and perspective. J Am Diet Assoc 85:455, 1985.

Crowley, L. V., Seay, J., and Mullin, G.: Late effects of gastric bypass for obesity. Am J Gastroenterol 79:850, 1984.

Graney, A. S., Smith, L. B., and Hammer, K. A.: Gastric partitioning for morbid obesity: Postoperative weight loss, technical complications, and protein status. J Am Diet Assoc 86:630, 1986.

Raymond, J. L., Schipke, C. A., Becker, J. M., Lloyd, R. D., and Moody, F. G.: Changes in body composition and dietary intake after gastric partitioning for morbid obesity. Surgery 99:15, 1986.

POSTGASTRECTOMY

Bisballe, S., Buus, S., Lund, B., and Hessov, I.: Food intake and nutritional status after gastrectomy. Hum Nutr Appl Nutr 40:301, 1986.

Botta, D., Hugon, N., Excoffier, J. M., and Gauthier, A.: Post-operative nutrition in gastric surgery. In Luigi, G., Porro, G. B., Cheli, R., and Lipkin, M., eds.: Nutrition in Gastrointestinal Disease. New York: Raven Press, 1985.

Cristallo, M., Braga, M., Agape, D., Primignani, M., Zuliani, W., Vecchi, M., Murone, M., Sironi, M., Di Carlo, V., and De Franchis, R.: Nutritional status, function of the small intestine and jejunal morphology after total gastrectomy for carcinoma of the stomach. Surg Gynecol Obstet 163:225, 1986.

Floch, M. H.: Nutritional problems following gastric and small-bowel surgery. In Nutrition and Diet Therapy in Gastrointestinal Disease. New York: Plenum Medical Book Co., 1981.

Gudmand-Hoyer, E., and Jarnum, S.: Milk intolerance following gastric surgery. Scand J Gastroenterol 4:127, 1969.

Inoue, K., et al.: Release of cholecystokinin and gallbladder contraction before and after gastrectomy. Ann Surg 205:27, 1987.

Kozawa, K., Imawari, M., Shimazu, H., Kobori, O., Osuga, T., and Morioka, Y.: Vitamin D status after total gastrectomy. Dig Dis Sci 29:411, 1984.

Nishimura, O., Furumoto, T., Nosaka, K., Kouno, K., Sumikawa, M., Hisaki, T., Odachi, T., Mizumoto, K., Kishimoto, H., Yamamoto, K., and Koga, S.: Bone disorder following partial and total gastrectomy with reference to bone mineral content. Jpn J Surg 16:98, 1986.

Paakkonen, M., Alhova, E. M., and Karjalainen, P.: Bone mineral and intestinal calcium absorption after partial gastrectomy. Scand J Gastroenterol 17:369, 1982.

Raudin, I. S.: Symposium on fluid and electrolyte needs of surgical patients; hypoproteinemia and its relationship to surgical problems. Ann Surg 112:576, 1940.

HYPERINSULINISM

American Diabetes Association: Statement on hypoglycemia. Diabetes Care 5:72, 1982.

Bell, L. S., Tiglio, L. N., and Fairchild, M. M.: Dietary strategies in the treatment of reactive hypoglycemia. J Am Diet Assoc 85:1141, 1985.

Buss, R. W., Kansal, P. C., Roddam, R. F., Pino, J., and Boshell, B. R.: Mixed meal tolerance test and reactive hypoglycemia. Horm Metab Res 14:281, 1982.

Hogan, M. J., Service, F. J., Sharbrough, F. W., and Gerich, J. E.: Oral glucose tolerance test compared with a mixed meal in the diagnosis of reactive hypoglycemia: A caveat on stimulation. Mayo Clin Proc 58:491, 1983.

Sanders, L. R., Hofeldt, F. D., Kirk, M. C., and Levin, J.: Refined carbohydrate as a contributing factor in reactive hypoglycemia. South Med J 75:1072, 1982.

LACTOSE RESTRICTED

American Dietetic Association: Lactose Intolerance. Chicago: American Dietetic Association, 1985.

Bayless, T. M.: Disaccharidase deficiency. J Am Diet Assoc 60:478, 1972.

Fung, W., and Kho, K. M.: The importance of milk intolerance in patients presenting with chronic (nervous) diarrhoea. Aust NZ J Med 4:374, 1971.

In vivo digestion of yogurt lactose by yogurt lactase. Nutr Rev 42:216, 1984.

Katz, J., Spiro, H. M., and Herskovic, T.: Milk-precipitating substance in the stool in gastrointestinal milk sensitivity. N Engl J Med 278:1191, 1968.

Kolars, J. C., Levitt, M. D., Mostafi Aouji, D. A., and Savaiano, D. A.:Yogurt--an autodigesting source of lactose. N Engl J Med 310:1, 1984.

Newcomer, A. D., and McGill, D. B.: Clinical importance of lactase deficiency. N Engl J Med 310:42, 1984.

Newcomer, A. D., Park, H. S., O'Brien, P. C., and McGill, D. G.: Response of patients with irritable bowel syndrome and lactase deficiency using unfermented acidophilus milk. Am J Clin Nutr 38:257, 1983.

Paige, D. M., Bayless, T. M., Huang, S., and Wexler, R.: Lactose Intolerance and Lactose Hydrolyzed Milk. In James, A., and Hodge, J., eds.: Physiological Effects of Food Carbohydrates. Washington, DC: American Chemical Society 1975.

Payne, D. L., Welsh, J. D., Manion, C. V., Tsegaye, A., and Herd, L. D.: Effectiveness of milk products in dietary management of lactose malabsorption. Am J Clin Nutr 34:2711, 1981.

Savaiano, D. A., Abdiehak Abou El Anouar, D. A., Smith, D. E., and Levitt, M. D.: Lactose malabsorption from yogurt, sweet acidophilus milk, and cultured milk in lactase-deficient individuals. Am J Clin Nutr 40:1219, 1984.

Simoons, F. J., Johnson, J. D., and Kretchmer, N.: Perspective on milk-drinking and malabsorption of lactose. Pediatrics 59:98, 1977.

Stephenson, L. S, and Latham, M. C.: Lactose intolerance and milk consumption: The relation of tolerance to symptoms. Am J Clin Nutr 27:296, 1974.

Turner, S. J., Daly, T., Hourigan, J. A., Rand, A. G., and Thayer, W. R.: Utilization of a low-lactose milk. Am J Clin Nutr 29:739, 1976.

SECTION 6

ALLERGIES

American Academy of Allergy and Immunology, Committee on Adverse Reactions to Food and the National Institute of Allergy and Infectious Diseases: Adverse reactions to foods. HHS Publication 84:117, 1984.

Anderson, J. A.: Non-immunologically-mediated food sensitivity. Nutr Rev 42:109, 1984.

Bahna, S. L., and Heiner, D. C. (eds): Allergies to Milk. New York: Grune and Stratton, 1980.

Butkus, S. N., and Mahan, L. K.: Food allergies: Immunological reactions to food. J Am Diet Assoc 86:601, 1986.

Collins-Williams, C.: Clinical spectrum of adverse reactions to tartrazine. J Asthma 22:139, 1985.

Dahl, R.: Sodium salicylate and aspirin disease. Allergy 35:155, 1980.

Freedman, B. J.: Sulphur dioxide in foods and beverages: Its use as a preservative and its effect on asthma. Br J Dis Chest 74:128, 1980.

Fulton, L., and Davis, C.: Baking for People with Food Allergies. USDA Agriculture Handbook No. 147, Rev., Washington, DC, 1981.

Gibson, A., and Clancy, R.: Management of chronic idiopathic urticaria by the identification and exclusion of dietary factors. Clin Allergy 10:699, 1980.

Ibero, M., Eseverri, J. L., Barroso, C., and Botey, J.: Dyes, preservatives and salicylates in the induction of food intolerance and/or hypersensitivity in children. Allergol Immunopathol 10:263, 1982.

Jamieson, D. M., Guill, M. F., Wray, B. B., and May, J. R.: Metabisulfite sensitivity: case report and literature review. Ann Allergy 54:115, 1985.

Lessof, M. H.: Food intolerance. Proc Nutr Soc 44:121, 1985.

Lessof, M. H.: Food intolerance and allergy--a review. Q J Med 52:111, 1983.

Mathison, D. A., Stevenson, D. D., and Simon, R. A.: Precipitating factors in asthma: aspirin, sulfites, and other drugs and chemicals. Chest 87 (1 Suppl):505, 1985.

Noid, H. E., Schultze, T. W., and Winkelman, R. K.: Diet plan for patients with salicylate-induced urticaria. Arch Dertmatol 109:866, 1974.

Ortolani, C., Pastorello, E., Luraghi, M. T., Torre, F. D., Bellani, M., and Zanussi, C.: Diagnosis of intolerance to food additives. Ann Allergy 53:587, 1984.

Podell, R. N.: Unwrapping urticaria: The role of food additives. Postgrad Med 78:83, 1985.

Riggs, B. S., Harchelroad, F. P., and Poole, C.: Allergic reaction to sulfiting agents. Ann Emerg Med 15:129, 1986.

Rowe, A. H., and Rowe, A., Jr.: Food Allergy, Its Manifestations and Control and the Elimination Diets. Springfield, IL: Charles C. Thomas, 1972.

Settipane, G. A.: Adverse reaction to sulfites in drugs and foods. J Am Acad Dermatol 10:1077, 1984.

Stevenson, D. D., and Simon, R. A.: Sensitivity to ingested metabisulfites in asthmatic subjects. J Allerg Clin Immunol 68:26, 1981.

Sun, M.: Salad, house dressing, but hold the sulfites. Science 226:520, 1984.

Swain, A. R., Dutton, S. P., and Truswell, A. S.: Salicylates in foods. J Am Diet Assoc 85:950, 1985.

Taylor, S. I.: Food allergies and sensitivities. J Am Diet Assoc 86:599, 1985.

Zeiger, R. S., Heller, S., Mellon, M., O'Conner, R., and Hamburger, R. N.: Effectiveness of dietary manipulation in the prevention of food allergy in infants. J Allerg Clin Immunol 78:224, 1986.

GLUTEN RESTRICTED

Advisory Committee on Technology Innovation Board on Science and Technology for International Development: Amaranth, Modern Prospects for an Ancient Crop. Washington, DC: National Research Council, National Academy Press, 1984.

American Dietetic Association: Gluten Intolerance. Chicago: American Dietetic Association, 1985.

Auricchio, S., DeRitus, G., DeVincenzi, M., and Silano, V.: Toxicity mechanisms of wheat and other cereals in celiac disease and related enteropathies. J Pediatr Gastroenterol Nutr 4:923, 1985.

Becker, R., Wheeler, E. L., Lorenz, K., Stafford, A. E., Grosjean, O. K., Betschart, A. A., and Saunders, R. M.: A compositional study of amaranth grain. J Food Sci 46:1175, 1981.

Ciclitira, P. J., Ellis, H. J., Evans, D. J., and Lennox, E. S.: A radioimmunoassay for wheat gliadin to assess the suitability of gluten free foods for patients with coeliac disease. Clin Exp Immunol 59:703, 1985.

Colaco, B., Egan-Mitchell, F. M., Stevens, F. M., Fottrell, P. F., McCarthy, C. F., and McNicholl, B.: Compliance with gluten free diet in coeliac disease. Arch Dis Child 62:706, 1987.

Cornell, H. J., and Townley, R. R. W.: The toxicity of certain cereal proteins in coeliac disease. Gut 15:862, 1974.

McNicholl, B.: Coeliac disease: Ecology, life history and management. Hum Nutr Appl Nutr 40A, Suppl 1:55, 1986.

Sanchez-Marroquin, A., Domingo, M. V., Maya, S., and Saldana, C.: Amaranth flour blends and fractions for baking applications. J Food Sc 50:789, 1985.

Saunders, R. M., Research Leader, Cereals Research Unit, Western Regional Research Center, Albany, CA. Personal communication. 1989.

Saunders, R. M., and Becker, R.: Amaranthus: A potential food and feed resource. Adv Cereal Sci Tech 6:357, 1985.

Shiner, M.: Present trends in celiac disease. Postgrad Med 60:773, 1984.

LOW OXALATE, RESTRICTED ASCORBIC ACID

Briggs, M. H., Garcia-Webb, P., and Davies, P.: Urinary oxalate and vitamin C supplements. Lancet 2:201, 1973.

Brinkley, L., McGuire, J., Gregory, J., and Pak, C. Y.: Bioavailability of oxalate in foods. Urol 17:534, 1981.

Dobbins, J. W., Binder, H. J.: Importance of the colon in enteric hyperoxaluria. N Engl J Med 296:298, 1977.

Earnest, D. L., Williams, H. E., and Admirand, W. H.: A physicochemical basis for treatment of enteric hyperoxaluria. Trans Assoc Am Physicians 88:224, 1975.

Fassett, D. W.: Oxalates. In Committee on Food Protection, Food and Nutrition Board, National Research Council: Toxicants Occurring Naturally in Foods (2nd ed.). Washington, DC: National Research Council, 1973.

Finch, A. M., Kasidas, G. P., and Rose, G. A.: Urine composition in normal subjects after oral ingestion of oxalate-rich foods. Clin Sci 60:411, 1981.

Gelbart, D. R., Brewer, L. L., Fajardo, L. F., and Weinstein, A. B.: Oxalosis and chronic renal failure after intestinal bypass. Arch Intern Med 137:239, 1977.

Hodgkinson, A.: Comment: Is there a place for a low-oxalate diet? J Hum Nutr 35:136, 1981.

Hodgkinson, A.: Oxalic Acid in Biology and Medicine. New York: Academic Press, 1977.

Jaeger, P., Portmann, L., Jacquet, A., and Burchhardt, P.: Influence of the calcium content of the diet on incidence of mild hyperoxaluria in idiopathic renal stone formers. Am J Nephrol 5:40, 1985.

Kasidas, G. P., and Rose, G. A.: Oxalate content of some common foods: Determination by an enzymatic method. J Hum Nutr 34:255, 1980.

Kaul, S., and Verma, S. L.: Oxalate contents of foods commonly used in Kashmir. Ind J Med Res 55:274, 1967.

Marshall, R. W., Cochran, M., and Hodgkinson, A.: Relationship between calcium and oxalic acid intake in the diet and their excretion in the urine of normal and renal-stone-forming subjects. Clin Sci 43:91, 1972.

Pak, C. Y. C., Sakhaee, K., Crowther, C., and Brinkley, L.: Evidence justifying a high fluid intake in treatment of nephrolithiasis. Ann Intern Med 93:36, 1980.

Piepmeyer, J.: Planning diets controlled in oxalic acid content. J Am Diet Assoc 65:438, 1974.

Smith, L. H., Fromm, H., and Hofmann, A. F.: Acquired hyperoxaluria, nephrolithiasis, and intestinal disease. N Engl J Med 286:1371, 1972.

Stauffer, J. Q.: Hyperoxaluria and intestinal disease, the role of steatorrhea and dietary calcium in regulating intestinal oxalate absorption. Dig Dis 22:921, 1977.

LOW PURINE

Bollet, A. J.: Diagnostic and therapeutic aids in gout and hyperuricemia. Medical Times 109:23, 1981.

Emmerson, B. T.: Alteration of urate metabolism by weight reduction. Aust NZ J Med 3:410, 1973.

Khachadurian, A. K.: Hyperuricemia and gout: An update. Am Fam Physician 24:143, 1981.

Lieber, C. S., Jones, D. P., Losowsky, M. S., and Davidson, C. S.: Interrelation of uric acid and ethanol metabolism in man. J Clin Invest 41:1863, 1962.

Maclachlan, M. J., and Rodnan, G. P.: Effects of food, fast and alcohol on serum uric acid and acute attacks of gout. Am J Med 42:38, 1967.

Mikkelsen, W. M., and Robinson, W. D.: Physiologic and biochemical basis for the treatment of gout and hyperuricemia. Med Clin North Am 53:1331, 1969.

Pennington, J. A., and Church, H. N. (eds): Food Values of Portions Commonly Used (14th ed.). Philadelphia: Lippincott, 1985.

Rodnan, G. P., Robin, J. A., Tolchin, S. F., and Elion, G. B.: Allopurinol and gouty hyperuricemia, efficacy of a single daily dose. JAMA 231:1143, 1975.

Scott, J. T.: Food, drink, and gout. Br Med J 287:78, 1983.

Scott, J. T.: Long-term management of gout and hyperuricaemia. Br Med J 281:1164, 1980.

Turner, D.: Handbook of Diet Therapy (5th ed.). Chicago: University of Chicago Press, 1970.

Wyngaarden, J. B.: Metabolic defects of primary hyperuricemia and gout. Am J Med 56:651, 1974.

TYRAMINE RESTRICTED

McCabe, B. J.: Dietary tyramine and other pressor amines in MAOI regimens: A review. J Am Diet Assoc 86:1059, 1986.

Roberts, Robert: Pharmacology Department, University of Iowa Hospitals and Clinics, Iowa City, IA. Personal communication. 1986.

VEGETARIAN

Adams, C. F.: Nutritive Value of American Foods in Common Units. USDA Handbook 456. Washington, DC, 1975

Agricultural Research Service: Composition of Foods: Raw, Processed, Prepared. USDA Handbook 8, Sections 1-16. Washington, DC, 1976-1988.

American Dietetic Association: Position paper on the vegetarian approach to eating. J Am Diet Assoc 77:61, 1980.

Dwyer, J.: Health implications of vegetarian diets. Compr Ther 9:23, 1983.

Erhard, D.: Nutrition education for the "now" generation. J Nutr Ed 2:135, 1971.

ESHA Research: Sources of Vitamins and Minerals, Section D. Salem, OR, 1985.

Freeland-Graves, J. H., Ebangit, M. L., and Bodzy, P. W.: Zinc and copper content used in vegetarian diets. J Am Diet Assoc 77:648, 1980.

Harland, B. F., et al.: Calcium, phosphorus, iron, iodine, and zinc in the "total" diet. J Am Diet Assoc 77:16, 1980.

Hughes, J., and Sanders, T. A. B.: Riboflavin levels in the diet and breast milk of vegans and omnivores. Proc Nutr Soc 38:95A, 1979.

Immerman, A. M.: Vitamin B_{12} status on a vegetarian diet, a critical review. Wld Rev Nutr Diet 37:38, 1981.

King, J. C., Stein, T., and Doyle, M.: Effect of vegetarianism on the zinc status of pregnant women. Am J Clin Nutr 34:1049, 1981.

Krey, S. H.: Alternate dietary lifestyles. Prim Care 9:595, 1982.

Leveille, G. A., Zabik, M. E., and Morgan, K. J.: Nutrients in Foods. Cambridge, MA: The Nutrition Guild, 1983.

Levin, N., Rattan, J., and Gilat, T.: Mineral intake and blood levels in vegetarians. Isr J Med Sc 22:105, 1986.

Pennington, J. A. and Church, H. N. (eds): Food Values of Portions Commonly Used (14th ed.). Philadelphia: Lippincott, 1985.

Register, U. D., and Sonnenberg, L. M.: The vegetarian diet. J Am Diet Assoc 62:253, 1973.

Skipper, A.: Specialized formulas for enteral nutrition support. J Am Diet Assoc 86:654, 1986.

Trace Elements in Human and Animal Nutrition, Vol. 2. 5th ed. Edited by Walter Mertz. Orlando, FL: Academic Press, 1986.

Truesdell, D. D., Whitney, E. N., and Acosta, P. B.: Nutrients in vegetarian foods. J Am Diet Assoc 84:28, 1984.

SECTION 7

CHILDREN'S GENERAL DIET, ADVANCED BABY SOFT AND BABY SOFT DIETS, INFANT FORMULAS AND FEEDINGS

American Academy of Pediatrics: Pediatric Nutrition Handbook (2nd ed.). Elk Grove Village, IL: American Academy of Pediatrics, 1985.

Arnon, S. S., Midura, T. F., Damus, K., Thompson, B., Wood, R. M., and Chin, J.: Honey and other environmental risk factors for infant botulism. J Pediatrics 94:331, 1979.

Brady, M. S., Rickard, K. A., Fitzgerald, J. F., and Lemons, J. A.: Specialized formulas for infants with malabsorption or formula intolerance. J Am Diet Assoc 86:191, 1986.

Brady, M. S., Rickard, K. A., Fitzgerald, J. F., and Lemons, J. A.: Specialized formulas and feedings for infants with malabsorption or formula intolerances. J Am Diet Assoc 86:191, 1986.

Brown, K. H., and MacLean, W. C.: Nutritional management of acute diarrhea: An appraisal of the alternatives. Pediatrics 73:119, 1984.

Buissert, P. D.: Common manifestations of cow's milk allergy in children. Lancet 1:304, 1978.

Committee on Nutrition: The use of whole cow's milk in infancy. Pediatrics 72:253, 1983.

Fahey, P. J., Boltri, J. M., and Monk, J. S.: Key issues in nutrition from conception through infancy. Postgrad Med 81:301, 1987.

Fomon, S. J.: Bioavailability of supplemental iron in commercially prepared dry infant cereals. J Pediatr 110:660, 1987.

Fomon, S. J.: Infant Nutrition. Philadelphia: Saunders, 1974.

Fomon, S. J.: Reflections on infant feeding in the 1970's and 1980's. Am J Clin Nutr 46:171, 1987.

Fomon, S. J., Filer, L. J., Anderson, T. A., and Ziegler, E. E.: Recommendations for feeding normal infants. Pediatrics 63:52, 1979.

Georgieff, M. K., and Sasanow, S. R.: Nutritional assessment of the neonate. Clin Perinatal 13:73, 1986.

Greene, H. L., and Ghishan, F. K.: Excessive fluid intake as a cause of chronic diarrhea in young children. J Pediatr 102:836, 1983.

Kohler, J. A., and Rolles, C. J.: Cystic Fibrosis. J Clin Hosp Pharm 11:21, 1986.

Laing, S. C.: The nutrition management of children with cystic fibrosis. Hum Nutr Appl Nutr 40A:24, 1986.

Lo, C. W., and Walker, W. A.: Chronic protracted diarrhea of infancy: A nutritional disease. Pediatrics 77:786, 1983.

Parsons, H. G., and Beaudry, P.: Energy needs: Growth in children with cystic fibrosis. J Pediatr Gastroenterol Nutr 2:44, 1983.

Pipes, P. L.: Nutrition in Infancy and Childhood. St. Louis: Times Mirror/Mosby College Publishing, 1985.

Position of the American Dietetic Association: Promotion of breast feeding. J Am Diet Assoc 86:1580, 1986.

Position of The American Dietetic Association: Promotion of breast feeding: Technical support paper. J Am Diet Assoc 86:1581, 1986.

Satter, E. M.: Child of Mine--Feeding with Love and Good Sense. Palo Alto, CA: Bull Publishing Company, 1986.

Satter, E. M.: Childhood eating disorders. J Am Diet Assoc 86:357, 1986.

Satter, E. M.: The feeding relationship. J Am Diet Assoc 86:352, 1986.

Weidman, W., Kwiterovich, P., Jesse, M. J., and Nugent, E.: Diet in the healthy child. News from the American Heart Association 67:1411A, 1983.

WEIGHT CONTROL FOR CHILDREN

Frankle, R. T.: Obesity a family matter: Creating new behavior. J Am Diet Assoc 85:597, 1985.

Mellin, L. M., Slinkard, L. A., and Irwin, C. E.: Adolescent obesity intervention: Validation of the SHAPEDOWN program. J Am Diet Assoc 87:333, 1987.

Paige, D. M.: Obesity in childhood and adolescence, special problems in diagnosis and treatment. Postgrad Med 79:233, 1986.

Stark, O., and Lloyd, J. K.: Some aspects of obesity in childhood. Postgrad Med 62:87, 1986.

CONSTANT CARBOHYDRATE

Luther, T., Broubard, B., and Schreiner, B. J.: Dietary Management, Diabetes Mellitus in Children and Adolescents. Philadelphia: W.B. Saunders Co., 1987.

DISACCHARIDE RESTRICTED

Ament, M. E., Perera, D. R., and Ester, L. J.: Sucrase-isomaltose deficiency--a frequently misdiagnosed disease. J Pediatr 83:721, 1973.

Arnon, S. S., Midura, T. F., Damus, K., Thompson, B., Wood, R. M., and Chin, J.: Honey and other environmental risk factors for infant botulism. J Pediatrics 94:331, 1979.

Davidson, G. P.: Cow's milk protein intolerance: Diagnosis and management. Aust Fam Physician 15:204, 1986.

Fisher, S. E., Leone, G., and Kelly, R. H.: Chronic protracted diarrhea: Intolerance to dietary glucose polymers. Pediatrics 67:271, 1981.

Lifshitz, F.: Carbohydrate problems in pediatric gastroenterology. Clin Gastroenterol 6:415, 1977.

Lindquist, B., and Meeuwisse, G.: Diets in disaccharidase deficiency and defective monosaccharide absorption. J Am Diet Assoc 48:307, 1966.

GALACTOSE FREE

Elsas, L. J., and Acosta, P. B.: Nutrition support of inherited metabolic diseases. In Shils, M. E., and Young, V. R.: Modern Nutrition in Health and Disease. Philadelphia: Lea and Febiger, 1988.

Fanning, A. P.: Dietary treatment of galactosemia and other inherited disorders of carbohydrate metabolism. Top Clin Nutr 2:64, 1987

Fishler, K., Koch, R., Donnell, G. N., and Wenz, E.: Developmental aspects of galactosemia from infancy to childhood. Clin Pediatr 19:38, 1980.

Galactosemia health professional fact sheet. Bureau of Health Promotion and Disease Prevention. Michigan Department of Public Health.

Hansen, R. G.: Hereditary galactosemia. JAMA 208:2077, 1969.

Roberts, R. S., and Myer, B. A.: Living with Galactosemia: A Handbook for Families. Indianapolis, IN: Metabolism Clinic, Indiana University Foundation, 1983.

Segal, S.: Disorder of galactose metabolism. In Stanbury, J. B., Wyngaarden, J. B., Fredrickson, D. S., Goldstein, J. L., and Brown, M. S., eds.: The Metabolic Basis of Inherited Disease (5th ed.). New York: McGraw Hill, 1983.

Sinclair, L.: Metabolic Disease in Childhood. St. Louis: Blackwell-Mosby, 1979.

Wenz, E., and Michell, M.: Galactosemia. In Palmer, S., and Ekvall, S.: Pediatric Nutrition in Developmental Disorders. Springfield, IL: Thomas, 1978.

PHENYLKETONURIA

Acosta, P. B., and Wenz, E.: Diet Management of PKU for Infants and Preschool Children. DHHS Publication No. (HSA) 78-5209. Rockville, MD: Public Health Service, Bureau of Community Services, 1978.

Bickel, H.: Phenylketonuria: Past, present, future. J Inherited Metab Dis 3:123, 1980.

Ernest, A. E., McCabe, E., Neifert, M. R., and O'Flynn, M. E.: Guide to Breastfeeding the Infant with PKU. DHHS Publication No. (HSA) 79-5110. Rockville, MD: Public Health Service, Bureau of Community Services, 1979.

Hunt, M. M., Berry, H. K., and White, P. P.: Phenylketonuria, adolescence, and diet. J Am Diet Assoc 85:1328, 1985.

Koch, R., Wenz, E., Steinberg, M. S., Fishler, K., and Acosta, P. B.: A Guide to Dietary Management. Evansville, IN: Mead Johnson Nutritional Division, 1981.

Lenke, R. R., and Levy, H. L.: Maternal phenylketonuria and hyperphenylalaninemia: An international survey of the outcome of untreated and treated pregnancies. N Engl J Med 303:1202, 1980.

O'Flynn, M. E., Holtzman, N. A., Blaskovics, M., Azen, C., and Williamson, M. L.: The diagnosis of phenylketonuria. Am J Dis Child 134:769, 1980.

Ross Metabolic Formula System. Columbus, OH: Ross Laboratories, 1987.

Schuett, V. E.: Low Protein Food List for Phenylketonuria and Metabolic Diseases Requiring a Low Protein Diet. Madison, WI: University of Wisconsin Press, 1981.

Schuett, V. E., Brown, E. S., and Michals, K.: Reinstitution of diet therapy in PKU patients from twenty-two U.S. clinics. Am J Public Health 75:39, 1985.

Tourian, A., Sidbury, J. B.: Phenylketonuria and hyperphenylalaninemia. *In* Stanbury, J. B., Wyngaarden, J. B., Frederickson, D. S., Goldstein, J. L., and Brown, M. S., eds.: The Metabolic Basis of Inherited Disease (5th ed.). New York: McGraw Hill, 1983.

SECTION 8

GLUCOSE TOLERANCE TEST

Anderson, J. W., and Herman, R. H.: Effects of carbohydrate restriction on glucose tolerance of normal men and reactive hypoglycemic patients. Am J Clin Nutr 28:748, 1975.

Anderson, J. W., Herman, R. H., and Zakim, D.: Effect of high glucose and high sucrose diets on glucose tolerance of normal men. Am J Clin Nutr 26:600, 1973.

Himsworth, H. P.: The dietetic factor determining the glucose tolerance and sensitivity to insulin of healthy men. Clin Sci 2:67, 1935.

Owens, D. R., Wragg, K. G., Briggs, P. I., Luzio, S., Kimber, G., and Davies, C.: Comparison of the metabolic response to a glucose tolerance test and a standardized test meal and the response to serial test meals in normal healthy subjects. Diabetes Care 2:409, 1979.

Wilkerson, H. L. C., Hyman, H., Kaufman, M., McCuistion, A. C., and Francis, J. O'S.: Diagnostic evaluation of oral glucose tolerance tests in non-diabetic subjects after various levels of carbohydrate intake. N Engl J Med 262:1047, 1960.

FATS

Bentley, S. J., Eastham, R. D., and Lane, R. F.: Oral butter fat test meal with serum nephelometry in suspected fat malabsorption. J Clin Pathol 28:80, 1975.

Chaun, H., Mullinger, M. A., Solvonuk, P., Ediss, I., and Bogoch, A.: The butterfat absorption test in adults. Dig Dis 20:914, 1975.

Gardner, F. H., and Santiago, E. P.: Oral absorption tolerance tests in tropical sprue. Arch Int Med 98:467, 1956.

Goldbloom, R. B., Blake, R. M., and Cameron, D.: Assessment of three methods for measuring intestinal fat absorption in infants and children. Pediatrics 34:814, 1964.

Hashim, S. A., and Babayan, V. K.: Studies in man of partially absorbed dietary fats. Am J Clin Nutr 31:S273, 1978.

Hodgson, J. R.: The technical aspects of cholecystography. Radiol Clin North Am 8:85, 1970.

Laufer, I., and Gledhill, L.: The value of the fatty meal in oral cholecystography. Radiology 114:525, 1975.

Luey, K., Pattinson, N. R., Hinton, D., Cook, H. B., and Campbell, C. B.: Comparison of three methods to estimate steatorrhoea. NZ Med J 93:36, 1981.

Osmon, K. L., Zinn, W. J., and Wharton, G. K.: Simplified test of fat absorption, JAMA 164:633, 1957.

Steen, G., and Holthuis, N.: The fat meal test of malabsorption: Some further experience. Clinica Chimica Acta 162:291, 1987.

West, P. S., Levin, G. E., Griffin, G. E., and Maxwell, J. D.: Comparison of simple screening tests for fat malabsorption. Br Med J 282:1501, 1981.

FAT-FREE TEST MEAL

Parkin, G. J. S.: Dietary preparation for oral cholecystography--a critical reappraisal. Br J Radiol 47:452.

Saxton, H. M., and Strickland, B.: Practical Procedures in Diagnostic Radiology. London: H.K. Lewis, 1972.

5-HYDROXYINDOLE-ACETIC ACID TEST

The American Dietetic Association: Manual of Clinical Dietetics. Chicago: The American Dietetic Association, 1988.

The American Dietetic Association: Handbook of Clinical Dietetics. New Haven and London: Yale University Press, 1981.

Anderson, J. A., Ziegler, M. R., and Doeden, D.: Banana feeding and urinary excretion of 5-Hydroxyindoleacetic acid. Science 127:236, 1958.

Bruce, D. W.: Carcinoid tumours and pineapples. J Pharm Pharmacol 13:256, 1961.

Cardon, P. V., and Guggenheim, F. G.: Effects of large variations in diet on free catecholamines and their metabolites in urine. J Psychiat Res 7:263, 1970.

Crout, J. R., and Sjoerdsma, A.: The clinical and laboratory significance of serotonin and catecholamines in bananas. N Engl J Med 261:23, 1959.

Deanovic, Z., Iskric, S., and Dupelj, M.: Fluctuation of 5-Hydroxy-indole compounds in the urine of migrainous patients. Biomedicine 23:346, 1975.

Feldman, J. M., Lee, E. M., and Castleberry, C. A.: Catecholamine and serotonin content of

282

foods, effect on urinary excretion of homovanillic and 5-hydroxyindoleacetic acid. J Am Diet Assoc 87:1031, 1987.

Lovenberg, W.: Some vaso- and psychoactive substances in foods: Amines, stimulants, depressants, and hallucinogens. *In* Committee on Food Protection, Food and Nutrition Board, National Research Council: Toxicants Occurring Naturally in Foods (2nd ed.). Washington, DC: National Research Council, National Academy of Sciences, 1973.

Oates, J. A., and Butler, T. C.: Pharmacologic and endocrine aspects of carcinoid syndrome. *In* Garattini, S., and Shore, P. A., eds.: Advances in Pharmacology. New York and London. Academic Press, 1967.

Shaw, K. N. F., and Trevarthen, J.: Exogenous sources of urinary phenol and indole acids. Nature 182:797, 1958.

Shihabi, Z. K., and Scaro, J.: Liquid-chromatographic assay of urinary 5-hydroxy-3-indoleacetic acid, with electrochemical detection. Clin Chem 26:907, 1980.

Udenfriend, S., Lovenberg, W., and Sjoerdsma, A.: Physiologically active amines in common fruits and vegetables. Arch Biochem Biophy 85:487, 1959.

Waalkes, T. P., Sjoerdsma, A., Creveling, C. R., Weissbach, H., and Udenfriend, S.: Serotonin, norephinephrine, and related compounds in bananas. Science 127:648, 1958.

West, G. B.: Trytamines in edible fruits. J Pharm Pharmacol 10:589, 1958.

Yamaguchi, Y., and Hayashi, C.: Simple determination of high urinary excretion of 5-hydroxyindole-3-acetic acid with ferric chloride. Clin Chem 24:149, 1978.

VANILLYLMANDELIC ACID TEST

American Dietetic Association: Handbook of Clinical Dietetics. New Haven and London: Yale University Press, 1981.

Amery, A., and Conway, J.: A critical review of diagnostic tests for pheochromocytoma. Am Heart J 73:129, 1967.

Anderson, J. A., Ziegler, M. R., and Doeden, D.: Banana feeding and urinary excretion of 5-hydroxy-indoleacetic acid. Science 127:236, 1958.

Cardon, P. V., and Guggenheim, F. G.: Effects of large variations in diet on free catecholamines and their metabolites in urine. J Psychiat Res 7:263, 1970.

Feldman, J. M., Lee, E. M., and Castleberry, C. A.: Catacholamine and serotonin content of foods: Effect on urinary excretion of homovanillic and 5-hydroxyindoleacetic acid. J Am Diet Assoc 87:1031, 1987.

National Institutes of Health Clinical Staff: Pheochromocytoma: Current concepts of diagnosis and treatment. Ann Intern Med 65:1302, 1966.

Page, L. B., and Copeland, R. B.: Pheochromocytoma. Disease a Month 1:1, 1968.

Pisano, J. J., Crout, J. R., and Abraham, D.: Determination of 3-methoxy-4-hydroxymandelic acid in urine. Clin Chim Acta 7:285, 1962.

Rayfield, E. J., Caine, J. P., Casey, M. P., Williams, G. H., and Sullivan, J. M.: Influence of diet on urinary VMA excretion. JAMA 221:704, 1972.

Remine, W. H., Chong, G. C., Van Heerden, J. A., Sheps, S. G., and Harrison, E. G.: Current management of pheochromocytoma. Ann Surg 179:740, 1974.

Shaw, K. N., and Trevarthen, J.: Exogenous sources of urinary phenol and indole acids. Nature 182:797, 1958.

Smith, P.: Significance of urinary vanillic acid. Nature 182:1741, 1958.

Sjoerdsma, A., Engelman, K., Waldmann, T. A., Cooperman, L. H., and Hammond, W. G.: Pheochromocytoma: Current concepts of diagnosis and treatment. Ann Intern Med 65:1302, 1966.

Udenfriend, S., Lovenberg, W., and Sjoerdsma, A.: Physiologically active amines in common fruits and vegetables. Arch Biochem Biophys 85:487, 1959.

Weise, V. K., McDonald, R. K., Labrosse, E. H.: Determination of urinary 3-methoxy-4-hydroxymandelic acid in man. Clin Chim Acta 6:79, 1961.

Young, R. B., Steiker, D. D., Bongiovanni, A. M., Koop, C. E., and Eberlein, W. R.: Urinary vanilmandelic acid (VMA) excretion in children: use of simple semiquantitative test. J Pediatr 62:844, 1963.

PRIMARY ALDOSTERONISM TEST

Conn, J. W.: Primary aldosteronism and primary reninism. Hosp Pract 9:131, 1974.

Lauler, D. P.: Preoperative diagnosis of primary aldosteronism. Am J Med 41:855, 1966.

Espiner, E. A., and Donald, R. A.: Aldosterone regulation in primary aldosteronism: Influence of salt balance, posture and ACTH. Clin Endocrinol 12:277, 1980.

Robertson, J. I.: The Franz Gross Memorial Lecture. The renin-aldosterone connection: Past, present and future. J Hypertens Suppl. 1984.

SECTIONS 9 AND 10

NUTRITIONAL ASSESSMENT, CRITICAL
CARE NUTRITION, AND ENTERAL
FORMULAS AND SUPPLEMENTS

Adler, W.: Immune status and aging. *In* Calvert, S., et al., eds.: Assessing the Nutritional Status of the Elderly--State of the Art. Columbus, OH: Ross Laboratories, 1982.

American Dietetic Association: Handbook of Clinical Dietetics. New Haven, CT: Yale University Press, 1981.

A.S.P.E.N. Board of Directors: Guidelines for use of total parenteral nutrition in the hospitalized adult patient. JPEN 10:441, 1976.

Baker, J. P., and Detsky, A. S., et al.: Nutritional assessment: A comparison of clinical judgement and objective measurements. N Engl J Med 306:969, 1982.

Bell, S. J., Bistrian, B. R., Wade, J. E., and Blackburn, G. L.: Modular enteral diets: cost and nutritional value comparisons. J Am Diet Assoc 87:1526, 1987.

Blackburn, G. L., Bistrian, B., Maini, B., Schlamm, H. T., and Smith, M. F.: Nutritional and metabolic assessment of the hospitalized patient. JPEN 1:111, 1977.

Cerra, F., Shronts, E., Olson, G., et al.: Practical aspects of metabolic and nutritional assessment. Am Soc Parenteral Enteral Nutr Update 4:1-3, 1982.

Chernoff, R.: Nutritional support: Formulas and delivery of enteral feeding: II. Delivery systems. J Am Diet Assoc 79:430, 1981.

Del Rio, D., Williams, K., and Esvelt, B.: Handbook of Enteral Nutrition. El Segundo, CA: Medical Specifics Publishing, 1982.

Dickerson, R. N.: Clinical utility of intravenous lipid emulsion. Hosp Pharm 21:564, 1986.

Dietary Department, The University of Iowa Hospitals and Clinics: Enteral Nutrition Handbook. Iowa City: University of Iowa Hospitals and Clinics, 1989.

Dudrick, S., Jensen, T., Englert, A., et al.: Interpretation of nutritional assessment data, Nutr Support Serv 1:14, 1981.

Frank, H., and Green, L. C.: Successful use of a bulk laxative to control the diarrhea of tube feeding. Scand J Plast Reconstr Surg 13:193, 1979.

Grant, A.: Nutritional Assessment Guidelines. Berkeley, CA: Cutter Laboratories, Inc., 1979.

Grills, N., and Bosscher, M. (eds.): Manual of Nutrition and Diet Therapy. New York: Macmillan, 1981.

Harris, J. A., and Benedict, F. G.: A Biometric Study of Basal Metabolism in Man. Washington, DC: Carnegie Institution of Washington, 1919.

Hermann-Zaidins, M. G.: Malabsorption in adults: Etiology, evaluation, and management. J Am Diet Assoc 86:1171, 1986.

Jensen, T. G.: Home enteral nutrition. Dietetic Currents 9:15, 1982.

Logan, R. F. A., Gillon, J., Ferrington, C., and Ferguson, A.: Reduction of gastrointestinal protein loss by elemental diet in Crohn's disease of the small bowel. Gut 22:383, 1981.

Moss, G.: Malabsorption associated with extreme malnutrition: Importance of replacing plasma albumin. J Am Coll Nutr 1:89, 1982.

Mullen, J. L., et al.: Prediction of operative morbidity and mortality by preoperative nutritional assessment. Surg Forum 30:80, 1979.

Pathology Laboratory Services Handbook. Iowa City: The University of Iowa Hospitals and Clinics, 1986.

Roe, D.: Geriatric Nutrition. Englewood Cliffs, NJ: Prentice-Hall, 1983.

Roesner, M., and Grant, J. P.: Intravenous lipid emulsions. Nutr Clin Prac 2:96, 1987.

Segar, W. E.: Parenteral fluid therapy. Curr Probl Pediatr 3:3-40, 1972.

Solomons, N. W., and Allen, L. H.: The functional assessment of nutritional status: Principles, practice and potential. Nutr Rev 41:33, 1983.

NUTRITION MANAGEMENT OF BURN
PATIENTS

Bell, S. J., Molnar, J. A., Krasker, W. S., and Burke, J. F.: Weight maintenance in pediatric burned patients. J Am Diet Assoc 86:207, 1986.

Bell, S. J., and Wyatt, J.: Nutrition guidelines for burned patients. J Am Diet Assoc 86:648, 1986.

Burdge, J. J., Conkright, J. M., and Ruberg, R. L.: Nutritional and metabolic consequences of thermal injury. Clin Plast Surg 13:49, 1986.

Curreri, P. W., Richmond, D., Marin, J., and Baxter, C. S.: Dietary requirements of patients with major burns. J Am Diet Assoc 65:415, 1974.

Ireton, C. S., Turner, Jr., W. W., Hunt, J. L., and Liepa, G. U.: Evaluation of energy expenditures in burn patients. J Am Diet Assoc 86:331, 1986.

Turner, W. W., Ireton, C. S., Hunt, J. L., and Baxter C. R.: Predicting energy expenditures in burned patients. J Trauma 25:11, 1985.

Wilmore, D. W.: Nutrition and metabolism following thermal injury. Clin Plast Surg 1:603, 1974.

Wilmore, D. W., and Aulick, L. H.: Metabolic changes in burned patients. Surg Clin North Am 58:1173, 1978.

Wilmore, D. W., Curreri, P. W., Spitzer, K. W., Spitzer, M. E., and Pruitt, B. A.: Supranormal dietary intake in thermally injured hypermetabolic patients. Surg Gynecol Obstet 132:881, 1971.

NUTRITION AND CANCER

Arnold, C.: Nutrition intervention in the terminally ill cancer patient. J Am Diet Assoc 86:522, 1986.

Bell, S. J., Coffey, L. M., and Blackburn, G. L.: Use of total parenteral nutrition in cancer patients. Top Clin Nutr 1:37, 1986.

Carter, P., Carr, D., van Eys, J., Ranirez, I., Coody, D., and Taylor, G.: Energy and nutrient intake of children with cancer. J Am Diet Assoc 82:610, 1983.

Carter, P., Carr, D., van Eys, J., and Coody, D.: Nutritional parameters in children with cancer. J Am Diet Assoc 82:616, 1983.

Enig, B., Winther, E., and Hessov, I.: Energy and protein intake and nutritional status in non-surgically treated patients with small cell anaplastic carcinoma of the lung. Acta Radio Oncol 25:19, 1986.

Flombaum, C., Isaacs, M., Scheiner, E., and Vanamee, P.: Management of fluid retention in patients with advanced cancer. JAMA 245:611, 1981.

Hearne, B. E., Dunaj, J. M., Daly, J. M., Strong, E. W., Bhadrasain, V., LePorte, B. J., and DeCosse, J. J.: Enteral nutrition support in head and neck cancer: Tube vs. oral feeding during radiation therapy. J Am Diet Assoc 85:669, 1985.

Moloney, M., Moriarty, M., and Daly, L.: Controlled studies of nutritional intake in patients with malignant disease undergoing treatment. Hum Nutr Appl Nutr 37A:30, 1983.

Ross Laboratories: Dietary Modifications in Disease. Cancer. Columbus, OH: Ross Laboratories, 1983.

Walsh, T. D., Bowman, K. B., and Jackson, G. P.: Dietary intake of advanced cancer patients. Hum Nutr Appl Nutr 37A:41, 1983.

ANOREXIA NERVOSA, BULIMIA

Andersen, A. E.: Anorexia nervosa and bulimia: Diagnosis and comprehensive treatment. Comp Ther 9:9, 1983.

Boskind-White, M., and White, W. C.: "Bulimarexia": The Binge/Purge Cycle. New York: Norton, 1983.

Dally, P.: Anorexia nervosa. Br J Clin Pract 26:509, 1972.

Drossman, D. A., Ontjes, D. A., and Heizer, W. D.: Anorexia nervosa. Gastroenterol 77:1115, 1979.

Garfinkel, P. E., and Garner, D. M.: Anorexia Nervosa, a Multidimensional Perspective. New York: Brunner/Mazel, 1982.

Halmi, K. A., Brodland, G., and Loney, J.: Prognosis in anorexia nervosa. Ann Int Med 78:907, 1973.

Halmi, K. A., Powers, P., and Cunningham, S.: Treatment of anorexia nervosa with behavior modification. Arch Gen Psychiatry 32:93, 1975.

Herzog, D. B., and Copeland, P. M.: Eating disorders. N Engl J Med 313:295, 1985.

Huse, D. M., and Lucas, A. R.: Dietary patterns in anorexia nervosa. Am J Clin Nutr 40:251, 1984.

Kirkley, B. G.: Bulimia: Clinical characteristics, development, and etiology. J Am Diet Assoc 86:468, 1986.

Omizo, S. A., and Oda, E.: Anorexia nervosa: Psychological considerations for nutrition counseling. J Am Diet Assoc 88:49, 1988.

Position of the American Dietetic Association: Nutrition intervention in the treatment of anorexia nervosa and bulimia nervosa. J Am Diet Assoc 88:68, 1988.

Ross Laboratories: Report of the Fourth Ross Conference on Medical Research, Understanding Anorexia Nervosa and Bulimia. Columbus, OH: Ross Laboratories, 1983.

Schwabe, A. D., et al.: Anorexia nervosa. Ann Intern Med 94:371, 1981.

Silverman, J. A.: Anorexia nervosa: Clinical observations in a successful treatment plan. J Pediatr 84:68, 1974.

Squire, S.: The Slender Balance: Causes and Cures for Bulimia, Anorexia and the Weight-Loss/Weight-Gain Seesaw. New York: Putnam Publishing Group, 1983.

Wells, S., Wells, J. E., McKenzie, J. M., and Hornblow, A. R.: Eating and weight problems among women attending their general practitioner. NZ Med J 99:671, 1986.

Wilson, C. P., and Mintz, I.: Abstaining and bulimic anorexics, two sides of the same coin. Prim Care 9:517, 1982.

SPORTS NUTRITION

Brotherhood, J. R.: Nutrition and sports performance. Sports Med 1:350, 1984.

Buskirk, E. R.: Some nutritional considerations in the conditioning of athletes. Ann Rev Nutr 1:319, 1981.

Clement, D. B., and Sawchuk, L. L.: Iron status and sports performance. Sports Med 1:65, 1984.

Costill, D. L.: Carbohydrate nutrition before, during and after exercise. Fed Proc 44:364, 1985.

Costill, D. L., and Saltin, B.: Factors limiting gastric emptying during rest and exercise. J Appl Physiol 37:679, 1974.

Costill, D. L.: Sports nutrition: The role of carbohydrates. Nutrition News 41:1, 1978.

Ehn, L., Carlmark, B., and Hoglund, S.: Iron status in athletes involved in intense physical activity. Med Sci Sports Exerc 12:61, 1980.

Foster, C., Costill, D. L., and Fink, W. J.: Effects of pre-exercise feedings on endurance performance. Med Sci Sports Exerc 11:1, 1979.

Fox, E. L., and Matthew, D. K.: The Physiological Basis of Physical Education and Athletics. Philadelphia: Saunders, 1981.

Getchell, B.: Being Fit. New York: Wiley, 1982.

Jackson, A. S., and Pollock, M. L.: Generalized equations for predicting body density in men. Br J Nutr 40:497, 1978.

Jackson, A. S., Pollock, M. L., and Ward, A.: Generalized equations for predicting body density in women. Med Sci Sports Exerc 12:175, 1980.

Katch, F. I., Katch, V. L., and McArdle, W. D.: Exercise Physiology: Energy, Nutrition, and Human Performance. Philadelphia: Lea and Febiger, 1981.

Katch, F. I., and McArdle, W. D.: Nutrition, Weight Control, and Exercise (2nd ed.). Philadelphia: Lea and Febiger, 1983.

Lemon, P. W., Yarasheski, K. E., and Dolny, D. G.: The importance of protein for athletes. Sports Med 1:474, 1984.

McCutcheon, M. L.: The athlete's diet: A current view. J Fam Prac 16(3):529, 1983.

Nelson, R. A.: Nutrition and physical performance. Physic Sports Med 10:55, 1982.

Nutrition and physical fitness: A statement by the American Dietetic Association. J Am Diet Assoc 76:437, 1980.

O'Neil, F. T., Hynak-Hankinson, M. T., and Gorman, J.: Research and application of current topics in sports nutrition. J Am Diet Assoc 86:1007, 1986.

Parizkova, J.: Total body fat and skinfold thickness in children. Metabolism 10:794, 1961.

Position of the American Dietetic Association: Nutrition for physical fitness and athletic performance for adults. J Am Diet Assoc 87:933, 1987.

Position paper: Nutrition for physical fitness and athletic performance for adults: Technical support paper. J Am Diet Assoc 87:934, 1987.

Sherman, W. M., and Costill, D. L.: The marathon: Dietary manipulation to optimize performance. Am J Sports Med 12:44, 1984.

Sherman, W. M., Costill, D. L., Fink, W. J., and Miller, J. M.: Effect of exercise-diet manipulation on muscle glycogen and its subsequent utilization during performance. Int J Sports Med 2:114, 1981.

APPENDIXES

Appendix C

Brunnstrom, S.: Clinical Kinesiology. Philadelphia: F. A. Davis, 1981.

Campbell, S. M.: Practical Guide to Nutritional Care for Dietitians and Other Health Care Professionals. Birmingham, AL: University of Alabama, 1984.

Frequency of Overweight and Underweight: Metrop Life Insur Co Stat Bull 41:4, 1960.

1983 Metropolitan Height and Weight Tables. Metrop Life Insur Co Stat Bull 64:1, 1983.

Peiffer, S. C., Blust, P., Leyson, J. F.: Nutritional assessment of the spinal cord injured patient. J Am Diet Assoc 78:501, 1981.

Wilkens, K.: Suggested guidelines for nutrition care of renal patients. Renal Dietitians Practice Group, The American Dietetic Association, 1986.

Williams, M., and Lissner, H. R.: Biomechanics of Human Motion, Philadelphia: W. B. Saunders, 1977.

Appendix D

Hamill, P. V., Moore, W. M.: Contemporary growth charts: Needs, construction and application (newsletter). Ross Timesaver Diet Curr 3:1976.

Hamill, P. V., Drizd, T. A., Johnson, C. L., Reed, R. B., Roche, A. F., and Moore, W. M.: Physical growth: National center for health statistics percentiles. Am J Clin Nutr 32:607, 1979.

Appendix E

Boothby, W. M., and W. M., and Berkson, J.: Food Nomogram. October 1933. (Copyright 1959 Mayo Association.)

Woodbury, R. E.: Statures and Weights of Children under Six Years of Age. U.S. Children's Bureau publication 87. Washington, D.C.: U.S. Government Printing Office, 1921.

Appendix G

Food and Nutrition Board, National Research Council, National Academy of Sciences: Recommended Dietary Allowances (9th ed). Washington, DC: U.S. Government Printing Office, 1980.

Appendix H

Hardinge, M. G., Swarner, J. B., and Crooks, H.: Carbohydrates in foods. J Am Diet Assoc 46:197, 1965.

Appendix I

Bickel, J. H., and Gray, J. C.: The Low Cholesterol Diet Manual. Iowa City: University of Iowa Press, 1968.

University of Iowa Hospitals and Clinics: Formulary and Handbook-1988, Iowa City, 1988.

Per 1000 cc	CHO gms/L	PRO gms/L	FAT gms/L	Cal/cc	Carbohydrate	Protein	Fat	mOsm/ Kg H_2O	Na mEq/L	K mEq/L
BLENDERIZED										
Compleat	128	43	43	1.07	Hydrolyzed cereal solids, pureed green beans, pureed pea, maltodextrin, peach puree, orange juice	Beef puree, nonfat milk	Beef puree, corn oil, mono- and diglycerides	405	56	36
Compleat Modified	141	43	37	1.07	Hydrolyzed cereal solids, green beans, pea and peach puree, orange juice	Beef puree, calcium caseinate	Beef puree, corn oil, mono- and diglycerides	300	30	36
Vitaneed	125	35	40	1.0	Maltodextrin, pureed green beans, pureed peaches, pureed carrots, mono- and diglycerides	Pureed beef	Partially hydrogenated soy oil	310	22	32
MILK-BASED FORMULAS										
Carnation Instant Breakfast	139	69	34	1.2	Sucrose, corn syrup solids, lactose	Nonfat dry milk, sweet dairy whey, calcium caseinate, isolated soy protein, sodium caseinate		NA	45	71
Meritene (liquid)	110	58	32	1.0	Skim milk, corn syrup solids, sucrose	Skim milk, sodium caseinate	Corn oil	505[a]	38	41
Meritene Powder/ Whole Milk (8 oz)	119	69	34	1.0	Whole milk, nonfat dry milk, sucrose, corn syrup solids, fructose	Whole milk, nonfat dry milk, calcium caseinate	Whole milk	690[a]	47	72
Sustagen	300	107	16	1.7	Corn syrup solids, dextrose	Nonfat milk, powdered whole milk, calcium caseinate	Powdered whole milk	1100[a]	43	82
Sustacal Powder/ Whole Milk (8 oz)	48	21	9	1	Sucrose, corn syrup solids	Nonfat milk	Whole milk	1010[a]	14	23
LACTOSE-FREE FORMULAS (1.0 to 1.2 calories/cc)										
Apricot Cooler	127	42	35	1.0	Apricot concentrate, frutose, orange juice concentrate, maltodextrin	Egg albumin	Partially hydrogenated soybean oil, lecithin	NA	34	62
Enrich	153	38	35	1.1	Hydrolyzed cornstarch, sucrose	Sodium and calcium caseinates	Corn oil	480[a]	37	40

Ca mg/L	P mg/L	Vit. A mcg(RE)	Vit. D mcg	Vit. E mg -TE	Vit. K mcg	Vit. C mg	Fe mg	Zn mg	I mcg	Cu mg	Mg mg	Reference	Cost/ 2000/Kcal	cc/USRDA
680	1320	1000	6.8	20	68	60	12	10	100	1.3	268	10	Moderate	1500
680	920	1000	6.7	13.42	68	60	12.0	10.0	100	1.3	268	10	Moderate	1500
500	500	750	5.0	45	150	150	9	15	75	1.0	200	6	Moderate	1470
2389	1833	2821	393	NA	NA	44	14	15.6	147	1.1	204	2	Low	1400
1200	1200	1200	8.0	16.11	77	72	14.4	12	120	1.6	320	10	Low	1250
2192	1923	1442	9.63	19.33	NA	58	17.3	14.4	146	1.9	385	10	Low	1040
3200	2400	1500	10	67	250	300	18	20	150	2.0	400	4	Low	1000
580	480	501	3	15	NA	20	6	5	50	0.7	135	4	Low	800
268	226	1080	NA	31	NA	21	3.5	NA	7	0.7	212	5	Low	---
714	714	1416	7.2	47	50	126	13.0	16.0	110	1.4	288	9	Low	1390

APPENDIX A. Nutrient Analysis of Enteral Formulas and Supplements

Per 1000 cc	CHO gms/L	PRO gms/L	FAT gms/L	Cal/cc	Carbohydrate	Protein	Fat	mOsm/ Kg H_2O	Na mEq/L	K mEq/L
Ensure	137	35	35	1	Hydrolyzed cornstarch sucrose	Sodium and calcium caseinates, soy protein isolate	Corn oil	450	35	38
Ensure HN	134	42	34	1.0	Hydrolyzed cornstarch, sucrose	Sodium and calcium caseinates	Corn oil	470[a]	38	38
Entrition	136	35	35	1.0	Maltodextrin	Sodium and calcium caseinates	Corn oil, soy lecithin	300	31	31
Attain	120	40	40	1.0	Maltodextrin	Sodium and calcium caseinates	Corn oil	300	30	29
Isocal	132	34	44	1.06	Maltodextrin	Calcium and sodium caseinates, soy protein isolate	Soy oil, MCT	300	23	34
Isocal HN	124	44	45	1.0	Maltodextrin	Sodium and calcium caseinates	Soy oil, MCT	270	40	40
Isosource	175	43	42	1.25	Maltodextrin	Sodium and calcium caseinates	MCT, corn oil	300	31	43
Isosource HN	171	53	43	1.28	Maltodextrin	Sodium and calcium caseinates	MCT, corn oil	300	31	43
Nutren	127	40	38	1.0	Maltodextrin, corn syrup, sucrose	Potassium and calcium caseinates	MCT, corn oil	300	21	32
Nutri-Aid	140	39	37	1.05	Corn syrup solids, sucrose	Potassium and sodium caseinates	Corn oil	290[a]	30	31
Osmolite	137	35	36	1.06	Hydrolyzed cornstarch	Sodium and calcium caseinates, soy protein isolate	MCT, corn oil, soy oil	300	23	24
Osmolite HN	141	44	37	1.06	Hydrolyzed cornstarch	Sodium and calcium caseinates, soy protein isolate	MCT, corn oil, soy oil	310	40	40
Pre-Attain	60	20	20	0.5	Maltodextrin	Sodium and calcium caseinates	Corn oil	150	15	15
Profiber	132	40	40	1.0	Hydrolyzed cornstarch	Sodium and calcium caseinates	Corn oil	300	32	32
Replete	113	62	33	1.0	Maltodextrin, sucrose	Potassium and calcium caseinates	Corn oil	350	22	40
Resource	145	37	37	1.06	Maltodextrin, sucrose	Sodium caseinate, calcium caseinate, soy protein isolate	Hydrogenated soy oil, polyglycerol esters of fatty acids	450	37	40
Sustacal Liquid	140	61	23	1.0	Sucrose, corn syrup	Calcium caseinate, soy protein isolate, sodium caseinate	Partially hydrogenated soy oil	625[a]	41	53

Ca mg/L	P mg/L	Vit. A mcg(RE)	Vit. D mcg	Vit. E mg -TE	Vit. K mcg	Vit. C mg	Fe mg	Zn mg	I mcg	Cu mg	Mg mg	Reference	Cost/ 2000/Kcal	cc/USRDA
500	500	750	5.0	23	36	150	9.0	15.0	75	1.0	200	9	Low	1890
720	720	1080	7.2	47.68	52	132	13.2	16.4	108	1.4	288	9	Low	1320
500	500	750	5.0	44.7	100	150	9.0	7.5	75	1.0	200	13	Low	2000
625	625	938	6.3	20	35	60	11.25	15.0	100	1.5	250	3	Low	1600
634	528	793	5.28	26.64	131	159	9.5	10.6	80	1.1	211	4	Low	1890
833	833	1251	8.3	52	104	250	15	12.5	125	1.7	333	4	Low	1250
680	680	1001	6.7	36	48	200	12	17	100	1.3	267	10	Low	1500
680	680	1001	6.7	36	48	200	12	17	100	1.3	267	10	Low	1500
500	500	1129	5.0	24	124	100	9	10	76	1.0	250	11	Low	2000
500	500	781	5.2	47	1000	167	9.3	15.6	79	1.0	208	1	NA	2000
500	500	750	5.0	23	36	150	9.0	15.0	75	1.0	200	9	Low	1890
761	761	1141	7.6	33	80	139	13.9	17.3	114	1.5	304	9	Low	1320
312.5	312.5	938	6.3	20	35	60	11.25	15	100	1.5	250	3	Moderate	1600
667	667	1001	6.7	40	50	120	12	20	100	1.5	267	3	Low	1500
600	540	1129	5.0	24	124	100	9	10	76	1.0	300	11	Low	2000
555	555	802	5.3	24.1	38	161	9.5	15.9	80	1.1	211	10	Low	1895
1014	930	1412	9.38	42.01	235	56	16.9	14.1	141	2.0	380	4	Low	1080

Per 1000 cc	CHO gms/L	PRO gms/L	FAT gms/L	Cal/cc	Carbohydrate	Protein	Fat	mOsm/ Kg H$_2$O	Na mEq/L	K mEq/L
Travasorb MCT Diet	123	49	33	1.0	Corn syrup solids	Lactalbumin, potassium caseinate	MCT, sunflower oil	NA	15	45

HIGH CALORIC DENSITY FORMULAS
(1.5 calorie/cc)

Per 1000 cc	CHO gms/L	PRO gms/L	FAT gms/L	Cal/cc	Carbohydrate	Protein	Fat	mOsm/ Kg H$_2$O	Na mEq/L	K mEq/L
Comply	180	60	60	1.5	Maltodextrin, sucrose	Sodium and calcium caseinates	Corn oil	410	44	44
Ensure Plus	189	52	51	1.5	Hydrolyzed cornstarch, sucrose	Sodium and calcium caseinates, soy protein isolate	Corn oil	600	47	56
Ensure Plus HN	189	59	47	1.5	Hydrolyzed cornstarch, sucrose	Sodium and calcium caseinates	Corn oil	650	51	47
Nutren 1.5	170	60	68	1.5	Maltodextrin, corn syrup, sucrose	Potassium and calcium caseinates	MCT, corn oil	420	33	48
Sustacal HC	190	61	58	1.5	Corn syrup solids, sugar	Calcium and sodium caseinates	Partially hydrogenated soybean oil	650[a]	37	38

(2.0 calorie/cc)

Per 1000 cc	CHO gms/L	PRO gms/L	FAT gms/L	Cal/cc	Carbohydrate	Protein	Fat	mOsm/ Kg H$_2$O	Na mEq/L	K mEq/L
Isocal HCN	225	75	91	2.0	Corn syrup	Calcium and sodium caseinates	Soybean oil, MCT	740	35	36
Magnacal	250	70	80	2.0	Maltodextrin, sucrose	Sodium and calcium caseinates	Partially hydrogenated soy oil	590	44	32
Nutren 2.0	196	80	106	2.0	Maltodextrin, corn syrup, sucrose	Potassium and calcium caseinates	MCT, corn oil	800	43	64
Two Cal HN	214	83	90	2.0	Hydrolyzed cornstarch, sucrose	Sodium and calcium caseinates	Corn oil, MCT	NA	46	59

PEPTIDE FORMULATIONS

Per 1000 cc	CHO gms/L	PRO gms/L	FAT gms/L	Cal/cc	Carbohydrate	Protein	Fat	mOsm/ Kg H$_2$O	Na mEq/L	K mEq/L
Citrotein	122	41	2	0.7	Sucrose, maltodextrin	Pasteurized egg white solids	Partially hydrogenated soy oil	495[a]	31	18
Criticare HN	222	38	3.0	1.06	Maltodextrin, modified cornstarch	Enzymatically hydrolyzed casein, free amino acids	Safflower oil	NA	36	21
Isotein HN	156	68	34	1.2	Maltodextrin, fructose	Delactosed lactalbumin, sodium caseinate	Partially hydrogenated soybean oil, MCT	300	30	22
Nutrex	142	38	0.5	0.7	Corn syrup solids, sucrose, mono- and diglycerides	Dried egg whites		450	26	41
Precision HN	216	44	1.3	1.05	Maltodextrin, sucrose	Pasteurized egg white solids	MCT, partially hydrogenated soybean oil	500[a]	43	23

Ca mg/L	P mg/L	Vit. A mcg(RE)	Vit. D mcg	Vit. E mg -TE	Vit. K mcg	Vit. C mg	Fe mg	Zn mg	I mcg	Cu mg	Mg mg	Reference	Cost/ 2000/Kcal	cc/USRDA
500	500	750	5.0	45	75	150	9.0	15.0	75	1.0	200	11	NA	2000
938	938	1408	9.4	30	52.5	90	17	22.5	150	2.25	375	3	Low	1060
600	600	1068	7.0	46	52	152	13.5	22.5	100	1.5	300	9	Low	1600
1060	1060	1056	10.58	66.16	110	254	19.0	16.1	161	2.1	423	9	Low	950
752	752	1682	7.5	36	188	152	14	15	112	1.5	376	11	Low	1333
850	850	1260	8.5	37	210	76	15.0	13	130	1.7	340	4	Low	1180
668	668	1002	6.65	33.49	165	200	11.8	19.9	101	2.0	266	4	Low	1500
1000	1000	1500	10	89	300	300	18	30	150	2.0	400	3	Moderate	1000
1000	1000	2282	10	48	252	200	18	20	152	2.0	500	11	Low	1000
1060	1060	1579	10.5	72	76	189	18.9	24	160	2.1	421	9	Low	1900
900	900	399	10.8	31	NA	240	38.4	16.0	160	2.1	427	10	Low	70% in 3 servings
835	835	1251	8.3	47.8	30	75	15.0	19	125	1.7	355	9	High	1890
565	565	848	5.7	11.34	56	51	10.2	8.5	85	1.1	226	10	Moderate	1770
800	800	1469	9.55	40.23	NA	76	19	12.7	127	1.7	338	7	Low	---
351	351	526	3.5	7.05	35	32	6.3	5.3	53	0.7	140	10	Moderate	2850

Per 1000 cc	CHO gms/L	PRO gms/L	FAT gms/L	Cal/cc	Carbohydrate	Protein	Fat	mOsm/ Kg H$_2$O	Na mEq/L	K mEq/L
Precision Isotonic	144	29	30	0.96	Maltodextrin, sucrose	Egg white solids, sodium caseinate	Partially hydrogenated soybean oil	300	34	25
Precision LR	248	26	1.6	1.1	Maltodextrin, sucrose	Egg white solids	MCT, partially hydrogenated soybean oil	540[a]	31	22
Reabilan	131	31	39	1.0	Maltodextrin, tapicoa starch	Protein hydrolysate	MCT, linoleic acid	350	30	32
Ross SLD	137	38	0.5	0.7	Sucrose, hydrolyzed cornstarch	Egg white solids	None	650	27	34

ELEMENTAL

Per 1000 cc	CHO gms/L	PRO gms/L	FAT gms/L	Cal/cc	Carbohydrate	Protein	Fat	mOsm/ Kg H$_2$O	Na mEq/L	K mEq/L
Peptamen	127	40	39	1.0	Maltodextrin	Enzymatically hydrolyzed whey proteins	MCT (fractionated coconut oil), sunflower oil	242	22	32
Pepti-2000	189	40	10	1.0	Maltodextrin	Hydrolyzed lactalbumin	MCT, corn oil	490	29	29
Travasorb HN	175	45	13	1.0	Glucose oligo-saccharides	Enzymatically hydrolyzed lactalbumin	MCT (fractionated coconut oil), sunflower oil	560	40	30
Travasorb Standard	190	30	13	1.0	Glucose oligo-saccharides	Enzymatically hydrolyzed lactalbumin	MCT (fractionated coconut oil), sunflower oil	560	40	30
Vital HN	188	42	11	1.0	Hydrolyzed cornstarch, sucrose	Hydrolyzed whey, meat, and soy, free amino acids	Safflower oil, MCT	460	20	34
Tolerex	230	22	1.5	1.0	Glucose oligo-saccharides	Free L-amino acids	Safflower oil	550[a]	20	30
Vivonex HN	210	43	0.9	1.0	Glucose oligo-saccharides	Free L-amino acid	Safflower oil	810	23	30
Vivonex TEN	206	38	2.1	1.0	Predigested carbohydrate	Free L-amino acids (33.1% BCAA)	Safflower oil	630	20	20

SPECIALTY FORMULAS

Per 1000 cc	CHO gms/L	PRO gms/L	FAT gms/L	Cal/cc	Carbohydrate	Protein	Fat	mOsm/ Kg H$_2$O	Na mEq/L	K mEq/L
Amin-Aid	414	22	52	2.0	Maltodextrin sucrose	Crystalline amino acids plus histidine	Soybean oil, lecithin, mono- and diglycerides	1095	<15	<6
Hepatic Aid II	143	38	31	1.0	Maltodextrin, sucrose	Crystalline amino acids (46% BCAA)	Soybean oil, lecithin, mono- and diglycerides	560[a]	<15	<6
Lonalac	74	53	55	1.0	Lactose	Casein	Coconut oil	NA	150	48
Portagen	110	34	46	1.0	Corn syrup solids, sucrose	Sodium caseinate	MCT, corn oil	320	20	31
Pulmocare	104	62	91	1.5	Hydrolyzed cornstarch, sucrose	Sodium and calcium caseinates	Corn oil, soy lecithin	490	56	48

Ca mg/L	P mg/L	Vit. A mcg(RE)	Vit. D mcg	Vit. E mg -TE	Vit. K mcg	Vit. C mg	Fe mg	Zn mg	I mcg	Cu mg	Mg mg	Reference	Cost/ 2000/Kcal	cc/USRDA
641	641	962	6.4	12.89	64	58	11.5	9.6	96	1.3	256	10	Moderate	1560
585	585	877	8.1	11.74	58	53	10.5	8.8	88	1.2	234	10	Moderate	1710
500	848	800	5.1	18	51	101	10	10	75	1.6	235	12	Moderate	2000
530	530	780	5.3	60	132	159	9.5	10.6	79	1.1	210	9	Moderate	2000
600	500	1125	5.0	29.8	125	100	9.0	10.0	75	1.0	300	11	Moderate	2000
625	625	938	6.3	20	35	60	11.25	15	100	1.5	250	3	Moderate	1600
500	500	750	5.0	22.4	75	45	9.0	7.5	75	1.0	200	11	NA	2000
500	500	750	5.0	22.4	75	45	9.0	7.5	75	1.0	200	11	NA	2000
667	667	1000	6.7	29.8	47	60	12.0	10.0	100	1.3	267	9	Moderate	1500
556	556	833	5.55	11.21	37	33	10.0	8.3	83	1.1	222	6	Moderate	1800
333	333	600	3.3	14.9	22	20	6.0	5.0	50	0.7	133	6	High	3000
500	500	750	5.0	22.3	22	60	9.0	10.0	75	1.0	200	6	High	2000
Negl.	Negl.	-	-	-	-	-	tr	tr	tr	tr	-	1	High	---
Negl.	Negl.	-	-	-	-	-	-	-	-	-	-	1	Extremely high	---
1760	1562	-	-	-	-	-	-	-	-	-	-	4	Low	---
900	675	2250	18.75	20.13	150	78	18.0	9.0	70	1.5	200	4	Moderate	---
1041	1041	1562	10.4	47	75	250	18.8	23.3	158	2.08	417	9	Low	960

Per 1000 cc	CHO gms/L	PRO gms/L	FAT gms/L	Cal/cc	Carbohydrate	Protein	Fat	mOsm/ Kg H_2O	Na mEq/L	K mEq/L
Stresstein	170	70	28	1.2	Maltodextrin	Free L-amino acids (44% BCAA)	MCT, soybean oil, and polyglycerol esters of fatty acids	910	28	28
Trauma-Aid HBC	166	56	12	1.0	Mono- and diglycerides	Free L-amino acids (50% BCAA)	Soybean oil, MCT, lecithin	675	23	30
Traum-cal	143	83	69	1.5	Corn syrup, sucrose	Calcium and sodium caseinates	Soybean oil, MCT, lecithin	550	52	36
Travasorb Hepatic	209	29	15	1.1	Glucose, oligo-saccharides, sucrose	Crystalline L-amino acids (50% BCAA)	MCT, sun-flower oil	690	19	29
Travasorb Renal	271	23	18	1.3	Glucose oligo-saccharides	Crystalline L-amino acid	MCT, sun-flower oil	590	Negl.	Negl.

MODULAR COMPONENTS
Carbohydrate Supplements

Per 1000 cc	CHO gms/L	PRO gms/L	FAT gms/L	Cal/cc	Carbohydrate	Protein	Fat	mOsm/ Kg H_2O	Na mEq/L	K mEq/L
Moducal/T (1T = 8 gm)	8	-	-	32/T	Maltodextrin	None	None	28	0.24	Negl.
Polycose Liquid/T	8	0	0	2	Cornstarch	None	None	13	0.03	Negl.
Polycose Powder/T	8	0	0	32	Cornstarch	None	None	68	9	0.8
Pro-Mix Liquid Carbohydrate Supplement (1T = 15 cc)	9	-	-	38/T	Cornstarch	None	None	315	0.4	0.07
Pro-Mix Pure Carbo-hydrate Supplement/T (1T = 8 gm)	8	-	-	32/T	Cornstarch	None	None	131	0.05	Negl.
Sumacal/T	5	0	0	19	Maltodextrin	None	None	-	0.2	-

Protein Supplements

Per 1000 cc	CHO gms/L	PRO gms/L	FAT gms/L	Cal/cc	Carbohydrate	Protein	Fat	mOsm/ Kg H_2O	Na mEq/L	K mEq/L
Casec/T (1T = 5gm)	0	4	0	19	None	Calcium caseinate from skim milk	NA	-	0.3 mg	0.01 mg
Pro-Mix R.D.P./T	0.25	4	0.2	18	Trace	Whey protein	Lecithin	30	0.5	1.05
Promod/T (1T = 3 gm)	0.40	17	0.36	17/T	Trace	Whey protein concentrate	Soy lecithin	30	0.34	0.1
Propac/T (1T = 4 gm)	0.2	3	0.3	16/T	Trace	Whey	None	-	0.4	0.5

Fat Supplements

Per 1000 cc	CHO gms/L	PRO gms/L	FAT gms/L	Cal/cc	Carbohydrate	Protein	Fat	mOsm/ Kg H_2O	Na mEq/L	K mEq/L
MCT Oil/T	0	0	14	115	None	None	Coconut oil	-	0	0
Microlipid/T	0	0	7.5	4.5	None	None	Safflower oil, poly-glycerol	80	0	0
Pro-Mix High Fat	3.24	tr	3.8	48/T	Corn syrup, sucrose	None	Partially hydrogenated coconut oil, mono and diglycerides	-	0.6	tr

Ca mg/L	P mg/L	Vit. A mcg(RE)	Vit. D mcg	Vit. E mg -TE	Vit. K mcg	Vit. C mg	Fe mg	Zn mg	I mcg	Cu mg	Mg mg	Reference	Cost/ 2000/Kcal	cc/USRDA
507	507	750	5.0	15	35	30	9.0	7.5	75	1.0	200	10	High	2000
400	400	500	3.3	30	50	33	6.0	6.7	50	0.67	133	1	High	3000
750	750	750	5.0	56	125	150	9.0	15	75	1.5	200	4	Moderate	2000
380	471	477	4.8	4.8	50	43	8.6	7.1	71	0.95	186	11	NA	2100
Negl.	Negl.	0	0	0	0	32	0	0	0	0	0	11	High	2100
-	-	-	-	-	-	-	-	-	-	-	-	4	Low/T	---
-	-	-	-	-	-	-	-	-	-	-	-	4	Low/T	---
-	-	-	-	-	-	-	-	-	-	-	-	9	Low/T	---
2.8	0.9	-	-	-	-	-	-	-	-	-	-	8	Low/T	---
16	0.8	-	-	-	-	-	-	-	-	-	-	8	Low/T	---
-	-	-	-	-	-	-	-	-	-	-	-	3	Low/T	---
80	40	-	-	-	-	-	-	-	-	-	-	4	Low/T	---
18	16	-	-	-	-	-	-	-	-	-	-	8	Low/T	---
13.8	13	-	-	-	-	-	-	-	-	-	-	9	Low/T	---
24	12	-	-	-	-	-	-	-	-	-	-	3	Low/T	---
0	0	-	-	-	-	-	-	-	-	-	-	4	Low/T	---
0	0	-	-	-	-	-	-	-	-	-	-	3	Low/T	---
tr	tr	-	-	-	-	-	-	-	-	-	-	8	Low/T	---

	CHO gms	PRO gms	FAT gms	Cal	Carbohydrate	Protein	Fat	mOsm/ Kg H_2O	Na mEq	K mEq
MODULAR SYSTEM										
Nutrisource Amino Acids (per packet)	0	15	0	60/ pkt	None	Amino acids	None	-	-	-
Nutrisource Amino Acids High Branched Chain (per packet)	0	15	0	60/ pkt	None	Amino acids	None	-	-	-
Nutrisource Protein (Intact) (per packet)	2	15	1	80/ pkt	Mono- and diglycerides, polysorbate 80	Delactosed lactalbumin, egg white solids	None	-	2	3
Nutrisource Carbohydrate (per can)	200	0	0	3.2	Deionized corn syrup solids	None	None	-	5 mg	3 mg
Nutrisource Lipid-Long-Chain Triglycerides (per can)	0	0	61	549/ can	None	None	Soybean oil, polyglycerol esters of fatty acids	-	-	-
Nutrisource Lipid-Medium-Chain Triglycerides (per can)	0	0	61	510/ can	None	None	MCT, poly-glycerol esters of fatty acids hydroxylated lecithin	-	-	-
Nutrisource Minerals for Amino Acid Formulas (per packet)	3	0	0	12/ pkt	Magnesium gluconate, calcium gly-cerophosphate, manganese and copper gluconate	None	None	-	33	56
Nutrisource Minerals for Amino Acid Formulas Electrolyte Restricted (per packet)	12	0	0	48/ pkt	Maltodextrin, magnesium gluconate, calcium gly-cerophosphate, manganese and copper gluconate	None	None	-	<15 mg	<5 mg
Nutrisource Minerals for Protein Formulas (per packet)	6	0	0	24/ pkt	Magnesium gluconate, maltodextrin, calcium gly-cerophosphate	None	None	-	43	45
Nutrisource Minerals for Protein Formulas Electrolyte Restricted (per packet)	13	0	0	52/ pkt	Maltodextrin, magnesium gluconate, calcium gly-cerophosphate, manganese and copper gluconate	None	None	-	<15 mg	<5 mg
Nutrisource Vitamins	9	0	0	36/ pkt	Maltodextrin	None	None	-	-	-

Notes: I.U. Vitamin A ÷ 3.33 = mcg retinol; I.U. Vitamin D x 0.025 = mcg cholecalciferol; I.U. Vitamin E ÷ 1.49 = mg d-alpha-tocopherol.

Cost: Low = up to $10 per 2000 kcal; Moderate = $10-20 per 2000 kcal; High = $20-35 per 2000 kcal; Extremely High = $50-80 per 2000 kcal.

Reference: 1 = Kendall McGaw, Division of American Hospital Supply Corporation, Irvine, CA 92714; 2 = Carnation Company, Healthcare Services, Department 282, P.O. Box 550, Pico Rivera, CA 90665; 3 = Sherwood Medical, St. Louis, MO 63103; 4 = Bristol-Myers Institutional Products. Mead Johnson Nutritionals, Evansville, IN 47721; 5 = MLG Labs, Inc., 175 Derby Street, Hingham, MA 02043; 6 = Norwich Eaton Pharmaceuticals, Inc., Norwich NY 13815; 7 = Nutrex Corporation, 1168 Aster Avenue, Building C, Sunnyvale, CA 94086; 8 = Pro-Mix, Navaco Laboratories, P.O. Box 23162, Phoenix, AZ 85063; 9 = Ross Laboratories,

Ca mg	P mg	Vit. A mcg(RE)	Vit. D mcg	Vit. E mg -TE	Vit. K mcg	Vit. C mg	Fe mg	Zn mg	I mcg	Cu mg	Mg mg	Reference	Cost/ 2000/Kcal	cc/USRDA
-	-	-	-	-	-	-	-	-	-	-	-	10	Moderate[b]	---
-	-	-	-	-	-	-	-	-	-	-	-	10	Moderate[b]	---
70	60	-	-	-	-	-	-	-	-	-	-	10	Moderate[b]	---
1	5	-	-	-	-	-	-	-	-	-	-	10	Moderate[b]	---
-	-	-	-	-	-	-	-	-	-	-	-	10	Moderate[b]	---
-	-	-	-	-	-	-	-	-	-	-	-	10	Moderate[b]	---
800	800	-	-	-	-	-	18	15	150	2	350	10	Moderate[b]	---
800	800	-	-	-	-	-	18	15	150	2	350	10	Moderate[b]	---
650	650	-	-	-	-	-	18	15	150	2	350	10	Moderate[b]	---
650	650	-	-	-	-	-	18	15	150	2	350	10	Moderate[b]	---
-	-	1000	5	10	70	60	-	-	-	-	-	10	Moderate[b]	---

625 Cleveland Ave., Columbus, OH 43216; 10 = Sandoz Nutrition, 5320 W. 23rd St., P.O. Box 370, Minneapolis, MN 55440; 11 = Baxter, Clintec Nutrition Division, Baxter Laboratories, Inc., Deerfield, IL 60015; 12 = O'Brien Pharmaceuticals, Inc., Parsippany, NJ 07054; 13 = Biosearch, 35 Industrial Parkway, P.O. Box 1700, Somerville, NJ 08876.

[a]Varies with flavors.
[b]Moderate when combined.
NA = Information not available.

THE UNIVERSITY OF IOWA HOSPITALS AND CLINICS
Dietary Department

PATIENT DIET HISTORY

Admitting Problem _____

Problem List   1. _____

              2. _____   Addressograph Stamp

              3. _____   Today's date _____

Diet Order _____   Ht(cm) _____

Food Allergies (egg, milk, etc.):   Present Wt(kg) _____

_____   Suggested Wt for Ht _____

Est Needs _____   Usual Wt _____

Medications/Vitamins/Minerals

  1. _____

  2. _____

  3. _____

  4. _____

Additional Information/Activity:

Lab Date \ Lab	Lab Data				

Previous Diets _____

Previously Seen by Dietitian: Yes   No

Change in Appetite _____

Constipation _____ Nausea _____ Vomiting _____

Diarrhea _____ Other _____

Visual Observation: Hair

                  Skin

                  Eye

                  Nails

(over)

APPENDIX B. Patient Diet History Forms

Breakfast + A.M. Snack	C	P	F	Lunch + P.M. Snack	C	P	F	Dinner + H.S. Snack	C	P	F
Total											

	C	P	F
Daily Total			
Calories			

Food Frequency/Amount:

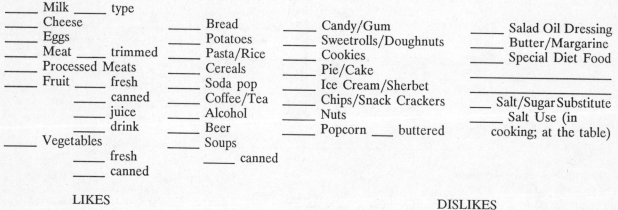

_____ Milk _____ type
_____ Cheese
_____ Eggs
_____ Meat _____ trimmed
_____ Processed Meats
_____ Fruit _____ fresh
         _____ canned
         _____ juice
         _____ drink
_____ Vegetables
         _____ fresh
         _____ canned

LIKES

_____ Bread
_____ Potatoes
_____ Pasta/Rice
_____ Cereals
_____ Soda pop
_____ Coffee/Tea
_____ Alcohol
_____ Beer
_____ Soups
         _____ canned

_____ Candy/Gum
_____ Sweetrolls/Doughnuts
_____ Cookies
_____ Pie/Cake
_____ Ice Cream/Sherbet
_____ Chips/Snack Crackers
_____ Nuts
_____ Popcorn _____ buttered

_____ Salad Oil Dressing
_____ Butter/Margarine
_____ Special Diet Food
_____
_____
_____ Salt/Sugar Substitute
_____ Salt Use (in cooking; at the table)

DISLIKES

Weekend Variation: .
Meals Out:
Who Prepares Meals: Teeth Condition:

302

DIET HISTORY
WITH EMPHASIS ON CHOLESTEROL AND FAT

	Amount	Chol (mg)	Total Fat (g)	Sat Fat (g)	Poly Fat (g)	Minimum Significant Amount
Eggs	_____	_____	_____	_____	_____	½ mo
Bacon	_____	_____	_____	_____	_____	4 strips/mo
Sausage	_____	_____	_____	_____	_____	2 oz/mo
Meat L	_____	_____	_____	_____	_____	
D	_____	_____	_____	_____	_____	
Luncheon meat	_____	_____	_____	_____	_____	See sausage
Shrimp	_____	_____	_____	_____	_____	2 oz/mo
Liver, pork, beef, calf,	_____	_____	_____	_____	_____	3 oz/6 mo (or)
chicken	_____	_____	_____	_____	_____	1 oz/2 mo
Gravy	_____	_____	_____	_____	_____	1 cup/mo
Milk, whole	_____	_____	_____	_____	_____	½ cup/wk
2%	_____	_____	_____	_____	_____	1 cup/wk
Cheese	_____	_____	_____	_____	_____	1 oz/2 wks
Cottage cheese	_____	_____	_____	_____	_____	½ cup/2 wks
Cream — light, sour	_____	_____	_____	_____	_____	1 tbsp/wk
heavy	_____	_____	_____	_____	_____	1 tbsp/wk
half-and-half	_____	_____	_____	_____	_____	1 tbsp/mo
non-dairy creamer	_____	_____	_____	_____	_____	1 tbsp/wk
Ice cream	_____	_____	_____	_____	_____	½ cup/mo
Ice milk	_____	_____	_____	_____	_____	1 cup/mo
Butter	_____	_____	_____	_____	_____	1 tsp/2 wks
Margarine (as spread)	_____	_____	_____	_____	_____	1 tsp/wk
(in cooking)	_____	_____	_____	_____	_____	1 tsp/wk
Salad dressing	_____	_____	_____	_____	_____	1 tbsp/wk
*Breaded fried foods	_____	_____	_____	_____	_____	1 tsp/wk
*Fried potatoes	_____	_____	_____	_____	_____	1 tsp/wk
*Baked products	_____	_____	_____	_____	_____	1 serving/mo
*Snack foods	_____	_____	_____	_____	_____	
Chocolate	_____	_____	_____	_____	_____	½ oz/wk
Peanut butter	_____	_____	_____	_____	_____	1 tbsp/mo
Nuts	_____	_____	_____	_____	_____	14 tbsp/mo
TOTAL		_____	_____	_____	_____	
				P/S =		_____

_____

*For calculations use:

1 tbsp of salad dressing . . . . 1½ tsp of oil

3 oz meat . . . . 2 tsp fat

½ cup potatoes. . . . . 2 tsp fat

cake with frosting (1 piece, 2″ × 3″ × 2″) . . . 3 tsp fat

pie (1 piece, 1/7th of 9″) . . . . 4 tsp fat

cookies (4 pieces, 3″ diam) . . . . 3 tsp fat

doughnuts and sweet rolls (1 piece, 4″ diam) . . . 2 tsp fat

crackers and chips

(excluding low fat crackers) (12 pieces) . . . . . 3 tsp fat

Height (in shoes)[b]			Weight (in indoor clothing)[a]					
			Small Frame		Medium Frame		Large Frame	
feet	in.	cm	lb	kg	lb	kg	lb	kg
			Men					
5	2	158	112-120	51-55	118-129	54-59	126-141	57-64
5	3	160	115-123	52-56	121-133	55-60	129-144	59-65
5	4	163	118-126	54-57	124-139	56-62	132-148	60-67
5	5	165	121-129	55-59	127-139	58-63	135-152	61-69
5	6	168	124-133	56-60	130-143	59-65	138-156	63-71
5	7	170	128-137	58-62	134-147	61-67	142-161	64-73
5	8	173	132-141	60-64	138-152	63-69	147-166	67-75
5	9	176	136-145	62-66	142-156	64-71	151-170	69-77
5	10	178	140-150	64-68	146-160	66-73	155-174	70-79
5	11	180	144-154	65-70	150-165	68-75	159-179	72-81
6	0	183	148-158	67-72	154-170	70-77	164-184	74-84
6	1	185	152-162	69-74	158-175	72-79	168-189	76-86
6	2	188	156-167	71-76	162-180	74-82	173-194	79-88
6	3	191	160-171	73-78	167-185	76-84	178-199	81-90
6	4	193	164-175	74-79	172-190	78-86	182-204	83-93
			Women					
4	10	147	92-98	42-45	96-107	44-49	104-119	47-54
4	11	150	94-101	43-46	98-110	45-50	106-122	48-55
5	0	152	96-104	44-47	101-113	46-51	109-125	49-57
5	1	155	99-107	45-49	104-116	47-53	112-128	51-58
5	2	158	102-110	46-50	107-119	49-54	115-131	52-59
5	3	160	105-113	48-51	110-122	50-55	118-134	54-61
5	4	163	108-116	49-53	113-126	51-57	121-138	55-63
5	5	165	111-119	50-54	116-130	53-59	125-142	57-64
5	6	168	114-123	52-56	120-135	55-61	129-146	59-66
5	7	170	118-127	54-58	124-139	56-63	133-150	60-68
5	8	173	122-131	55-59	128-143	58-65	137-154	62-70
5	9	175	126-135	57-61	132-147	60-67	141-158	64-72
5	10	178	130-140	59-64	136-151	62-69	145-163	66-74
5	11	180	134-144	61-65	140-155	64-70	149-168	68-76
6	0	183	138-148	63-67	144-159	65-72	153-173	69-79

Source: Adapted from Frequency of overweight and underweight (1960, 5).
Note: This table is used instead of the more recent 1983 table, because the consensus in the medical and dietetic literature is that the lower 1960 values are closer to ideal.
[a]Indoor clothing weighing 5 pounds for men and 3 pounds for women.
[b]Shoes with 1-in. heels.

1983 HEIGHT AND WEIGHT TABLES FOR MEN AND WOMEN
ACCORDING TO FRAME, AGES 25-59

Height (in shoes)[b]			Weight (in indoor clothing)[a]					
			Small Frame		Medium Frame		Large Frame	
feet	in.	cm	lb	kg	lb	kg	lb	kg
Men								
5	2	158	128-134	58.3-61.0	131-141	59.6-64.2	138-150	62.8-68.3
5	3	160	130-136	59.0-61.7	133-143	60.3-64.9	140-153	63.5-69.4
5	4	163	132-138	60.0-62.7	135-145	61.3-66.0	142-156	64.5-71.1
5	5	165	134-140	60.8-63.5	137-148	62.1-67.0	144-160	65.3-72.5
5	6	168	136-142	61.8-64.6	139-151	63.2-68.7	146-164	66.4-74.7
5	7	170	138-145	62.5-65.7	142-154	64.3-69.8	149-168	67.5-76.1
5	8	173	140-148	63.6-67.3	145-157	65.9-71.4	152-172	69.1-78.2
5	9	176	142-151	64.7-68.9	148-160	67.5-73.0	155-176	70.7-80.3
5	10	178	144-154	65.4-70.0	151-163	68.6-74.0	158-180	71.8-81.8
5	11	180	146-157	66.1-71.0	154-166	69.7-75.1	161-184	72.8-83.3
6	0	183	149-160	67.7-72.7	157-170	71.3-77.2	164-188	74.5-85.4
6	1	185	152-164	68.7-74.1	160-174	72.4-78.6	168-192	75.9-86.8
6	2	188	155-168	70.3-76.2	164-178	74.4-80.7	172-197	78.0-89.4
6	3	191	158-172	72.1-78.4	167-182	76.1-84.8	181-202	80.3-92.1
6	4	193	162-176	73.5-79.8	171-187	77.6-84.8	181-207	82.1-93.9
Women								
4	10	147	102-111	46.4-50.6	109-121	49.6-55.1	118-131	53.7-59.8
4	11	150	103-113	46.7-51.3	111-123	50.3-55.9	120-134	54.4-60.9
5	0	152	104-115	47.1-52.1	113-126	51.1-57.0	122-137	55.2-61.9
5	1	155	106-118	48.1-53.6	115-129	52.2-58.6	125-140	56.8-63.6
5	2	158	108-121	49.3-55.2	118-132	53.8-60.2	128-143	58.4-65.3
5	3	160	111-124	50.3-56.2	121-135	54.9-61.2	131-147	59.4-66.7
5	4	163	114-127	51.9-57.8	124-138	56.4-62.8	134-151	61.0-68.8
5	5	165	117-130	53.0-58.9	127-141	57.5-63.9	137-155	62.0-70.2
5	6	168	120-133	54.6-60.5	130-144	59.2-65.5	140-159	63.7-72.4
5	7	170	123-136	55.7-61.6	133-147	60.2-66.6	143-163	64.8-73.8
5	8	173	126-139	57.3-63.2	136-150	61.8-68.2	146-167	66.4-75.9
5	9	175	129-142	58.3-64.2	139-153	62.8-69.2	149-170	67.4-76.9
5	10	178	132-145	60.0-65.9	142-156	64.5-70.9	152-173	69.0-78.6
5	11	180	135-148	61.0-66.9	145-159	65.6-71.9	155-176	70.1-79.6
6	0	183	138-151	62.6-68.5	148-162	67.1-73.5	158-179	71.7-81.2

Source: Adapted from 1983 Metropolitan Height and Weight Tables. Basic data from Build Study, 1979.
[a]Indoor clothing weighing 5 pounds for men and 3 pounds for women.
[b]Shoes with 1-in. heels.

APPENDIX C. Height and Weight Tables and Information

305

HOW TO DETERMINE BODY FRAME BY ELBOW BREADTH

To make a simple approximation of frame size:

Extend the arm and bend the forearm upwards at a 90-degree angle. Keep the fingers straight and turn the inside of the wrist toward the body. Place the thumb and index finger of the other hand on the two prominent bones on either side of the elbow. Measure the space between the fingers against a ruler or a tape measure. (For the most accurate measurement, have a trained person measure the elbow breadth with calipers.) Compare this measurement with the measurements shown below.

These tables list the elbow measurements for men and women of medium frame at various heights. Measurements lower than those listed indicate a small frame, while higher measurements indicate a large frame.

Men				
Height[a] (in shoes)		Elbow Breadth (in.)	Height[a] (in shoes) (cm)	Elbow Breadth (cm)
Feet In.	Feet In.			
5 2 -	5 3	2-1/2 - 2-7/8	158-161	6.4 - 7.2
5 4 -	5 7	2-5/8 - 2-7/8	162-171	6.7 - 7.4
5 8 -	5 11	2-3/4 - 3	172-181	6.9 - 7.6
6 0 -	6 3	2-3/4 - 3-1/8	182-191	7.1 - 7.8
6 4		2-7/8 - 3-1/4	192-193	7.4 - 8.1
Women				
4 10 -	4 11	2-1/4 - 2-1/2	148-151	5.6 - 6.4
5 0 -	5 3	2-1/4 - 2-1/2	152-161	5.8 - 6.5
5 4 -	5 7	2-3/8 - 2-5/8	162-171	5.9 - 6.6
5 8 -	5 11	2-3/8 - 2-5/8	172-181	6.1 - 6.8
6 0		2-1/2 - 2-3/4	182-183	6.2 - 6.9

Source: Adapted from Metrop Life Insur Co Stat Bull (1983). Basic data from data tape, HANES I - Anthropometry, goniometry, skeletal age, bone density, and cortical thickness, ages 1-74, National Health and Nutrition Examination Survey, 1971-75, National Center for Health Statistics.

[a]Shoes with 1-in. or 2.5 cm heels.

ADJUSTMENT IN BODY WEIGHT FOR OBESE PATIENTS

The basal energy expenditure formula (see page 246) should be modified for the patient who is at more than 125% of ideal body weight. Since the obese person has a greater percentage of body fat, which is much less metabolically active, using actual body weight for an obese person will skew the caloric needs very high. Conversely, using ideal body weight for a person who is at more than 125% of ideal body weight does not take into account the increased caloric expenditure required for moving this excess weight, as well as the increase in body protein for structural support of extra fat tissue. Because of these factors, the following formula is suggested for patients whose body weight is greater than 125% of ideal body weight.

[Actual Body Weight* - Ideal Body Weight* x 0.25] + Ideal Body Weight* = Weight for BEE and protein requirements

*Kg Values
(0.25 = 25% of body fat tissue is metabolically active)

Source: Wilkens (1986).

ADJUSTMENT IN BODY WEIGHT FOR AMPUTEES

Body proportions vary considerably among individuals. The chart below can be used to estimate the weights of body parts.

Body Part	% of Total Body Weight	Average Weight in Young Adult Male (Kg)
Entire upper extremity	4.8	3.3
Upper arm	2.8	1.9
Forearm without hand	1.6	1.1
Hand	.6	.4
Entire lower extremity	15.6	10.6
Thigh	9.7	6.6
Leg without foot	4.6	3.1
Foot	1.5	1.0

Sources: Brunnstrom (1981) and Williams and Lissner (1977).

ADJUSTMENTS IN BODY WEIGHT FOR PATIENTS WITH PARAPLEGIA OR QUADRIPLEGIA

For patients with paraplegia, an estimated ideal weight can be calculated by subtracting 5 to 10% from the appropriate values given in the chart on page 304. For patients with quadriplegia, 10 to 15% can be subtracted. These adjustments allow for decreased muscle mass and bone weight.

Sources: Campbell (1984) and Peiffer, et al. (1981).

BOYS: BIRTH TO 36 MONTHS
PHYSICAL GROWTH
NCHS PERCENTILES*

NAME _____ RECORD # _____

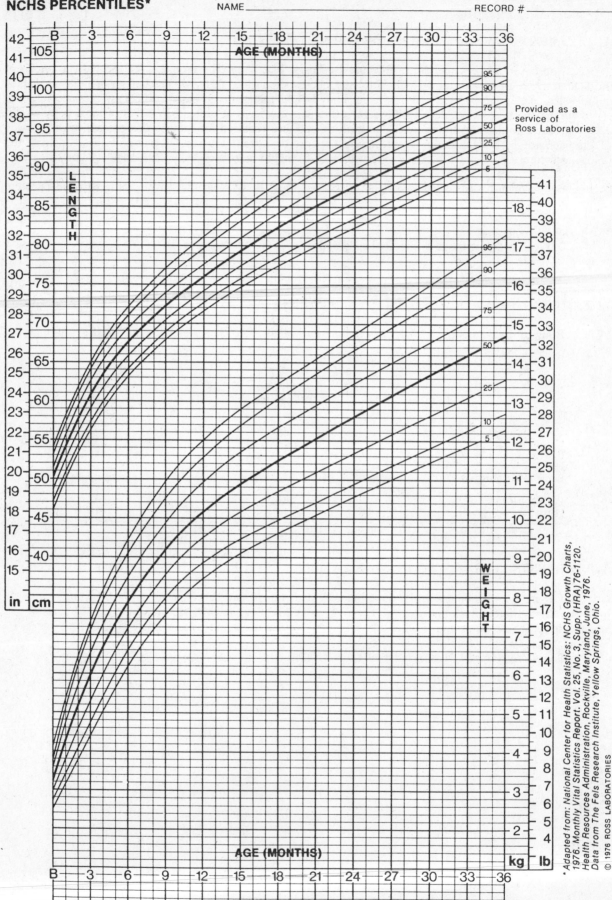

Provided as a service of Ross Laboratories

* Adapted from: National Center for Health Statistics: NCHS Growth Charts, 1976. Monthly Vital Statistics Report. Vol. 25, No. 3, Supp. (HRA) 76-1120. Health Resources Administration, Rockville, Maryland, June, 1976. Data from The Fels Research Institute, Yellow Springs, Ohio.

BOYS: BIRTH TO 36 MONTHS
PHYSICAL GROWTH
NCHS PERCENTILES*

NAME _____ RECORD # _____

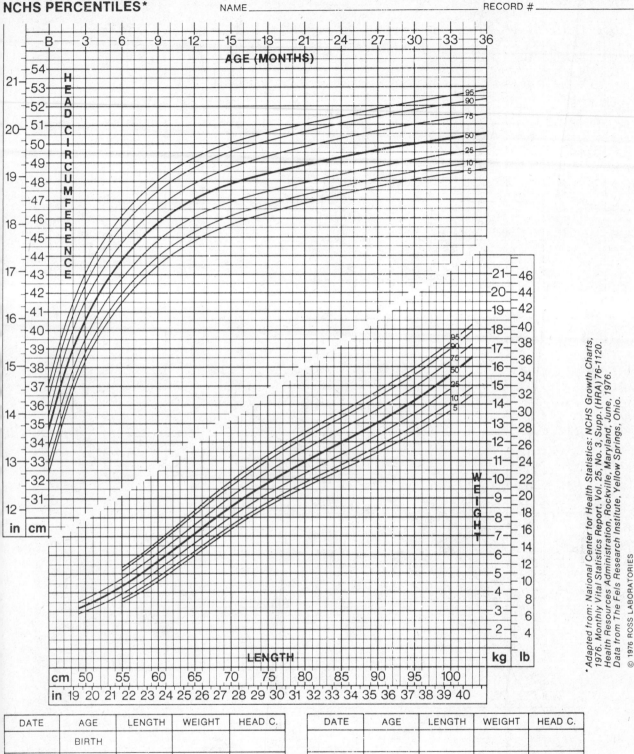

DATE	AGE	LENGTH	WEIGHT	HEAD C.
	BIRTH			

DATE	AGE	LENGTH	WEIGHT	HEAD C.

*Adapted from: National Center for Health Statistics: NCHS Growth Charts, 1976. Monthly Vital Statistics Report. Vol. 25, No. 3, Supp. (HRA) 76-1120. Health Resources Administration, Rockville, Maryland, June, 1976. Data from The Fels Research Institute, Yellow Springs, Ohio.

© 1976 ROSS LABORATORIES

APPENDIX D. **Growth Charts**

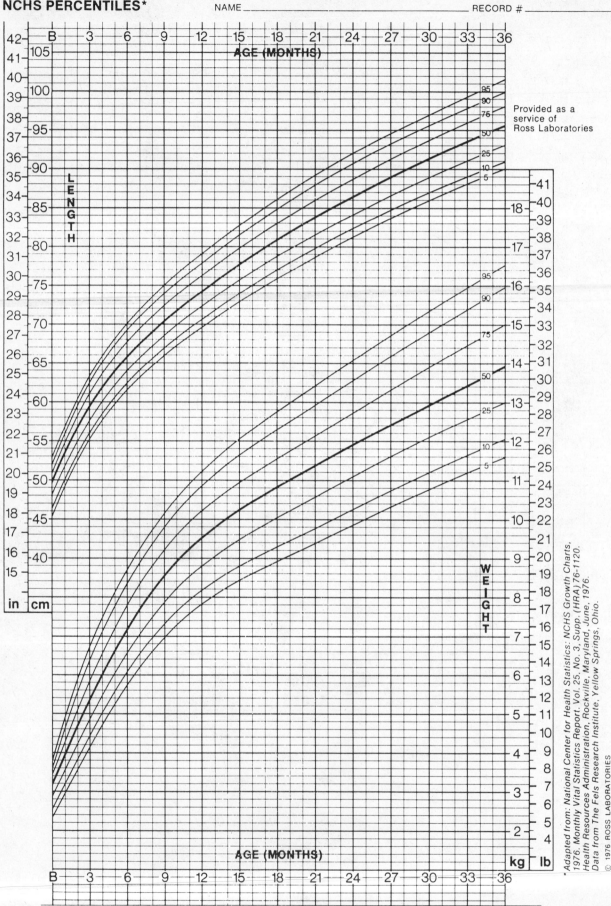

GIRLS: BIRTH TO 36 MONTHS
PHYSICAL GROWTH
NCHS PERCENTILES*

NAME _____ RECORD # _____

AGE (MONTHS)

LENGTH

Provided as a
service of
Ross Laboratories

WEIGHT

AGE (MONTHS)

*Adapted from: National Center for Health Statistics: NCHS Growth Charts, 1976. Monthly Vital Statistics Report. Vol. 25, No. 3, Supp. (HRA) 76-1120. Health Resources Administration, Rockville, Maryland, June, 1976. Data from The Fels Research Institute, Yellow Springs, Ohio.

GIRLS: BIRTH TO 36 MONTHS
PHYSICAL GROWTH
NCHS PERCENTILES*

NAME _____   RECORD # _____

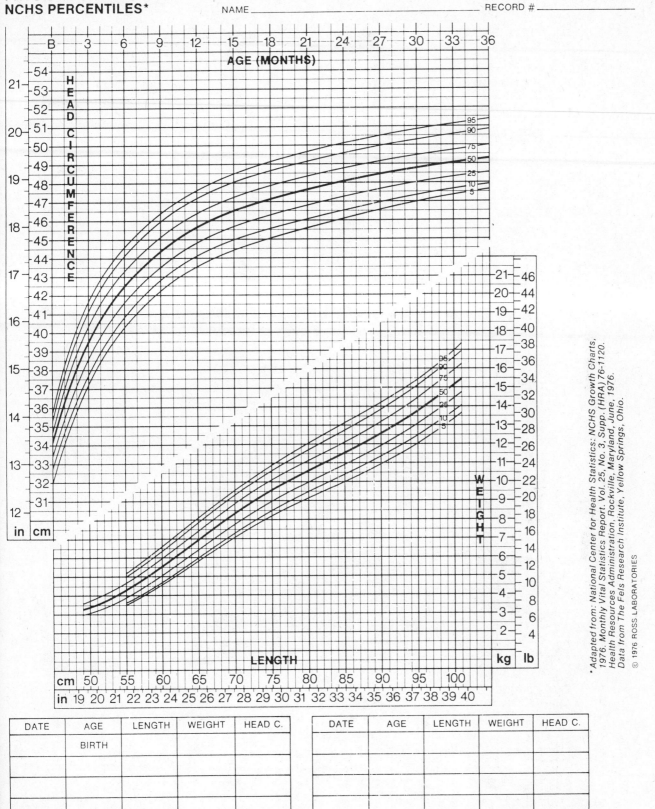

*Adapted from: National Center for Health Statistics: NCHS Growth Charts, 1976. Monthly Vital Statistics Report. Vol. 25, No. 3, Supp. (HRA) 76-1120. Health Resources Administration, Rockville, Maryland, June, 1976. Data from The Fels Research Institute, Yellow Springs, Ohio.

© 1976 ROSS LABORATORIES

DATE	AGE	LENGTH	WEIGHT	HEAD C.
	BIRTH			

DATE	AGE	LENGTH	WEIGHT	HEAD C.

311

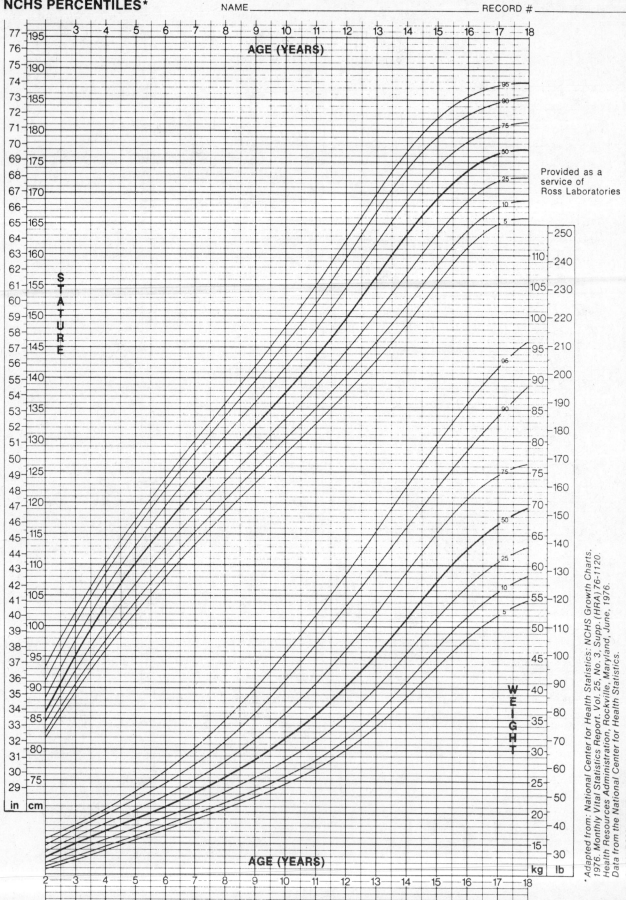

BOYS: 2 TO 18 YEARS
PHYSICAL GROWTH
NCHS PERCENTILES*

NAME _____ RECORD # _____

AGE (YEARS)

STATURE

Provided as a
service of
Ross Laboratories

* Adapted from: National Center for Health Statistics: NCHS Growth Charts, 1976. Monthly Vital Statistics Report. Vol. 25, No. 3, Supp. (HRA) 76-1120. Health Resources Administration, Rockville, Maryland, June, 1976. Data from the National Center for Health Statistics.

WEIGHT

AGE (YEARS)

BOYS: PREPUBESCENT
PHYSICAL GROWTH
NCHS PERCENTILES*

NAME _____ RECORD # _____

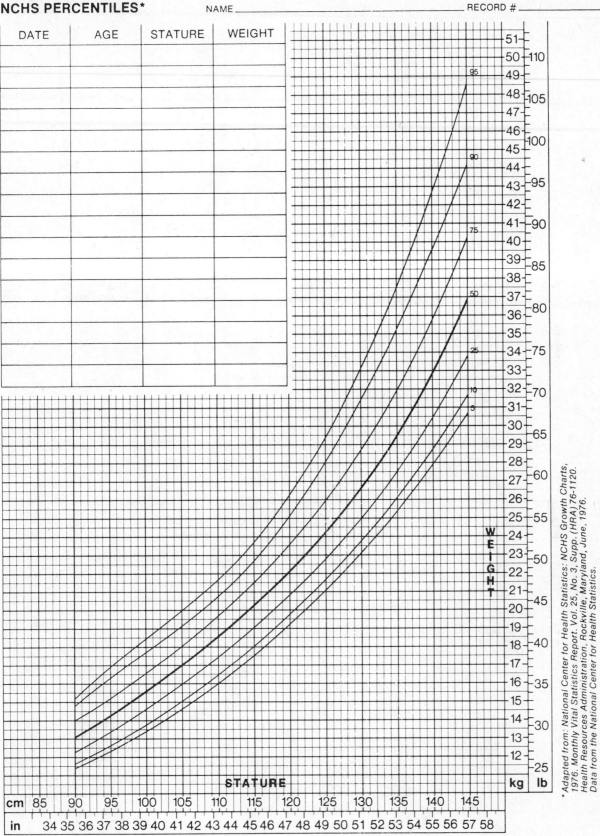

DATE	AGE	STATURE	WEIGHT

*Adapted from: National Center for Health Statistics: NCHS Growth Charts, 1976. Monthly Vital Statistics Report. Vol. 25, No. 3, Supp. (HRA) 76-1120. Health Resources Administration, Rockville, Maryland, June, 1976. Data from the National Center for Health Statistics.

© 1976 ROSS LABORATORIES

GIRLS: 2 TO 18 YEARS
PHYSICAL GROWTH
NCHS PERCENTILES*

NAME _____ RECORD # _____

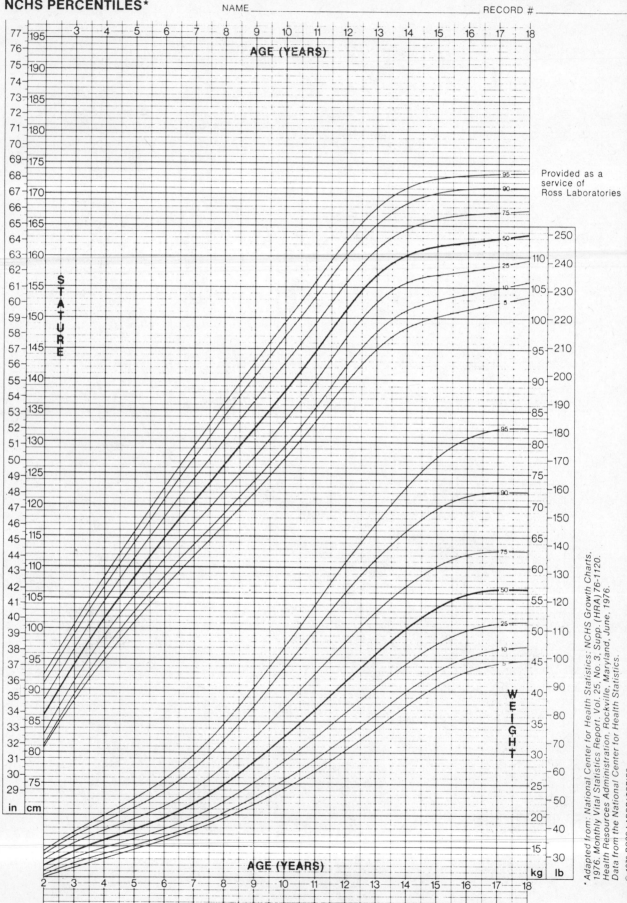

Provided as a
service of
Ross Laboratories

* Adapted from: National Center for Health Statistics: NCHS Growth Charts,
1976. Monthly Vital Statistics Report. Vol. 25, No. 3, Supp. (HRA) 76-1120.
Health Resources Adminstration. Rockville, Maryland, June, 1976.
Data from the National Center for Health Statistics.

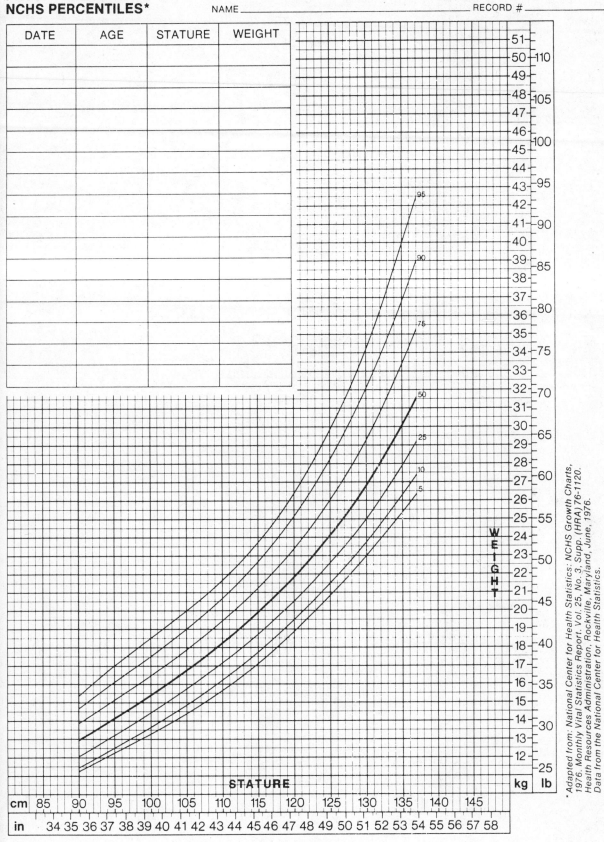

GIRLS: PREPUBESCENT
PHYSICAL GROWTH
NCHS PERCENTILES*

NAME _____ RECORD # _____

DATE	AGE	STATURE	WEIGHT

STATURE

| cm | 85 | 90 | 95 | 100 | 105 | 110 | 115 | 120 | 125 | 130 | 135 | 140 | 145 |

in 34 35 36 37 38 39 40 41 42 43 44 45 46 47 48 49 50 51 52 53 54 55 56 57 58

WEIGHT

* Adapted from: National Center for Health Statistics: NCHS Growth Charts, 1976. Monthly Vital Statistics Report. Vol. 25, No. 3, Supp. (HRA) 76-1120. Health Resources Administration. Rockville, Maryland, June, 1976. Data from the National Center for Health Statistics.

© 1976 ROSS LABORATORIES

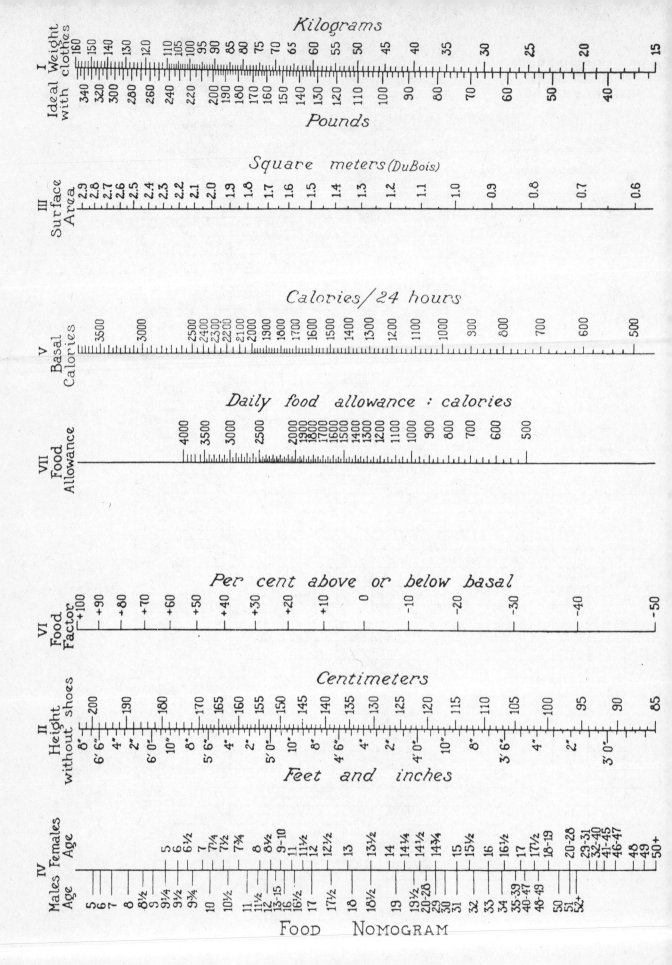

FOOD NOMOGRAM

ions for Estimating Caloric Requirement: To determine the desired allowance of calories, proceed as follows: 1. Locate the ideal
...on Column I by means of a common pin. 2. Bring edge of one end of a 12 or 15-inch ruler against the pin. 3. Swing the other end
...ruler to the patient's height on Column II. 4. Transfer the pin to the point where the ruler crosses Column III. 5. Hold the ruler
...the pin in Column III. 6. Swing the left hand end of the ruler to the patient's sex and age (measured from last birthday) given in
...a IV (these positions correspond to the Mayo Clinic's metabolism standards for age and sex). 7. Transfer the pin to the point where
...r crosses Column V. This gives the basal caloric requirement (basal calories) of the patient for 24 hours and represents the calories
...d by the fasting patient when resting in bed. 8. To provide the extra calories for activity and work, the basal calories are increased
...rcentage. To the basal calories for adults add: 50 to 80 per cent for manual laborers, 30 to 40 per cent for light work or 10 to 20
...t for restricted activity such as resting in a room or in bed. To the basal calories for children add 50 to 100 per cent for children
...to 15 years. This computation may be done by simple arithmetic or by the use of Columns VI and VII. If the latter method is
...locate the "per cent above or below basal" desired in Column VI. By means of the ruler connect this point with the pin on Col-
..., Transfer the pin to the point where the ruler crosses Column VII. This represents the calories estimated to be required by the pa-

W. M. Boothby and J. Berkson
October, 1933

v. 10-59

BASAL REQUIREMENT FOR CALORIES
PER POUND PER 24 HOURS

Age	Calories	
	Boys	Girls
6 months	25	25
1 year	25.5	25.5
2 years	25	24.5
3 years	23.5	23.5
4 years	23	22

For a child less than 5 years of age, the basal caloric requirement for 24 hours
is computed by multiplying the standard weight for the measured height by the
basal requirement for calories per pound per 24 hours for the appropriate age (see
accompanying table). The height is that of the child measured without shoes; the
weight to be used is that in the "Woodbury Height-Weight-Age Table," which
corresponds to the measured height and age of the child; the age to be used is that
of the child to the nearest half or full year.

APPENDIX E.   Food Nomogram

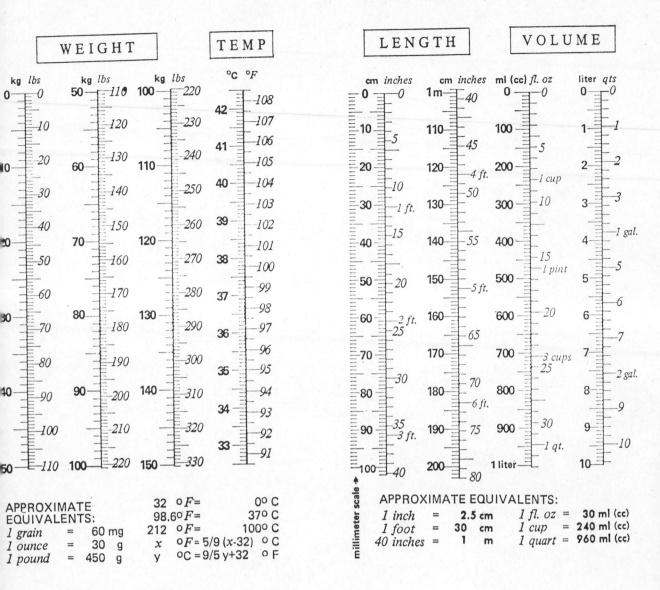

WEIGHT

kg	lbs	kg	lbs	kg	lbs
0	0	50	110	100	220
	10		120		230
10	20	60	130	110	240
	30		140		250
	40	70	150	120	260
20	50		160		270
	60		170		280
30	70	80	180	130	290
	80		190		300
40	90	90	200	140	310
	100		210		320
50	110	100	220	150	330

TEMP

°C	°F
	108
42	107
	106
41	105
40	104
	103
39	102
	101
38	100
37	99
	98
36	97
	96
35	95
	94
34	93
	92
33	91

LENGTH

cm	inches	cm	inches
0	0	1m	40
10		110	45
	5	120	4 ft.
20			50
	10	130	
30	1 ft.	140	55
40	15	150	5 ft.
50	20	160	65
60	2 ft. 25	170	
70	30	180	70 6 ft.
80		190	75
90	35 3 ft.	200	80
100	40		

VOLUME

ml (cc)	fl. oz	liter	qts
0	0	0	0
100	5	1	1
200	1 cup	2	2
300	10	3	3
400	15 1 pint	4	1 gal.
500		5	5
600	20	6	6
700	3 cups 25	7	7 2 gal.
800		8	8
900	30	9	9 10
1 liter	1 qt.	10	

millimeter scale →

APPROXIMATE
EQUIVALENTS:

1 grain	=	60 mg	32	°F=	0° C
1 ounce	=	30 g	98.6	°F=	37° C
1 pound	=	450 g	212	°F=	100° C
			x	°F = 5/9 (x-32)	°C
			y	°C = 9/5 y+32	°F

APPROXIMATE EQUIVALENTS:

1 inch	=	2.5 cm	1 fl. oz	=	30 ml (cc)
1 foot	=	30 cm	1 cup	=	240 ml (cc)
40 inches	=	1 m	1 quart	=	960 ml (cc)

Source: University of Iowa Hospitals and Clinics, Iowa City, Iowa.

APPENDIX F. Metric Conversion Scales

FOOD AND NUTRITION BOARD, NATIONAL ACADEMY OF SCIENCES–NATIONAL RESEARCH COUNCIL
RECOMMENDED DAILY DIETARY ALLOWANCES, Revised 1980
Designed for the maintenance of good nutrition of practically all healthy people in the U.S.A.

	Age (years)	Weight (kg)	Weight (lb)	Height (cm)	Height (in.)	Protein (g)	Fat-Soluble Vitamins Vita-min A (μg RE)[a]	Vita-min D (μg)[b]	Vita-min E (mg α-TE)[c]	Water-Soluble Vitamins Vita-min C (mg)	Thia-min (mg)	Ribo-flavin (mg)	Niacin (mg NE)[d]	Vita-min B-6 (mg)	Fola-cin[e] (μg)	Vitamin B-12 (μg)	Minerals Cal-cium (mg)	Phos-phorus (mg)	Mag-nesium (mg)	Iron (mg)	Zinc (mg)	Iodine (μg)
Infants	0.0-0.5	6	13	60	24	kg×2.2	420	10	3	35	0.3	0.4	6	0.3	30	0.5[f]	360	240	50	10	3	40
	0.5-1.0	9	20	71	28	kg×2.0	400	10	4	35	0.5	0.6	8	0.6	45	1.5	540	360	70	15	5	50
Children	1-3	13	29	90	35	23	400	10	5	45	0.7	0.8	9	0.9	100	2.0	800	800	150	15	10	70
	4-6	20	44	112	44	30	500	10	6	45	0.9	1.0	11	1.3	200	2.5	800	800	200	10	10	90
	7-10	28	62	132	52	34	700	10	7	45	1.2	1.4	16	1.6	300	3.0	800	800	250	10	10	120
Males	11-14	45	99	157	62	45	1000	10	8	50	1.4	1.6	18	1.8	400	3.0	1200	1200	350	18	15	150
	15-18	66	145	176	69	56	1000	10	10	60	1.4	1.7	18	2.0	400	3.0	1200	1200	400	18	15	150
	19-22	70	154	177	70	56	1000	7.5	10	60	1.5	1.7	19	2.2	400	3.0	800	800	350	10	15	150
	23-50	70	154	178	70	56	1000	5	10	60	1.4	1.6	18	2.2	400	3.0	800	800	350	10	15	150
	51+	70	154	178	70	56	1000	5	10	60	1.2	1.4	16	2.2	400	3.0	800	800	350	10	15	150
Females	11-14	46	101	157	62	46	800	10	8	50	1.1	1.3	15	1.8	400	3.0	1200	1200	300	18	15	150
	15-18	55	120	163	64	46	800	10	8	60	1.1	1.3	14	2.0	400	3.0	1200	1200	300	18	15	150
	19-22	55	120	163	64	44	800	7.5	8	60	1.1	1.3	14	2.0	400	3.0	800	800	300	18	15	150
	23-50	55	120	163	64	44	800	5	8	60	1.0	1.2	13	2.0	400	3.0	800	800	300	18	15	150
	51+	55	120	163	64	44	800	5	8	60	1.0	1.2	13	2.0	400	3.0	800	800	300	10	15	150
Pregnant						+30	+200	+5	+2	+20	+0.4	+0.3	+2	+0.6	+400	+1.0	+400	+400	+150	g	+5	+25
Lactating						+20	+400	+5	+3	+40	+0.5	+0.5	+5	+0.5	+100	+1.0	+400	+400	+150	g	+10	+50

Note: The allowances are intended to provide for individual variations among most normal persons as they live in the United States under usual environmental stresses. Diets should be based on a variety of common foods in order to provide other nutrients for which human requirements have been less well defined.

[a] Retinol equivalents. 1 retinol equivalent = 1 μg retinol or 6 μg β carotene.

[b] As cholecalciferol. 10 μg cholecalciferol = 400 I.U. of Vitamin D.

[c] α-tocopherol equivalents. 1 mg d-α tocopherol = 1 α-TE.

[d] 1 NE (niacin equivalent) is equal to 1 mg niacin or 60 mg dietary tryptophan.

[e] The folacin allowances refer to dietary sources as determined by Lactobacillus casei assay after treatment with enzymes (conjugases) to make polyglutamyl forms of the vitamin available to the test organism.

[f] The recommended dietary allowance for vitamin B-12 in infants is based on average concentration of the vitamin in human milk. The allowances after weaning are based on energy intake (as recommended by the American Academy of Pediatrics) and consideration of other factors such as intestinal absorption.

[g] The increased requirement during pregnancy cannot be met by the iron content of habitual American diets nor by the existing iron stores of many women; therefore the use of 30-60 mg supplemental iron is recommended. Iron needs during lactation are not substantially different from those of nonpregnant women, but continued supplementation of the mother for 2-3 months after parturition is advisable in order to replenish stores depleted by pregnancy.

APPENDIX G.   Recommended Daily Dietary Allowances

COMMON CARBOHYDRATES IN FOODS PER 100 g EDIBLE PORTION

Food	Fructose	Glucose	Reducing Sugars[a]	Lactose	Maltose	Sucrose	Cellulose	Dextrins	Hemicellulose	Pectin	Pentosans	Starch
	Monosaccharides			Disaccharides			Polysaccharides					
Fruits												
						(grams)						
Agave juice	17		19									
Apple	5	1.7	8.3			3.1	0.4		0.7	0.6		0.6
Apple juice			8			4.2						
Apricots	0.4	1.9				5.5	0.8		1.2	1		
Banana												
Yellow green			5			5.1						8.8
Yellow			8.4			8.9						1.9
Flecked	3.5	4.5				11.9						1.2
Powder			32.6			33.2		9.6				7.8
Blackberries	2.9	3.2				0.2						
Blueberry juice, commercial			9.6			0.2						
Boysenberries			5.3			1.1				0.3		
Breadfruit												
Hawaiian			1.8			7.7						
Samoan			4.9			9.7						
Cherries												
Eating	7.2	4.7	12.5			0.1				0.3		
Cooking	6.1	5.5	11.6			0.1						
Cranberries	0.7	2.7				0.1						
Currants												
Black	3.7	2.4				0.6						
Red	1.9	2.3				0.2						
White	2.6	3										
Dates												
Invert sugar, seedling type	23.9	24.9				0.3						
Deglet Noor			16.2			45.4						
Egyptian			35.8			48.5						3
Figs, Kadota												
Fresh	8.2	9.6				0.9						0.1
Dried	30.9	42				0.1						0.3
Gooseberries	4.1	4.4				0.7						
Grapes												
Black	7.3	8.2										
Concord	4.3	4.8	9.5			0.2						
Malaga			22.2			0.2						
White	8	8.1										
Grapefruit	1.2	2				2.9					1.3	
Guava			4.4			1.9						
Lemon												
Edible portion			1.3			0.2				3	0.7	
Whole	1.4	1.4				0.4						
Juice	0.9	0.5				0.1						
Peel			3.4			0.1						
Loganberries	1.3	1.9				0.2						
Loquat												
Champagne		12				0.8						
Thales		9				0.9						
Mango			3.4			11.6						0.3
Melon												
Cantaloupe	0.9	1.2	2.3			4.4				0.3		
Cassaba												
Vine ripened			2.8			6.2						
Picked green			3.2			3.9						
Honeydew												
Vine ripened			3.3			7.4						
Picked green			3.6			3.3						
Yellow	1.5	2.1				1.4						

Food	Mono-saccharides			Disaccharides			Polysaccharides					
	Fructose	Glucose	Reducing Sugars[a]	Lactose	Maltose	Sucrose	Cellulose	Dextrins	Hemicellulose	Pectin	Pentosans	Starch
						(grams)						
Mulberries	3.6	4.4										
Orange												
Valencia (Calif.)	2.3	2.4	4.7			4.2						
Composite values	1.8	2.5	5			4.6	0.3		0.3	1.3	0.3	
Juice												
Fresh	2.4	2.4	5.1			4.7						
Frozen, reconstituted			4.6			3.2						
Palmyra palm, tender kernel	1.5	3.2				0.4						
Papaw *(Asimina triloba)*												
(North America)			5.9			2.7						
Papaya *(Carica papaya)*												
(tropics)			9			0.5						
Passion fruit juice	3.6	3.6				3.8						1.8
Peaches	1.6	1.5	3.1			6.6	0.7		0.7			
Pears												
Anjou			7.6			1.9				0.7		
Bartlett	5	2.5	8			1.5				0.6		
Bose	6.5	2.6				1.7				0.6		
Persimmon			17.7									
Pineapple												
Ripened on plant	1.4	2.3	4.2			7.9						
Picked green			1.3			2.4						
Plums												
Damson	3.4	5.2	8.4			1						
Green gage	4	5.5				2.9						
Italian prunes			4.6			5.4				0.9		
Sweet	2.9	4.5	7.4			4.4	0.5			1	0.1	
Sour	1.3	3.5				1.5				1		
Pomegranate			12			0.6						
Prunes, uncooked	15	30	47			2	2.8		10.7	0.9	2	0.7
Raisins, Thompson												
seedless			70							1		
Raspberries	2.4	2.3	5			1				0.8		
Sapote	3.8	4.2		0.7								
Strawberries												
Ripe	2.3	2.6				1.4						
Medium ripe			3.8			0.3						
Tangerine			4.8			9						
Tomatoes	1.2	1.6	3.4				0.2		0.3	0.3		
Canned			3			0.3						
Seedless pulp			6.5			0.4	0.4	•		0.5		
Watermelon												
Flesh red and firm, ripe			3.8			4				0.1		
Red, mealy, overripe			3			4.9				0.1		
Vegetables												
Asparagus, raw			1.2							0.3		
Bamboo shoots			0.5			0.2	1.2					
Beans												
Lima												
Canned						1.4						
Fresh						1.4						
Snap, fresh			1.7			0.5	0.5	0.3	1	0.5	1.2	2
Beets, sugar						12.9	0.9		0.8			
Broccoli							0.9		0.9		0.9	1.3
Brussels sprouts							1.1		1.5			
Cabbage, raw			3.4			0.3	0.8		1			

Food	Mono-saccharides			Disaccharides			Polysaccharides					
	Fructose	Glucose	Reducing Sugars[a]	Lactose	Maltose	Sucrose	Cellulose	Dextrins	Hemicellulose	Pectin	Pentosans	Starch
						(grams)						
Carrots, raw			5.8			1.7	1		1.7	0.9		
Cauliflower		2.8				0.3	0.7		0.6			
Celery												
Fresh			0.3			0.3						
Hearts			1.7			0.2						
Corn												
Fresh		0.5				0.3	0.6	0.1	0.9		1.3	14.5
Bran									77.1		4	
Cucumber			2.5			0.1						
Eggplant			2.1			0.6			0.5			
Lettuce			1.4			0.2	0.4		0.6			
Licorice root		1.4				3.2						22
Mushrooms, fresh			0.1				0.9		0.7			2.5
Onions, raw			5.4			2.9			0.3	0.6		
Parsnips, fresh						3.5						7
Peas, green						5.5	1.1		2.2			4.1
Potatoes, white	0.1	0.1	0.8			0.1	0.4		0.3			17
Pumpkin			2.2			0.6			0.5			0.1
Radishes			3.1			0.3			0.3	0.4		
Rutabagas		5				1.3					0.8	
Spinach			0.2				0.4		0.8			
Squash												
Butternut	0.2	0.1				0.4						2.6
Blue hubbard	1.2	1.1				0.4	0.7					4.8
Golden crookneck			2.8			1						
Sweet potato												
Raw	0.3	0.4	0.8		1.6	4.1	0.6		1.4	2.2		16.5
Baked			14.5			7.2						4
Mature Dry Legumes												
Beans												
Mung												
Black gram						1.6						
Green gram						1.8						
Navy							3.1	3.7	6.4		8.2	35.2
Soy			1.6			7.2	2.6	1.4	6.6		4	1.9
Cow pea						1.5	5.4		4.8			
Garbanzo (chick peas)						2.4						
Garden pea *(Pisum salivum)*[c]						6.7	5		5.1			38
Horse gram *(Dolichos biplorus)*						2.7						
Lentils						2.1						28.5
Pigeon pea (red gram)						1.6						
Soybean												
Flour						6.8						
Meal						6.8						
Milk and Milk Products												
Buttermilk												
Dry			39.9									
Fluid, genuine and cultured			5									
Casein		0.1	4.9									
Ice cream (14.5% cream)			3.6		16.6							
Milk												
Ass			6									
Cow			4.9									
Dried												
Skim			52									
Whole			38.1									

Food	Monosaccharides		Reducing Sugars[a]	Disaccharides			Polysaccharides					
	Fructose	Glucose		Lactose	Maltose	Sucrose	Cellulose	Dextrins	Hemicellulose	Pectin	Pentosans	Starch
						(grams)						
Milk, cow *(continued)*												
Fluid												
Skim				5								
Whole				4.9								
Sweetened, condensed				14.1		43.5						
Ewe				4.9								
Goat				4.7								
Human												
Colostrum				5.3								
Mature				6.9								
Whey				4.9								
Yogurt				3.8								
Nuts and Nut Products												
Almonds, blanched			0.2			2.3					2.1	
Chestnuts			2.2			3.6					1.2	18
Virginia			1.2			8.1		0.3			2.8	18.6
French			3.3			3.6					2.5	33.1
Coconut milk, ripe						2.6						
Copra meal, dried	1.2	1.2				14.3	15.6	0.6			2.2	0.9
Macadamia			0.3			5.5						
Peanuts			0.2			4.5	2.4	2.5	3.8			4
Peanut butter			0.9									5.9
Pecans						1.1					0.2	
Cereals and Cereal Products												
Barley												
Grain, hulled							2.6		6		8.5	62
Flour						3.1					1.2	69
Corn, yellow							4.5		4.9		6.2	62
Flaxseed							1.8		5.2			
Millet grain									0.9		6.5	56
Oats, hulled											6.4	56.4
Rice												
Bran			1.4			10.6	11.4		7		7.4	
Brown, raw			0.1			0.8		2.1			2.1	69.7
Polished, raw		2	trace[d]			0.4	0.3	0.9			1.8	72.9
Polish			0.7								3.8	
Rye												
Grain							3.8		5.6		6.8	57
Flour											4.1	71.4
Sorghum grain											2.5	70.2
Soya-wheat (cereal)											3.3	46.4
Wheat												
Germ, defatted						8.3					6.2	
Grain		2				1.5	2	2.5	5.8		6.6	59
Flour, patent		2			0.1	0.2		5.5			2.1	68.8
Spices and Condiments												
Allspice (pimenta)			18			3						
Cassia			23.3									
Cinnamon			19.3									
Cloves			9									2.7
Nutmeg			17.2									14.6
Pepper, black			38.6									34.2

Food	Mono-saccharides		Reducing Sugars[a]	Disaccharides			Polysaccharides					
	Fructose	Glucose		Lactose	Maltose	Sucrose	Cellulose	Dextrins	Hemicellulose	Pectin	Pentosans	Starch
Syrups and Other Sweets												
							(grams)					
Corn syrup		21.2			26.4			34.7				
High conversion		33			23			19				
Medium conversion		26			21			23				
Corn sugar		87.5			3.5			0.5				
Chocolate, sweet dry						56.4						
Golden syrup			37.5			31						
Honey	40.5	34.2				1.9			1.5			
Invert sugar			74			6						
Jellies, pectin						40–65						
Royal jelly	11.3	9.8				0.9						
Jellies, starch						25–60						7–12
Maple syrup			1.5			62.9						
Milk chocolate				8.1		43						
Molasses	8	8.8				53.6						
Blackstrap	6.8	6.8	26.9			36.9						
Sorghum syrup			27			36						
Miscellaneous												
Beer			1.5					2.8			0.3	
Cacao beans, raw, Arriba	0.6	0.5	1.1			1.9						
Carob bean												
Pod			11.2			23.2				1.4		
Pod and seeds			11.1			19.4						
Soy sauce	0.9											

Source: Hardinge et al. (1965).
[a]Mainly monosaccharides plus the disaccharides, maltose and lactose.
[b]Blanks indicate lack of acceptable data.
[c]Also known as Alaska pea, field pea, and common pea.
[d]Trace = less than 0.05 g.

LESS COMMON CARBOHYDRATES IN FOODS
PER 100 g EDIBLE PORTION

Food	Carbohydrates		
	(grams)		
	Arabinose	Araban	
Beet sugar	0.6	...	
Soybean meal	...	4.7	
Soybean flour	...	3.6	
Soy sauce	0.3	...	
	Galactose	Galactans	
Peach	0.2	...	
Sapote	0.6	...	
Beet sugar	0.3	...	
Rutabaga	...	0.3	
Navy bean	...	1.3	
Soybeans	...	2.3	
Soybean flour	...	4.2	
Soybean meal	...	4.1	
Soybean sauce	0.4	...	
Casein	0.2	...	
Pear	0.2	...	
Apple	0.2	...	
	Glycogen (phytoglycogen)		
Corn, fresh	4.4		
Mushrooms, fresh	0.6		
	Mannose	Mannans	
Egg albumin	0.3	...	
Casein	0.1	...	
Brewer's yeast	...	14	
	Pentose		
Copra meal	2.4		
Corn kernel	0.2		
	Raffinose	Stachyose	Verbascose
Beans, black mung, dry	0.5	1.8	3.7
Beans, green mung, dry	0.8	2.5	3.8
Beans, soy, dry	1.9	5.2	...
Cacao seeds, raw	...	1.9	...
Copra meal	2.4	...	...
Cow peas	0.4	2	3.1
Field beans *(Dolichos lablab)*	0.5	2.1	3.6
Garbanzo (chick pea)	1	2.5	4.2
Horse gram	0.7	2	3.1
Lentils	0.6	2.2	3
Lima beans, canned	...	0.2	...
Molasses, beet	1.8	...	...
Pigeon peas	1.1	2.7	4.1
Wheat germ, defatted	6.6	...	...
	Sorbitol		
Apple	1		
Apple juice	0.3		
Apricot	1		
Hawthorn	4.7		
Hawthorn, English	7.6		
Loquat	0.2		
Pear, small, green	2.4		
Pear, large, green	1.9		
Pear, ripe	2.3		
Pear, Bose	3.5		
Peach	0.2		
Plum, Kelsey	2.8		
Pyracantha berries	4		
Rowan berries (mountain ash)	8.7		
Toyon berries, green	2.5		

Source: Hardinge et al. 1965.

MISCELLANEOUS INFORMATION

ENERGY VALUES (calories/g):

Carbohydrate	4
Protein	4
Fat	9
Alcohol	7

PROTEIN-NITROGEN CONVERSION:

Protein contains approximately 16% nitrogen. To convert grams of nitrogen to grams of protein, multiply total nitrogen by 6.25.

100-200 calories per gram of nitrogen are required for optimal use of amino acids.

COEFFICIENTS OF DIGESTIBILITY:

Carbohydrate	97-98%
Protein	92%
Fat	95%

ESSENTIAL FATTY ACIDS:

Linoleic
Arachidonic (can be formed from linoleic acid)

ESSENTIAL AMINO ACIDS:

Histidine	Phenylalanine
Isoleucine	Threonine
Leucine	Tryptophan
Lysine	Valine
Methionine	

CENTRAL VENOUS NUTRIENT (CVN) SOLUTION (STERILE):

Various CVN solutions are available for adults and children from the Pharmacy Department, University of Iowa Hospitals and Clinics. Crystalline amino acids and anhydrous dextrose can be compounded in differing concentrations to achieve the desired calorie and protein amounts. The standard adult CVN at UIHC is as follows:

Approximate calorie density: 1 cal/ml
Approximate osmolarity: 1620 milliosmols/l

CONTENT OF STANDARD ADULT CVN SOLUTION PER LITER:

Base	Adult
Crystalline amino acids	4.25%
Dextrose, anhydrous	25%

Electrolytes	
Sodium, mEq	35
Potassium, mEq	15
Calcium, mEq	4.7
Chloride, mEq	35
Magnesium, mEq	5
Phosphate, mEq	30
(Phosphorus, millimoles)	15

Essential Amino Acids	
Leucine, mg	2630
Valine, mg	1950
Lysine, mg	2460
Isoleucine, mg	2030
Phenylalanine, mg	2630
Threonine, mg	1780
Methionine, mg	2460
Histidine, mg	1860
Tryptophan, mg	760

Non-Essential Amino Acids	
Alanine, mg	8800
Arginine, mg	4400
Proline, mg	1780
Tyrosine, mg	170
Glycine, mg	8800

Multivitamin and Trace Element Injection - 10 ml	
Vitamin C, mg	100
Vitamin A, I.U.	3300
Vitamin D, I.U.	200
Thiamin, mg	3.0
Riboflavin, mg	3.6
Pyridoxine, mg	4.0
Niacin, mg	40
Pantothenic Acid, mg	15
Vitamin E, I.U.	10
Biotin, mcg	60
Folic Acid, mcg	400
Cyanocobalamin, mcg	5.0
Zinc, mg	4.0
Copper, mg	1.0
Manganese, mg	0.5
Chromium, mcg	10

DRUG ADMINISTRATION TIMES AT UNIVERSITY HOSPITALS

```
q 3 hr - 0900-1200-1500-1800-2100-2400-0300-0600
q 4 hr - 0800-1200-1600-2000-2400-0400
q 6 hr - 1200-1800-2400-0600
q 8 hr - 0800-1600-2400
q 12 hr - 0800-2000
TID(pc) -- 0730-1230-1730
TID(ac) -- 0630-1130-1630
q HS -- 2000
q d -- 0800
BID -- 0800-1600
TID -- 0800-1200-1600
QID -- 0800-1200-1600-2000
```

APPENDIX I.   Miscellaneous Information

CALORIC CONTENT OF ALCOHOLIC AND CARBONATED BEVERAGES

	Calories
Beer, alcohol 4.5% by volume	
(3.6% by weight), 12 oz	144
Carbonated, nonalcoholic	
Sweetened (quinine, sodas), 10 oz	88
Unsweetened (club sodas)	0
Cola type, 12 oz	133
10 oz	111
Ginger ale, 7 oz	62
Root beer, 12 oz	140
10 oz	117
Tom Collins mixer, 10 oz	130
Champagne, 4 oz	84
Creme de menthe, 2/3 oz	67
Daiquiri, 3 1/2 oz	122
Gin, Rum, Vodka, Whiskey 1 1/2 oz	
86 proof (36.0% alcohol by weight)	107
100 proof (42.5% alcohol by weight)	127
Highball, 8 oz	166
Manhattan, 3 1/2 oz	164
Martini, 3 1/2 oz	140
Old-Fashioned, 4 oz	179
Pop (fruit-flavored sodas,	
10-13% sugar) 12 oz	158
10 oz	130
Diet pop	0-3
Sherry, 2 oz	84
Tom Collins, 10 oz	180
Wines, 3 1/2 oz	
Dessert, alcohol 18.8% by volume	
(15.3% by weight)	137
Table, alcohol 12.2% by volume	
(9.9% by weight)	85

Source: Bickel and Gray (1968).

SPECIAL RECIPES

Low Protein Recipes
Blended Recipes
High Protein, Clear Liquid Recipes
Medium-chain Triglyceride Recipes
Low Calorie, Low Sodium, Low Cholesterol Salad Dressings and Sauces
Low Sodium Recipes
Reduced Sodium-Low Cholesterol and Low Cholesterol Cookbooks
Low Calorie Cookbooks

Low Protein Recipes

Low Protein Bread

Yield: 16-slice loaf

1/4 cup shortening
1 1.4 oz package
  Dream Whip
1 tbsp granulated sugar
1 tbsp boiling water
1 1/2 .6 oz packages
  refrigerated
  compressed yeast

2 drops almond flavor
2 drops rum flavor
1 tsp lecithin[1]
2 1/2 cups Ener-G-Low
  Protein & Gluten-Free Mix
2/3 cup warm water

Method: Cream the first 7 ingredients together. Whip in lecithin. Scrape down bowl. Add Low-Protein and Gluten-Free Mix and blend until dry mix is thoroughly mixed in. Add 2/3 cup warm water. Mix for 1 1/2 to 2 minutes. Place dough in a greased 8 1/2 in. by 4 1/2 in. pan. Let rise in warm oven containing a pan of hot water until bread is 1/2 in. from top of pan. Bake in preheated oven for 30 to 35 minutes at 425°F.

Per Slice: Calories   128
          Protein, g   0.4
          Carbohydrate, g   22.7
          Fat, g   0.6
          Sodium, mg   1
          Potassium, mg   11
          Phosphorus, mg   7
          Phenylalanine, mg   36

---

[1]Available from most health food stores.

Low Protein Cream Sauce
Yield: Two 1/4 cup servings

1/2 cup Poly Rich
1/2 tbsp grated onion
1 bay leaf
1/4 tsp white pepper
3 tbsp margarine, low sodium

2 tbsp Poly Rich
1 tbsp cornstarch
1 tsp dry mustard *or*
2 tbsp low sodium prepared mustard

Method: Bring Poly Rich to boil with the grated onion and bay leaf. Mix cornstarch and dry mustard and add 2 tbsp Poly Rich. Mix and add to boiling mixture. Cook 3-4 minutes, constantly stirring. Remove from heat; add pepper and margarine and prepared mustard (if used). Stir until blended.

Per 1/4 cup:
Calories	295
Protein, g	1.2
Carbohydrate, g	17
Fat, g	25
Sodium, mg	18
Potassium, mg	94
Phosphorus, mg	44
Phenylalanine, mg	50

Low Protein Applesauce Cake
Yield: 15 servings

1/4 cup margarine or butter,
  unsalted
1 cup light brown sugar
1 tsp ground cinnamon
1/2 tsp ground cloves
1/4 tsp ground nutmeg

1 3/4 cups dp Low Protein wheat
  starch
1 cup applesauce
3/4 tsp soda
1/2 cup seedless raisins

Method: Cream margarine, brown sugar, cinnamon, cloves, and nutmeg. Beat until well blended. Stir in wheat starch, applesauce, and soda; beat well. Add raisins and pour into a nonstick 8 1/2 in. x 4 1/2 in. x 2 1/2 in. loaf pan or 15 cupcake tins. Bake at 350°F about 25 minutes or until done. Let stand in pan 10 minutes before removing.

Per serving:
Calories	174
Protein, g	0.5
Carbohydrate, g	37
Fat, g	3
Sodium, mg	48
Potassium, mg	107
Phosphorus, mg	10
Phenylalanine, mg	8.4

Low Protein Orange Coffee Cake

Yield: 9 servings

2 eggs
7 tbsp margarine, low sodium,
  softened
1/2 cup sugar
1 tsp vanilla
2 tbsp water

1 cup dp Low Protein Baking Mix
3 tsp low sodium baking powder *or*
1 tsp regular double-action
  baking powder
1 tbsp grated orange peel
Orange glaze

Method: Heat oven to 350°F. Grease 9 x 1 1/2 in. round layer pan; coat with baking mix. In small mixer bowl, beat eggs, margarine, sugar, and vanilla 4 minutes on high speed. Mix in water, baking mix, baking powder, and orange peel until blended. Spread batter in pan. Bake until wooden pick inserted in center comes out clean--25 to 30 minutes. While warm, spread Orange Glaze over top.

Orange Glaze: Mix 3/4 cup confectioners' sugar, 1 tsp grated orange peel, and 1 to 2 tbsp orange juice until smooth.

Per serving (using low sodium baking powder):

Calories	251
Protein, g	1.5
Carbohydrate, g	37
Fat, g	11
Sodium, mg	25
Potassium, mg	133
Phosphorus, mg	124
Phenylalanine, mg	71

Per serving (using 1 tsp regular double-action baking powder):

Calories	251
Protein, g	1.5
Carbohydrate, g	37
Fat, g	11
Sodium, mg	61
Potassium, mg	28
Phosphorus, mg	37
Phenylalanine, mg	71

Low Protein Sugar Cookies

Yield: 4 dozen 2 1/2 in. diameter cookies

1 package (300 g) Kingsmill Co. Sugar Cookie Base
1 cup sugar
2/3 cup margarine or butter
1 egg *or* 1 tsp Kingsmill Egg Replacer and 4 tbsp water
1 tsp vanilla

Method: Cream the sugar and margarine until light and fluffy. Add the egg and beat mixture until light and smooth. Gradually add cookie mix and blend until it forms a smooth dough. Roll into balls, place on greased cookie sheet, flatten with fork, and bake in preheated oven at 325°F for 10-12 minutes. Cool on rack.

Variations:

1. Chill the dough for at least 2 hours or until very firm. Roll out the dough 1/8" - 1/4" thick and cut in various shapes with cookie cutters on lightly floured board. Bake as above. Yield: 6 dozen 2 in. diameter cookies.

2. Orange or lemon extracts may be substituted for the vanilla.

3. For spice cookies add 1 tsp cinnamon, ginger, nutmeg, or allspice.

4. Decorate with colored icings and colored crystal sugars.

Per 2 1/2 in. diameter cookie:	
Calories	99
Protein, g	0.3
Carbohydrate, g	14
Fat, g	5
Sodium, mg	75
Potassium, mg	6
Phosphorus, mg	2
Phenylalanine, mg (with egg)	16
Phenylalanine, mg (without egg)	9.4

Low Protein Butter Cookies

Yield: 76 cookies

2 cups salt-free butter, margarine, or shortening
1 cup confectioners' sugar
2 tsp vanilla
5 cups dp Low Protein Baking Mix

Method: Cream shortening, sugar, and vanilla until fluffy. Add baking mix and stir until smooth. Form dough into roll and chill for 1 hour. Divide into 76 slices. Place each slice onto ungreased baking sheet. Bake at 350°F for 10-12 minutes.

Per cookie:	
Calories	91
Protein, g	0.1
Carbohydrate, g	10
Fat, g	6
Sodium, mg	6
Potassium, mg	2
Phosphorus, mg	6
Phenylalanine, mg	3

Low Protein Applesauce Cookies

Yield: 4 dozen cookies

1/2 cup shortening
3/4 cup brown sugar, packed
1 egg
2 cups dp Low Protein Baking Mix
2/3 cup applesauce

1 tsp low sodium baking powder
1/2 tsp cinnamon
1/2 tsp nutmeg
1/2 tsp cloves
1/2 cup raisins

Method: Heat oven to 400°F. In medium bowl, mix shortening, brown sugar, and egg thoroughly. Stir in remaining ingredients. Drop by teaspoonful about 2 inches apart onto an ungreased baking sheet. Bake 10-12 minutes. Store in a tightly covered container.

Per cookie:		
Calories		67
Protein, g		0.2
Carbohydrate, g		11
Fat, g		3
Sodium, mg		6
Potassium, mg		35
Phosphorus, mg		14
Phenylalanine, mg		8

Low Protein Frosted Orange Cookies

Yield: 4 dozen cookies

3/4 cup sugar
2/3 cup unsalted butter
2 tbsp grated orange rind
1/4 cup water

1 tbsp orange extract
1/2 tsp soda
1/2 tsp baking powder
2 1/2 cups dp Low Protein
Baking Mix

Method: Cream butter and sugar. Add orange rind, extract, and water. Blend in dry ingredients. Chill dough in covered bowl for 1-2 hours. Roll teaspoonsful of dough into balls. Bake on ungreased cookie sheet at 350°F for 10-12 minutes.

Frost with a mixture of: 3 tbsp unsalted butter
1 1/2 cups confectioners' sugar
1 tbsp orange juice
1 tbsp grated orange rind

Per cookie:		
Calories		89
Protein, g		0.1
Carbohydrate, g		14
Fat, g		4
Sodium, mg		18
Potassium, mg		3
Phosphorus, mg		5
Phenylalanine, mg		2

Butterballs

Yield: 10 balls

6 tbsp unsalted butter
3/4 tsp vanilla
1 cup powdered sugar

3 tbsp Polycose powder
4 drops peppermint, butter extract,
  or other flavoring

Method: Mix ingredients together and divide into 10 equal balls. Place in freezer to harden. Peppermint flavoring may be omitted and powdered soft drink used on the outside of the balls.

Per butterball: Calories   117
         Protein, g   0.1
         Carbohydrate, g   14
         Fat, g   7
         Sodium, mg   4
         Potassium, mg   2
         Phosphorus, mg   2
         Phenylalanine, mg   23

Lemon Creams

Yield: 48 candies, 1/2 in. diameter

2 cups Polycose powder
1 cup confectioners' sugar
2 tbsp fresh lemon juice

Method: Mix the sugar and Polycose powder together; add the lemon juice and mix thoroughly. Knead into a stiff dough and roll the dough into balls 1/2 inch in diameter. Wrap separately in airtight wrappers.

Per candy: Calories   31
         Protein, g   0
         Carbohydrate, g   8
         Fat, g   0
         Sodium, mg   7
         Potassium, mg   1
         Phosphorus, mg   1
         Phenylalanine, mg   0

Caramels

Yield: 50 caramels

1 cup white sugar
1 cup light corn syrup
1 cup cream, heavy

1/4 cup unsalted butter or
  margarine
1/2 tsp vanilla

Method: Cook sugar and corn syrup rapidly to the firm ball stage, stirring occasionally. Add butter and cream gradually. Mixture should *not* stop boiling. Cook over medium heat to firm ball stage, stirring constantly (approximately 25 minutes). Add vanilla and mix. When bubbling stops, pour into buttered 9 x 13 in. pan. Score when cooled to room temperature. Cut in 1/2 in. cubes and wrap in waxed paper.

Per 3 caramels:
Calories	174
Protein, g	0.3
Carbohydrate, g	27
Fat, g	8
Sodium, mg	19
Potassium, mg	12
Phosphorus, mg	13
Phenylalanine, mg	15

Low Protein Rice Pudding

Yield: Four 1/2 cup servings

2/3 cup Polycose powder
2 cups cold water
1/4 cup sugar

1/4 cup cooked rice
2 tbsp margarine
1/4 cup heavy whipping cream

Method: Mix Polycose powder with 1/4 cup water. Heat in a double boiler until dissolved. *Do not boil.* Add remaining ingredients, except cream. Cook in double boiler until thick and creamy, stirring frequently. Add cream just prior to serving.

Per 1/2 cup serving:
Calories	242
Protein, g	0.5
Carbohydrate, g	35
Fat, g	11
Sodium, mg	89
Potassium, mg	18
Phosphorus, mg	15
Phenylalanine, mg	32

Low Protein Vanilla Ice Cream
Yield: 3 cups

6 tbsp sugar
1/4 cup water
1 tbsp lemon juice

2 tbsp cornstarch
1 cup whipping cream
1 tbsp vanilla

Method: Mix together sugar, water, lemon juice, and cornstarch in double boiler and cook over boiling water until thick. Cool. Beat cream until it stands in peaks but is not buttery. Fold in vanilla and cornstarch mixture. Freeze.

Variation: For chocolate ice cream, delete the lemon juice, reduce the vanilla to 1 tsp, and add 1 tbsp chocolate syrup.

Per 1/3 cup serving:
Calories	129
Protein, g	0.6
Carbohydrate, g	11
Fat, g	10
Sodium, mg	10
Potassium, mg	22
Phosphorus, mg	17
Phenylalanine, mg	27

Low Protein Sherbet
Yield: 11 servings

1 1/2 cups water
2 tbsp cornstarch
1/2 cup sugar
1 pkg (.16 oz) unsweetened Kool-Aid
powder

1/4 tsp mint flavoring
3 cups nondairy whipped topping
(already whipped)

Method: Mix 1 cup water, sugar, and Kool-Aid powder in small saucepan. Mix 1/2 cup cold water with cornstarch; stir until smooth. Stir into Kool-Aid mixture. Heat to boiling over medium heat, stirring constantly, until thick. Boil 3-5 minutes. Cool to room temperature, stirring occasionally. Fold Kool-Aid mixture into whipped topping. Add 1/4 tsp mint flavoring (or to taste). Portion into 1/3 cup servings. Freeze.

Per serving:
Calories	143
Protein, g	0.4
Carbohydrate, g	18
Fat, g	8
Sodium, mg	8
Potassium, mg	6
Phosphorus, mg	17
Phenylalanine, mg	12

Blended Recipes

Blended Broccoli Cheese Soup

Yield: 3 3/4 cups (2-3 servings)

1 10 1/2 oz can cream of mushroom
  soup concentrate
1 10 oz package frozen broccoli,
  cooked and drained

4 tbsp margarine
1/4 cup cheese spread
5 oz whole milk

Method: Mix all ingredients and blend thoroughly. Heat.

Variations: Substitute cauliflower for broccoli. Substitute garlic cheese spread for plain.

Beef Stew

Yield: 2 cups

1 cup cubed cooked beef
1/4 cup cooked vegetables
1/4 cup cooked potatoes

1/2 cup liquid from cooked beef,
  or milk

Method: Cooked ingredients should be tender. Combine all ingredients in blender and blend to achieve desired consistency. Heat.

Blended Chili

Yield: 1 1/2 - 1 3/4 cups

1-1 1/4 cups canned or homemade chili
1/2 cup tomato juice

Method: Blend chili and tomato juice to achieve desired consistency. Heat.

Chicken-Rice Dinner

Yield: 2 cups

1 cup cubed cooked chicken
1/4 cup cooked brown rice
1/4 cup cooked vegetables

1/4 cup milk
1/4 cup chicken broth

Method: Cooked ingredients should be tender. Combine all ingredients in blender and blend to achieve desired consistency. Heat.

Blended Mashed Potatoes and Gravy

Yield: 1 1/3 cups

1/2 cup mashed potatoes
1/3 cup gravy, homemade, canned,
  or reconstituted dry

1/2 cup whole milk

Method: Combine ingredients in blender and blend to achieve desired consistency. Heat.

Blended Vegetables

Yield: 1 serving

1/2 cup drained well-cooked or
  canned vegetables

2 tbsp milk

Method: Combine ingredients and blend thoroughly.

Variations: Substitute vegetable juice, tomato juice, cream sauce, cheese sauce, or vegetable cooking liquid for milk. Heat.

Hawaiian Delight

Yield: 1 3/4 cups

1/2 cup pineapple juice
1/2 medium banana

3/4 cup vanilla ice cream

Method: Combine ingredients in blender and blend to achieve desired consistency.

Strawberry and Pear Cooler

Yield: 1 3/4 cups

1/2 cup strawberry yogurt
1/2 cup pureed pears
1/2 cup creamed cottage cheese
1/2 cup whole milk

1 tbsp sugar
1 tbsp strawberry jelly
1-2 drops almond extract

Method: Combine all ingredients in blender and blend to achieve desired consistency.

Creamy Orange Delight

Yield: 1 3/4 cups

1/2 cup whole milk
1/2 packet Creamy Vanilla Resource
1/4 cup orange juice
1 tbsp brown sugar

1/4 cup vanilla ice cream
1/4 cup orange sherbet
1/2 cup orange flavored yogurt
1-2 drops vanilla extract

Method: Combine milk and Resource powder in blender and blend for 15-20 seconds. Add remaining ingredients and blend until smooth.

Orange Julia

Yield: 1 1/2 cups

3/4 cup orange juice
1 cup vanilla ice cream

Method: Mix thoroughly.

Variation: Substitute orange or rainbow sherbet for vanilla ice cream.

Strawberry Julia

Yield: 2 1/2 cups

1 1/2 cups frozen unsweetened
   strawberries
1/4 cup canned, drained, unsweetened
   pineapple

5 oz whole milk
1/4 cup sugar
1 tsp lemon juice

Method: Combine all ingredients in blender and blend until smooth.

Variation: Use sweetened strawberries and pineapple and omit sugar. Drain berries or reduce milk.

Berry Buttermilk Shake

Yield: 2 1/2 cups

1 cup whole fresh or frozen
   strawberries
1 cup buttermilk

3 standard ice cubes or
   about 1/3 cup

Method: Put all ingredients in blender. Cover and blend at medium speed for about 20 seconds or until smooth.

Apricot Ambrosia

Yield: 2 1/2 cups

1 cup plain yogurt
1/4 cup instant nonfat dry milk
6 ice cubes or about 2/3 cup

1/2 cup drained, canned apricot
   halves
1 tsp honey

Method: Place all ingredients in an electric blender, cover, and blend at medium speed for 15 seconds. Stop machine and push mixture down. Cover and blend 15 seconds longer or until smooth.

Peaches 'n Cream

Yield: 3 cups

1 cup whole milk
1 cup canned, drained peaches
1 cup vanilla ice cream

1/4 tsp salt
1-2 drops vanilla extract

Method: Combine all ingredients in blender and blend until smooth.

Fruited Pudding

Yield: 3 cups

1 cup strawberries (if frozen, drain)
1 3 oz package vanilla pudding mix

Method: Make pudding according to package directions. Add fruit and blend. Top with whipped cream if desired.

Variations: Substitute another fruit such as peaches, pears, apricots, cherries, or crushed pineapple for strawberries. Use chocolate pudding and add 1 1/2 - 2 bananas.

Tolerex Gelatin

Yield: 2 cups (Four 1/2 cup servings)

3/4 cup cold water
1 cup hot water
1 pkg Tolerex

1 3 oz package flavored gelatin
powder

Method: Pour cold water into blender. Pour hot water into blender. Add package of Tolerex and blend until dissolved. Stir in gelatin. Chill until set.

Calories	154	Carbohydrate, g	36
Protein, g	3.5	Sodium, mg	103
Fat, g	--	Potassium, mg	133

Citrotein Gelatin

Yield: Four 4.5 oz servings

1 3-oz package flavored gelatin
powder
1 cup boiling water
1 cup cold water

1/2 cup or 2 1.18-oz packets
Citrotein powder

Method: Dissolve gelatin in boiling water. Add cold water to gelatin mixture. Add Citrotein powder and stir vigorously. Chill until set.

Calories	143	Carbohydrate, g	30
Protein, g	6	Sodium, mg	135
Fat, g	0.2	Potassium, mg	112

Medium-chain Triglyceride Recipes

MCT oil is a lipid fraction of coconut oil consisting primarily of the triglycerides of the C_8 and C_{10} saturated fatty acids. MCT is an easily absorbed fat which does not require bile salts or lipase for absorption.

MCT oil may be mixed with fruit juice; sprinkled on salads and vegetables; incorporated into sauces for use on fish, chicken, or lean meat; or used in cooking or baking.

MCT Oil Spread

Yield: 2 2/3 cups (1 lb, 5 oz)

1 tbsp cornstarch
2/3 cup instant nonfat dry milk
1 tsp salt
1 tbsp lemon juice

2/3 cup water
2 cups MCT oil
Few drops yellow food coloring
Few drops butter flavoring

Method: Sift dry ingredients together into top of double boiler. Combine lemon juice and water; gradually add to starch mixture, mixing until smooth. Cook over boiling water, stirring constantly until mixture thickens (about 4 minutes). Remove from heat. Add MCT oil, 1/2 cup at a time, beating with a rotary beater after each addition. Add coloring to give desired shade. Do not use electric blender. 1 tsp MCT Oil Spread equals 3.3 g MCT oil and 27 calories.

MCT French Dressing

Yield: 1 cup

2/3 cup MCT oil
1/3 cup vinegar or lemon juice

Season to taste with any of the following:
1 tsp salt
1/2 tsp pepper
1/2 tsp sugar
1/4 tsp paprika

Method: Combine ingredients in jar and shake well. Vary seasoning to taste with dry mustard, minced onion, or garlic. 1 tbsp MCT French Dressing equals 11 g MCT oil and 78 calories.

MCT Cream Sauce

Yield: 1 cup

1 cup skim milk (hot)
2 tbsp flour

2 tbsp MCT oil
1/4 tsp salt
1/8 tsp white pepper

Method: Heat MCT oil; slowly add flour to make a paste. Cook over low heat, stirring constantly until it bubbles. Slowly add milk, stirring constantly, and cook until thick and smooth. Cool; add salt and pepper. Serve over meats and vegetables. One cup contains 383 calories.

Low Calorie, Low Sodium, Low Cholesterol Salad Dressings and Sauces

Tomato Salsa

Yield: 3 cups

4 whole jalapeno peppers
1 fresh tomato, chopped
1 pound No Added Salt tomatoes
  with juice

1/4 tsp cumin
1/4 tsp cayenne

Method: Dice peppers and tomato into 1-inch pieces. Combine with spices. Chill.

Portion size: 2 tbsp

Calories	6	Carbohydrate, g	1.25
Protein, g	0.3	Sodium, mg	1
Fat, g	.05	Potassium, mg	65

Suggested ADA exchange: Free

Lemon Dressing

Yield: 1/4 cup

1/4 cup fresh lemon juice
1/4 tsp dry mustard

1/4 tsp ground pepper
1 tsp chopped fresh parsley

Method: Prepare dressing. Use at once.

Portion size: 2 tbsp

Calories	10	Carbohydrate, g	2.7
Protein, g	0.4	Sodium, mg	0.5
Fat, g	0.1	Potassium, mg	51

Suggested ADA exchange: Free

Lemon Dressing

Yield: 1/4 cup

Juice of 1 fresh lemon
1 tsp ground pepper

Method: Squeeze lemon over salad and sprinkle with freshly ground pepper.

Portion size: 2 tbsp

Calories	9	Carbohydrate, g	2.6
Protein, g	0.3	Sodium, mg	--
Fat, g	--	Potassium, mg	45

Suggested ADA exchange: Free

Russian Salad Dressing

Yield: 1 3/4 cups

1 can low sodium tomato soup
  (10 1/2 oz)
1/4 cup oil
Peel of 1/2 lemon, grated
2 tbsp freshly squeezed lemon juice

2 tbsp chopped green onion
1 tsp fresh horseradish
Dash ground cinnamon
1 clove garlic, crushed

Method: Combine all ingredients; mix well. Shake well before serving.

Portion size: 2 tbsp

Calories	52	Carbohydrate, g	3.2
Protein, g	0.4	Sodium, mg	13
Fat, g	4.3	Potassium, mg	49

Suggested ADA exchange: 1 fat

Herb Salad Dressing

Yield: 2/3 cup

1 packet Butter Buds, made into
  liquid
1 tbsp distilled white vinegar
1 tbsp lemon juice
1/4 tsp garlic powder

1/4 tsp oregano
1/4 tsp tarragon
1/4 tsp thyme
1/8 tsp freshly ground pepper

Method: Combine all ingredients. Mix until well blended.

Portion size: 2 tbsp

Calories	12	Carbohydrate, g	2.8
Protein, g	0.1	Sodium, mg	127
Fat, g	--	Potassium, mg	24

Suggested ADA exchange: Free

Coleslaw Dressing

Yield: 1 1/3 cups

3/4 cup plain nonfat yogurt
1/3 cup malt or red wine vinegar
1/4 cup water

8 packets Equal
1/8 tsp salt substitute *or*
   to taste
Dash freshly ground pepper

Method: Combine all ingredients and mix well. Chill.

Portion size: 2 tbsp

Calories	15	Carbohydrate, g	2.5
Protein, g	0.9	Sodium, mg	12
Fat, g	0.3	Potassium, mg	80

Suggested ADA exchange: Free

Creamy French Dressing

Yield: 1/2 cup

1/3 cup plain lowfat yogurt
1 packet Butter Buds
1 tbsp red wine vinegar
2 packets Equal

3/4 tsp paprika
1/8 tsp dry mustard
1/8 tsp garlic powder

Method: Combine all ingredients and mix well. Chill.

Portion size: 2 tbsp

Calories	28	Carbohydrate, g	5.3
Protein, g	1.1	Sodium, mg	184
Fat, g	0.4	Potassium, mg	77

Suggested ADA exchange: 1 vegetable

Yogurt Dressing

Yield: 1 1/4 cups

1 cup plain nonfat yogurt
1/4 cup low calorie mayonnaise

Method: Blend well. Add herbs, spices as desired.

Portion size: 2 tbsp

Calories	22	Carbohydrate, g	1.9
Protein, g	1.3	Sodium, mg	23
Fat, g	1.1	Potassium, mg	54

Suggested ADA exchange: 1/2 fat

Thousand Island Dressing

Yield: 1 cup

1/2 cup dry cottage cheese
2 tbsp plain nonfat yogurt
2 tbsp low calorie mayonnaise
2 tbsp low sodium catsup
Dash cayenne pepper

1/4 cup skim milk
1 tbsp finely chopped onion
1 tbsp low sodium, chopped dill
  pickle *or*
1 tbsp cucumber and 1 tsp vinegar

Method: Combine all ingredients and blend thoroughly.

Portion size: 2 tbsp

Calories	17	Carbohydrate, g	1.0
Protein, g	1.9	Sodium, mg	9
Fat, g	0.6	Potassium, mg	45

Suggested ADA exchange: Free

Zero Dressing

Yield: 1 3/4 cups

1 1/4 cups unsalted tomato juice
3 oz vinegar or lemon juice
2 tbsp chopped parsley, green pepper,
  or fresh horseradish

3/4 tsp liquid artificial sweetener
1/2 tsp dry mustard (optional)

Method: Combine all ingredients thoroughly.

Portion size: 2 tbsp

Calories	7	Carbohydrate, g	1.6
Protein, g	0.2	Sodium, mg	2
Fat, g	--	Potassium, mg	72

Suggested ADA exchange: Free

Low Sodium Recipes

Homemade Salt Substitute

3 tsp dry mustard	1 tsp garlic powder
3 tsp onion powder	1/2 tsp white pepper
3 tsp paprika	1/4 tsp ground basil

Method: Mix thoroughly. Store in a salt shaker and use in place of salt.

Sodium-Free Baking Powder

(May be prepared by a pharmacist)

7.5 g tartaric acid	39.8 g potassium bicarbonate
56.1 g potassium bitartrate	28 g cornstarch

Method: Use 1 1/2 tsp of the above mixture in place of 1 tsp of regular baking powder. Add this baking powder toward the end of the mixing time and beat only enough to mix.

Reduced Sodium-Low Cholesterol and Low Cholesterol Cookbooks

The American Heart Association: The American Heart Association Cookbook. New York: Ballantine Books, 1986.

The American Heart Association, Northeast Ohio Affiliate, Inc.: Cooking Without Your Salt Shaker. Dallas: American Heart Association, 1978.

Connor, S., and Connor, W.: The New American Diet. New York: Simon and Schuster, 1986.

Debakey, M., et al.: The Living Heart Diet. New York: Raven Press, Simon and Schuster, 1984.

Goor, R., and Goor, N.: Eater's Choice. Boston: Houghton Mifflin Co., 1989.

Low Calorie Cookbooks

The American Diabetes Association and The American Dietetic Association: Family Cookbook, Volume I. New York: Prentice Hall, 1987.

The American Diabetes Association and The American Dietetic Association: Family Cookbook, Volume II. New York: Prentice Hall, 1987.

The American Diabetes Association and The American Dietetic Association: Family Cookbook, Volume III. New York: Prentice Hall, 1987.

Caviani, M.: The New Diabetic Cookbook. Chicago: Contemporary Books, Inc., 1984.

Jones, J.: Cook It Light. New York: Macmillan, 1987.

Oxmoor House, Inc.: Cooking Light '87. Birmingham: Book Division of Southern Progress Co., 1987.

Revell, D.: Oriental Cooking for the Diabetic. Tokyo: Japan Publications, Inc., 1981.

Trollope, J., ed.: The Dieter's Cookbook. Des Moines: Meredith Corp., 1982.